The Encyclopedia of Alternative Medicine and Self-Help

Devised and edited
by Malcolm Hulke

Editorial assistant: Ann Walker
Alternative medicine adviser: John Newton
Medical adviser: Dr Philip Hopkins FRCGP, MRCS, LRCP

Rider and Company, London

While every effort has been made to ensure
accuracy neither the publisher nor the editor
nor any other party involved in its preparation
can be held responsible for any loss or
disappointment suffered by readers, contributors
or directory-entrants occasioned by omissions
from or errors in this encyclopedia

Rider and Company
3 Fitzroy Square, London W 1P 6JD

An imprint of the Hutchinson Publishing Group

London Melbourne Sydney Auckland
Wellington Johannesburg and agencies
throughout the world
First published 1978

Set in Monotype Times

Printed in Great Britain at The Anchor Press Ltd
and bound by Wm Brendon & Son Ltd
both of Tiptree, Essex

ISBN 0 09 132870 5 (Hardback)
ISBN 0 09 132871 3 (Paperback)

Health is the thing that makes you feel that now is the best time of the year.

FRANKLIN PIERCE ADAMS

It is quite salutary to bear in mind that only one-third of the world population has access to western-type medicine and that the rest rely entirely on acupuncture, homoeopathy, ayurdic medicine, unani, herbalism, naturopathy and various forms of spiritual and psychic healing.

Nursing Times

In some hospitals elderly patients are given so many pills every night you would need a computer to work out what is going on inside them, when in many cases they would do far better with a nip of whisky.

DR W. J. MACLENNAN, Senior Lecturer in Geriatric Medicine, University of Southampton, addressing the British Association for the Advancement of Science at Birmingham, 1977

Contents

The Encyclopedia of Alternative Medicine and Self-Help

Message from Jack Warner

'People these days,' say the stand-up comedians, 'are taking so many pills they die much healthier.'

That old chestnut hits on the truth. We're pill mad. We pour chemicals into our bodies when the cause of many health problems is that we don't know how to live properly.

Conventional medicine has saved millions of lives. It would be stupid to reject out of hand Pasteur, Lister, Fleming and the remarkable Dr Christiaan Barnard. But with the greatest respect to the medical profession they are sometimes rather hidebound in their attitudes.

An actor has to keep very fit. I have had three experiences of alternative medicines when orthodox medicine failed. Osteopathy, naturopathy and homoeopathy, in that order, and they all worked. On reflection it is strange that many members of the medical profession did not think much of osteopathy, yet the first thing a young medical student is asked to study is a skeleton. If that isn't a step towards osteopathy I don't know what is.

The question of diet too is all important. My wife and I had a health food shop for several years, and the number of health food shops growing up all over the country during the last few years is indicative of the new successful trend of eating wisely and not too much.

Not long ago in Scotland a man with terminal cancer was the subject of prayers in his local Catholic church. He got better. Can we positively deny that miracles no longer happen?

What is important is that we find what suits us – and acknowledge that there are more things in heaven and earth than are always understood by even our most eminent scientists.

Foreword

This book is neither a recommendation nor a critique. It is a platform from which people holding different views may address you. An orthodox doctor read every entry to see if, in his view, any discipline could prove harmful. He found none. However, as a professional doctor committed to conventional medicine, he naturally urges the reader not to delay in seeking conventional medical advice for symptoms that might arise from serious disease, such as cancer, where early diagnosis and treatment are vital.

No censorship was applied other than the inevitable censorship of omission. We included every alternative medical discipline we could find. You may know of others. Write to me: there may be a second edition one day.

The schism between orthodox western medicine and all others is recent. At one time myth, medicine, faith and magic were entwined. Contemporary orthodoxy emerged only two or three centuries ago. Some people regard it as a passing phase.

What we call orthodox medicine is allopathy, a Greek word translatable as 'other-suffering'. Other or alien influences attack the body. The intruder is defeated by chemical or surgical counter-attack. Allopathy gained prominence in the past 100 years because surgery became safer and drugs more powerful. The fear is that surgery is now so easy it may be used as a quick but not necessarily lasting cure; more powerful drugs may result in unwanted side-effects.

Whereas orthodox medicine is single-minded in its allopathic approach the principles of alternative medicine are diverse. Roughly they may be divided into spiritual, organic, and the presupposition of the existence of certain forces. If any thread can be drawn through them it is that many alternative therapies tend to treat the whole person – mind, body and spirit – whereas conventional medicine concentrates on local specifics. Equally, humanistic psychology involves the body along with the mind. Having said that it should be remembered that many good family doctors with the psychosomatic approach also view their patients as whole entities, with emotions and family problems and social backgrounds, as well as the acne or indigestion they came to the surgery about.

In some areas the dividing line between 'straight' and 'fringe' medicine is blurred. Qualified British osteopaths could, if they wished, apply to become part of the National Health Service. They do not wish to because they would not achieve parity with doctors and would at best become a Profession Supplementary to Medicine, which is a fancy way of saying they would lose their right to diagnose. One of Queen Elizabeth's physicians, Dr Margery Blackie, is a homoeopathic doctor. In his excellent account of colour therapy Theo Gimbel writes, 'This is an auxiliary to straight medicine and does in no way eliminate the help of a doctor.' One doctor we found firmly believes in miracles; unfortunately we could not persuade him to contribute to this book since he feared ridicule by other doctors. Yet, as I know from personal contacts, he is not the only doctor who believes in prayer as wel as penicillin.

Possibly what drives some people to alternative medicine is the austere image of orthodoxy. The idea that hospital is a place for old people to die remains prevalent in mass thinking. Doctors sit behind desks, put on rubber gloves before touching us, treat us like children and write meaningless prescriptions in an indecipherable hand. At least in America you stand more chance of being treated as an adult. A doctor in New Mexico told me, 'Once I'm sure a patient has terminal cancer I tell them straight. I say, "It's time to go visit with the grandchildren." They seem to appreciate it.' In Britain we still talk in hushed tones about growths; no one, until they are dead, is allowed to have cancer.

Albeit with good intentions, doctors try to convince us they have the cure for every ailment; they do it by affecting a remote, starchy reserve. Since the days of barber-shop surgery, when Dr Robert Dutton denounced rivals as 'Common Pretenders and Quacks' and happily went on to advertise his own cure for 'Ruptures, bursten or broken Bellies; Loose Teeth; Scorbutick Humours; Headaches, Vapours and Indispositions', all of which could be disposed of with a single elixir, the medical profession has become respectable and conservative to the point of suffocation. Still, pendulums have always swung madly. Editing this book we came across intense stuffiness from certain quarters of alternative medicine. X would not write in a book in which Y's name was to appear, even though Z – the orthodox medical profession – regards both X and Y as 'Common Pretenders'.

Maybe climate puts up the barrier between patient and orthodox doctor. Conventional medicine is very northern hemisphere-based. Reserve and protocol are our styles. Freewheeling chumminess, let alone love, doesn't do so well in a cold climate. Avicenna, the founder of traditional Islamic medicine, encouraged his students to embrace their patients lovingly. If a western doctor started to embrace patients he would probably be struck off the register. In Provence, though, I have seen hospital nurses kissing their patients good night – in a mixed ward with a bottle of wine and a packet of Gauloises by every bed.

Much of alternative medicine is preventive.

Most of us eat too much of the wrong things. We live to eat, destroying ourselves in the process. By over-fuelling our bodies we burn them up too quickly.

At the age of forty Luigi Cornaro, a fifteenth-century Italian nobleman, was so burnt up by over-eating and drinking that he was said to be dying. He resolved he would live on one meal a day of twelve ounces of vegetables, leaves and grain and a little wine. He did die eventually, at the age of 102. During his long and belatedly healthy life he wrote, 'He who would eat much must eat little; for eating little lengthens a man's life, and by living longer he may eat a great deal more.'

According to J. M. Scott's novel *Queen Boadicea*, the Roman legionaries, who carried 60 lb in armour and equipment and marched twenty miles a day, grumbled if they were given meat. The Roman Empire was built by vegetarians.

I wish to thank three people in particular for their help in compiling this book:

Ann Walker, who came in to do some typing and quickly developed the most remarkable editorial flair. Her drive in chasing contributors to write their articles was always tempered with diplomacy and charm. She should be snapped up right away by a busy publisher or a movie producer.

John Newton, journalist, whose encyclopedic knowledge of alternative medicine in all its diversity was of immense help.

Philip Hopkins, our unorthodox orthodox doctor who read all the articles and was a treasure trove of advice.

Many other people have helped whom I wish to thank very sincerely: Brad Ashton, Rita Carter, Jan de Vries, Cathy Gould, Mohammad Hami, Lee Harris, Ruth Harrison, Jack Hollands, Susan Hopkins, Paul Keeler, Ann Leslie, Michael Nightingale, Lauraine Palmeri, Corenza Roele, Harvey Unna, Jack Warner.

MALCOLM HULKE

How to use this encyclopedia

If you have heard about a particular alternative medicine (say, herbalism) and want to know more about it, see if it is listed under Contents on pages 7–8.

If you have an ailment and seek a cure, look at the Index (pages 199–208). If your ailment is there you will find listed all the treatments that this encyclopedia has to offer.

Most articles end with cross-references to the directory sections at the back of the book. You may find up to five such references:

Reference   *Directory*

ASSOCIATIONS   Names and addresses of bodies representing or associated with the treatment. If you want to find a practitioner in your town or county, these are the people to contact.

Reference   *Directory*

BIBLIOGRAPHY   Books about, or making major reference to, the treatment.

CONTRIBUTORS   Name and address of the author of the article. A few non-practitioner contributors did not wish to be listed. To find a practitioner see Associations.

PRODUCTS   Things you can buy by mail, all related to alternative medicine.

TRAINING   Places where you can learn to become a practitioner of the treatment covered in the article.

When writing to associations, contributors, or to a training establishment, please always enclose a stamped addressed envelope.

Abbreviations and Initials

A.F.A.S.	Associate of the Faculty of Astrological Studies	F.R.C.G.P.	Fellow of the Royal College of General Practitioners
A.F.Phys.	Associate of the Faculty of Physiatrics	F.R.C.P.	Fellow of the Royal College of Physicians
A.M.R.S.H.	Associate Member of the Royal Society of Health	F.R.C.Path.	Fellow of the Royal College of Pathologists
B.A.	Bachelor of Arts	F.S.M.	Fellow of the Society of Metaphysicians
(Birm.)	Birmingham University		
B.SC.	Bachelor of Science	G.P.	General practitioner
C.Eng.	Chartered Engineer	(H.C.)	Honoris Causa (Honorary)
D.C.	Doctor of Chiropractic (U.S.A.)	I.R.M.T.	International Register of Manipulative Therapists
D.C.E.	Diploma of Curative Education	K.B.E.	Knight Commander Order of the British Empire
D.D.	Doctor of Divinity	L.C.N.P.	Licentiate of the National Council of Psychotherapists
Dip.Ed.	Diploma of Education		
Dip.P.E.	Diploma of Physical Education	L.C.S.P. (Phys.)	London and Counties Society of Physiologists
D.M.	Doctor of Medicine	L.D.S.	Licentiate of Dental Surgery
D.N.Th.	Diploma in Natural Therapeutics	Lic.AC.	Licentiate in Acupuncture
		(Lond.)	London University
D.O.	Diploma in Osteopathy	L.R.C.P.	Licentiate of the Royal College of Physicians
D.Phys.	Diploma of Physiotherapy		
Dr	Doctor	L.T.C.L.	Licentiate of Trinity College London
D.SC.	Doctor of Science		
D.St J.	Dame of Grace of St John of Jerusalem	M.A.	Master of Arts
F.C.G.L.I.	Finalist City and Guilds of London Institute	M.AC.A.	Member of the Acupuncture Association
F.C.O.	Fellow of the College of Osteopathy	M.A.H.P.	Member of the Association of Hypnotists and Physiotherapists
F.G.S.M.	Fellow of the Guildhall School of Music	M.B.N.O.A.	Member of the British Naturopathic and Osteopathic Association
F.L.C.S.P.	Fellow of the London and Counties Society of Physiologists	M.Brit.I.R.E.	Member of the British Institute of Radio Engineers
F.N.I.M.H.	Fellow of the National Institute of Medical Herbalists	M.C.	Military Cross
		M.C.S.P.	Member of the Chartered Society of Physiotherapists

15

M.D.	Doctor of Medicine	M.P.S.	Member of the Pharmaceutical Society of Great Britain
M.E.O.E.R.	Member of the European Osteopathic Register		
M.F.Phys	Member of the Faculty of Physiatrists	M.Rad.A.	Member of the Radionic Association
M.I.E.E.	Member of the Institute of Electrical Engineers	M.R.C.S.	Member of the Royal College of Surgeons
M.I.H.E.	Member of the Institute of Health Education	M.R.O.	Member of the Register of Osteopaths
M.I.O.P.	Member of the Institute of Osteopathy and Physiotherapy	M.S.O.	Member of the Society of Osteopaths
		N.D.	Diploma in Naturopathy
M.I.Psi.Med.	Member of the Institute of Psionic Medicine	(Oxon.)	Oxford University
		Ph.D.	Doctor of Philosophy
M.N.I.M.H.	Member of the National Institute of Medical Herbalists	R.M.T.	Registered Music Therapist (U.S.A.)
		S.C.M.	State Certified Midwife
		S.R.N.	State Registered Nurse

Part One
Encyclopedia

The articles are arranged in alphabetical
order. You will find a complete list of
contents on pages 7–8.

Most articles relate to therapies and
treatments and have this style of heading:
ABSENT HEALING. A few relate to ailments
and have this style: *AUTISM.*

An → preceding word in **bold type** within an
article signifies that you will find an article
on that subject elsewhere in the book.

ABSENT HEALING

A letter drops into a postbox and one more request for absent healing is on its way. The writer may be desperate, someone is ill and not responding to medical treatment; they, themselves, may be torn with nerves, sleepless, or suffering constant pain. The letter is to a healer, an ordinary man or woman with no medical knowledge but with a gift that helps sick people. This letter is often a last resort, a last hope in a sea of stress and anxiety.

From the time the letter is posted, help begins. The healing love-flow starts to reach out as soon as the first act of contact is made, because someone has asked, someone needs help.

Thousands of people, sentenced as incurable, are today leading active normal lives as a result of absent healing. Doctors are often baffled by these amazing recoveries. What is this strange power that has no known scientific law and which helps the sick to get better? How can it cure disease a thousand miles away?

Spiritual healing is a great force of love that enables a divine therapy to restore harmony to spirit, mind and body and so provide a basis for physical restoration. Healing is so natural. It has no harmful side-effects and comes on an unknown wavelength, reaching out from the healer to the patient wherever they may be. By re-creating harmony healing accelerates the self-repair mechanism of the body; the reverse gear, which allows disease to become established and the body to deteriorate, is changed. The impetus goes on to a new forward gear, the return journey to good health. A vital spark touches the spirit and prompts the body to get well.

It is not the healer who creates the healing power. The healer acts as a distributor, in the same way that the electric cable transmits energy and the telephone wire transmits the human voice; long-distance, or absent healing, from constant and proper direction of positive, thoughtful prayer. The rate of success is high and even those who are not cured find they are helped in many ways, so that they are better able to cope with life. People at the receiving end find that pain begins to lessen, sleep improves and cheerful thoughts prevail. Some even start to sing along the way, when before all was despair and misery. Patients write to say life has taken on a new meaning, painkillers are discontinued, sleeping pills thrown out; and one woman confessed, 'I don't shout at the children so much.'

It is a multiplying process. A tiny spark of love and hope sets healing in motion and it grows, always fed by spiritual power. New life starts pulsing. As it strengthens, the disharmony of ill health retreats, for healing is a great take-over that is never forceful.

When did spiritual healing begin? It goes back to the dawn of man and there are records of healing in early civilizations. The mother rocking a crying child, a cat licking an injured kitten are examples of the basics of the healing process. The desire to comfort, the desire to make better are age-old instincts. People often write for a friend or relative seeking a cure for illness, disease, irrational behaviour or asking for help with smoking, drinking or drug taking. Changes come about through the healing even though the person concerned remains totally unaware that a healing has been requested. A wife wrote on behalf of her husband who had suffered indescribable pain from a stomach ulcer for two years. Despite medical treatment his agony often kept him awake at night and he suffered all day. When shaving, she related, he was literally on his knees. So the healing began. Within a few days he was expressing surprise that his ulcer was not bothering him so much. It was then she told him about the healing. He was amazed and they were both more amazed as more days went by and the pain completely went. Twelve months later she wrote, 'The ulcer agony had not returned.'

Healing can work in conjunction with medical treatment. Most people who ask for absent healing are receiving medical attention, and the number who ask is growing every year. This unusual therapy offers new hope when faced with the heart-break of having to 'live with it'. Many without hope write pleading for help, hardly daring to believe that a layman can cure when doctors fail.

Age is no barrier to the healing force. The old and the very young can receive benefit. Children usually respond particularly well, including small babies.

Animals, too, can receive help from healing. Owners write in despair after veterinary surgeons surrender all hope. It has been reported that fierce, unruly dogs become more tractable. Certainly cats are very much *en rapport* with healing power. These successes with very young infants and animals surely prove that faith is not a necessary ingredient for a good healing. Sceptics have been healed too, almost against their will!

Some people see beautiful colours during the time of the healing. So many write of the great peace they feel enveloping them and a wonderful surge of upliftment. This often happens before they have even had an answer to their first letter.

Material and emotional problems that cause ill health and mental anguish are often resolved through healing. Marriages have been saved, enemies have become friends, noisy neighbours have been quietened. When chances seemed slim, flats have been found; families have been re-united after long separations. A mother wrote to say that shortly after she had sent a request for absent healing for an ill condition, she heard, out of the blue, from her son for the first time for seven years. These things happen too often to be coincidental.

The spiritual and physical are so closely intertwined that they cannot be separated. As the healing reaches out, a very powerful therapy is set in motion which invigorates the spirit, brightens the mind so the physical opportunity for betterment can expand.

Healing can be given and accepted in a down to earth, matter of fact way. It is not necessary for the recipient to be religious, though religious rites and healing have gone hand in hand through the ages. There are instances of healing in the old and new testaments. Moses' short prayer, 'Lord, heal her now!' swept away leprosy from his sister Miriam.

But most healings are gradual. Patience is required during the initial period of strengthening. Nerves must be soothed, tensions eased, the mind has to be calmed and thoughts re-directed to happier channels. Some of the best healings have developed long after the time when apparent progress was not evident. Sometimes people do or think things which impede receptivity and this can cause temporary setbacks. But the healing can help to closer attunement which will enable them to accept again renewed benefit.

There is some humour attached to a healer's correspondence, such as the man who wanted his hair restored in an overnight miracle! Writers describe the healing as like a secret parcel of strength, like having their batteries re-charged, or like a cloud being lifted. One woman wrote from a West Indian island saying that the healing had touched her complaint better than those who were there examining her. Absent healing reaches out over land and ocean: there are no distance limits to this remarkable power, which is directed by positive prayer and divine determination.

Any ill condition can be transformed through spiritual power. We cannot limit this great therapy. Troubled cells within the physical body are just waiting for a soothing influence to remove the discordancy of disease. Happiness amongst the cells brings order out of confusion, re-activating natural growth and accelerating the repair process from which good health can again develop.

The heavy demands of modern living put an unacceptable burden on the people of today. Tension builds on tension and each difficulty starts to grow to giant proportions. A tired mind is an ideal receptacle for wrong thinking and this affects the physical system. Always the weakest part of the body is the area which attracts disease. With calm and happy thoughts, ill conditions can be overcome. Spiritual healing clears away the cobwebs in the mind and empties the physical attic of all toxic junk. With the dispersal of wrong thinking a clearer mind cleanses the physical body. That is what absent spiritual healing is all about.

Phil and Kath Wyndham

ASSOCIATIONS, p. 217
CONTRIBUTORS, p. 220

ACUPUNCTURE

The idea that a needle stuck into one's foot can improve the condition of one's liver may appear to be a startling concept. Yet sufferers from liver ailments can testify that a series of needle pricks have resulted in considerable improvement.

The ancient art of acupuncture offers many similar surprising results and any belief that it is an oriental illusion is belied by the fact that it has been the standard form of medical treatment in China for thousands of years. Because of its proven effectiveness acupuncture has been adopted as a therapy by many western physicians. In 1974 a World Acupuncture Congress was held at the University of Pennsylvania in Philadelphia at which practitioners from all over the world discussed acupuncture in relation to suffering ranging from toothache to cancer. In July 1977 the world's first out-patient clinic for the treatment of drug addicts by acupuncture was opened in Hong Kong. Clearly the 5000-year-old healing art has come a long way.

The earliest known reference to acupuncture is the *Nei Ching*, the Classic of Internal Medicine, attributed to Huang Ti, the legendary Yellow Emperor who was reputed to have lived during the period 2697–2596 B.C. The *Nei Ching* is still the basic reference on the subject and has served as the foundation for the development of acupuncture up to the present century. The precise origins of acupuncture are obscure but it seems that in some fashion the ancient Chinese became aware of increased sensitivity of certain areas of the skin when impairment of some body organ or function existed. By observing these hypersensitive skin areas they came to recognize that a series of points existed that could be linked to an organ dysfunction during a specific illness and that these acupuncture points (there are approximately 800) followed a definite pattern over the body. The line that linked a series of points associated with a particular organ was named a meridian. These meridians became identified with the various organs. Not only was it recognized that these imaginary lines became sensitive when there was an organic or functional disorder in the body but they were also considered to act as 'energy pathways'. Through them flowed the life-energy or 'ch'i'. It was believed that health existed when this energy flowed through the acupuncture points in a state of balance, but when there was either an excess or an insufficiency the result was illness. This latter state of imbalance refers to the two energies, yang and yin, which together make up the 'ch'i'. Yang and yin represent, in Chinese philosophy, the masculine and feminine, the sun and moon, or in terms more acceptable to a western mind, the positive and negative forces, such as in electricity. Imbalance in the relative amounts of yin and yang energy are seen as the root of all pathology. For health to be maintained the 'ch'i' must flow without hindrance and the skill of the acupuncturist lies in his ability to free the meridians so that there is an even energy flow.

This is done by the light insertion of needles of pure copper, silver or gold into the flesh at specific points along the lines of the meridians. The prick of the needle at these points stimulates specific nerves which send electric impulses to the spinal cord and the lower centres of the brain, and on to the diseased area. In ancient times pointed wooden sticks were used for this purpose, later thorns and then iron or bronze needles. It was then observed that by using different metals, different effects could be achieved. For one disease a stimulating effect was required, for another sedation: to answer this need gold and silver needles were developed, gold acting as a stimulant, while silver sedated.

To select the appropriate meridians to treat, a 'pulse diagnosis' – the keystone of traditional Chinese diagnosis – is made. According to Chinese medicine each of the twelve main meridians is reflected in the radial artery and can be felt as a pulse at the wrist. The pulse at the radial artery is divided into three zones, each having a superficial and a deep position. By 'reading' these pulses (a subtle process in which three fingers are generally used) any excess or depletion of energy in the regular meridians can be detected. Pulse diagnosis is so sensitive that at times past illnesses will be registered and a virtual life history of the patient's health can be determined. It is also possible for the acupuncturist to identify disease long before any physical symptoms are present, an aspect of acupuncture that makes it invaluable as a preventive therapy. Treatment given at an early stage, it is claimed, will maintain health at a peak level. Regrettably, though, at least as far as western practitioners are concerned, most patients turn to acupuncture only as a last resort when orthodox methods have failed.

Among the many ailments that can be treated successfully are →migraine, ulcers and digestive troubles, arthritis, sciatica, psoriasis, anxiety and depression, asthma and bronchitis. Although acupuncture has a wide therapeutic range it should not be seen as a panacea; at times it needs to be combined with other therapies to be effective. In China and Japan the use of acupuncture is widespread. In Chinese hospitals it is not only used as a therapy but also as an anaesthetic agent. Operations for the removal of lungs and tumours have been performed while patients remained wide awake, even sipping tea or eating fruit while surgery was performed, the sole anaesthesia administered being acupuncture needles either twirled by hand or electrically stimulated by small machines. Acupuncture is practised in many hospitals in France and Germany where it can be obtained under the national health service. In the Soviet Union, where it is taught in several universities, there are over 1000 practitioners. In Europe alone there are well over 5000 acupuncturists and its use is spreading to the U.S.A. where it is now becoming widely accepted. In Britain the Acupuncture Association works to promote and encourage the study of acupuncture and publishes a register of qualified practitioners.

John Newton

ALEXANDER TECHNIQUE

Alexander technique is a form of re-education used primarily to get rid of faulty habits such as bad posture, over-tension, bad breathing and speech defects; secondarily, it is a means of helping people to become more aware of themselves, less bound by sheer mechanical habit, and hence having more control of their reactions and behaviour. As it is a re-educational procedure and therapeutic only indirectly, Alexander teachers regard those they teach as pupils who must co-operate and not expect to be merely passive patients. Although it is not a treatment for specific symptoms, many different kinds of disorders and malfunctioning, even intractable ones, often disappear in the re-educational process.

The inventor of the technique was F. M. Alexander, an Australian who started his working life as an actor at the end of the last century and soon developed a special talent for recitations of verse and ballads. He was already beginning to make a name for himself when his whole career was threatened by chronic trouble with his voice. In his third book *The Use of the Self*, he describes how this reached a climax when he was offered a very attractive engagement which he was keen to accept, but because of his voice he was uncertain whether he could fulfil it adequately. His doctor, however, encouraged him to accept, saying that if he continued to use throat sprays and rested his voice he would be all right on the day. Sure enough on the evening of the performance his voice seemed to have quite recovered and he began reciting confidently. Half-way through the performance the hoarseness began to recur and he only managed with great difficulty to complete the programme.

He returned to his doctor for advice. 'Continue the treatment,' was the answer. But Alexander replied that, as this had proved ineffective, the question he wanted answered was: since his voice was functioning satisfactorily when he started reciting and then gradually deteriorated, what was he doing with his voice that caused the trouble? As the doctor had no answer, Alexander decided he must find out for himself. He fixed up a mirror and observed himself in the act of ordinary speaking. At first he saw nothing unusual but when he recited he noticed that he involuntarily pulled back his head, depressed his larynx and sucked in breath, producing a gasping sound. This was the beginning of a long and incredibly patient investigation.

After months of experimenting and observing he entirely overcame the hoarseness. Ironically, having become so excited by the discovery of how his body worked and of the whole nature of habit, instead of resuming his career as an actor he became more interested in teaching other people what he called 'the proper use of themselves'.

What had he discovered? The first important thing was that his point of departure, namely the way he had used his voice, was the cause of his trouble. Many would have stopped there and become an elocution or singing instructor. But Alexander realized that his discovery could apply to all kinds of body misuse, and as his teaching experience increased he found that his technique filled a large gap in therapeutic and preventive medicine. It had been well known that bad posture predisposed to many disorders, yet no postural therapist had been capable of treating and curing his particular symptoms. To do this he had to evolve a technique which enabled him to control consciously and unlearn reactions and habits of which up to then he had been quite unaware.

One of the most important factors in the development of his method was his realization of the prime importance of the head–neck area and the relationship of this to the whole spine. He called this the Primary Control of Use because when the proper relationship was maintained it had an effect on the whole organism. He had found that ceasing to pull back his head had a good effect on his breathing and the functioning of his larynx. Later he realized even more clearly the importance of this area for the whole balance and poise of the body. If the neck was habitually stiffened and caused the head to be pulled back and down, this did not necessarily, as in his own case, lead to hoarseness, for as a professional reciter he was subjecting his vocal apparatus to more than usual strain. But it undoubtedly had a bad effect on breathing, was linked with harmful tensions in other parts of the body, and shortened the spine by exaggerating the dorsal or lumbar curves or both. Bad posture was the inevitable cause often leading to chronic backache, foot troubles and many other disorders.

The great advantage that Alexander derived from his discovery of the prime importance of the head–neck–back relationship was the unifying effect it had: it enabled him to deal with the body as a whole and not in a piecemeal way. He became very contemptuous of the advice still widely given, especially to women, 'pull your tummy in' or 'tuck in your tail'. Such instructions not merely set up harmful tensions, often adversely affecting respiratory movement, but also treated the body as a collection of unrelated parts. It is easily demonstrable that anyone standing upright at his full height with head high and level and back extended, with no undue dorsal or lumbar curves, finds his stomach no longer needs to be pulled in or his 'tail' tucked in.

It may seem strange that an Australian actor with very little anatomical knowledge should have hit upon a way of re-educating the human body more effectively than any system of physical education based on exercises hitherto devised. His strength lay partly in his ignorance, partly in his urgent feeling of need: 'If I don't cure myself then my career is finished.' His approach, in the absence of academic knowledge, had to be pragmatic. All his theories grew naturally out of his observation of what worked or failed. If he had had any training in anatomy he would not have approached the problem so practically or so free of preconceptions. An anatomist would not have been content to observe himself patiently in a mirror. More likely, he would have hurried off to the dissecting laboratory. Hence came Alexander's subsequent impatience with friendly doctors who tried to persuade him to study anatomy. Looking critically at the way they used themselves, he would say, 'Knowing anatomy doesn't seem to have done *you* much good!' (In this respect his successors do not follow him; knowledge of anatomy and physiology is included in the three-year training course.)

Another discovery, just as vital for the effectiveness of his re-educational method as the importance of the head–neck area, was the necessity to learn to inhibit his habitual reaction. When working on himself he found it impossible to change his habitual way of reciting unless he first inhibited the old pattern of use. He needed to inhibit even the intention to recite; otherwise the old reaction would always be more powerful than the new one which was still struggling to establish itself. Without unequivocally saying no – and remaining neutral and uncommitted – it was impossible to prevent the old pattern reasserting itself. People nowadays are frightened of inhibition in any form. But inhibition in this sense is quite different from the kind that psychoanalysts seek to eliminate: for Alexander inhibition meant the refusal to travel along the well-worn track that he knew led nowhere but to frustration. It meant remaining neutral about his end and attending solely to the means that he found enabled him to reach his objective – without really trying. He had to put his trust in the means he had worked out and let it take him where he wanted to go. He had to learn not to 'do' but just to let things happen. (This attitude of mind is akin to the way of Zen with its emphasis on not striving to achieve one's end.)

This was an extremely hard lesson for a man of his temperament, by nature very highly strung. He remarked how most of the misfortunes and disasters in his life had occurred because of his over-quick reactions and how after he had evolved his technique, and had learned the value of inhibition, the course of his life began to run more smoothly. He therefore put a very high value on it. For him it was a way of freedom of choice, freedom not to behave as he always had if he did not wish to.

His insistence on the need to concentrate on the means rather than end led him to coin the term 'end-gaining'. An end-gainer is someone who is so anxious to gain his end that he presses on regardless of the right means to attain it. The stammerer who increases tension when he has difficulty in getting out a word, the singer who tries too hard to reach her top notes, the pedestrian who is in such a hurry to cross a busy street that he fails to look both ways, are all end-gainers (the latter in more than one sense).

If one looks at different conditions of ill health one often finds end-gaining an important predisposing factor. The asthmatic with his understandable fear of not getting enough breath tends to make too much effort to breathe even when he is not in spasm so that he breathes too quickly and shallowly. Thereby he makes a spasm more likely instead of letting the breath come naturally. Picking up a heavy object with the knees straight and the back flexed can easily lead to disc trouble. Staring is an end-gaining habit because it involves trying too hard to see and so leads to eyestrain and defective vision instead, as the →**Bates method** teaches, of just allowing the visual field to appear. The perfectionist is an habitual end-gainer because he does everything with excessive tension at enormous cost to himself, thus making him liable to coronary thrombosis or other stress disorders.

End-gaining sometimes takes the form of trying to force the autonomic nervous system into behaviour which it may be quite willing to perform in its own way and time, but it refuses to be bullied and pushed around. The insomniac who tries hard to go to sleep succeeds only in prolonging his insomnia. A non-end-gaining approach is the only possible starting-point for the treatment of impotence. Trying to force an erection is futile. The best advice is: 'Don't try; be content to enjoy the naked propinquity of your partner. Play and caress if you feel like it. Then, if you can really give up trying, what you wish for will probably happen.'

Another important discovery surprised him a great deal: the fact that he could not rely upon the correctness of his feelings. Many times during his period of self-observation he believed that he was putting his head forward when the evidence in the mirror showed he was pulling it back. His feelings had become corrupted by prolonged misuse. Therefore, until his feelings corresponded with the true facts they were no better than blind guides. The restoration of trustworthy feeling was a necessary part of the re-educational process. Not merely did they not correspond with the true facts but they were addictive like drugs. One comes to 'enjoy' one's misuse in the same perverted way that one can come to 'enjoy' ill health. It feels nice and familiar and ministers to one's sense of security. How corrupted this feeling can be is vividly illustrated by the case of a small crippled girl who was brought to Alexander by her mother. To demonstrate what he might perhaps achieve over a period of time he gently pulled the child straight. The child said, 'Oh, mummy, he's pulled me all crooked.'

An important corollary of the unreliability of feelings is the doubt it raises about exercises. Every action one performs has a certain feel or, in more technical language, a kinaesthetic sensation connected with it. If the action is habitual it will feel natural, if non-habitual, unnatural. So as we inevitably prefer the natural to the unnatural it is almost certain that in doing exercises we will do them in as natural a way as we can. But if our feelings have become perverted it follows that our exercises may be exercising our worst faults and hence imprinting them even more deeply on our pattern of muscular behaviour. Just as the crooked man proverbially walks a crooked mile, so the hollow-backed man will do a hollow-backed exercise or the stiff-necked man a stiff-necked one. Exercises build up the muscular system on the basis of what is already present and hence may mean exercising existing defects. One expert in this field states simply that the keep-fit class is excellent only for the person who does not need it. Standard treatment for disc trouble is still a course of extension exercises although a recent investigation has shown that one in three of the patients were actually worse afterwards.

These figures are even more significant than they appear since there is always a tendency towards health and many people improve without any treatment at all.

Of course one can go too far in this direction – Alexander no doubt did – for exercises can be valuable as a means of building up weak muscles; in muscular atrophy they are indispensable. But as a way of changing habit they are not effective. They do not change the way a man walks to the telephone and picks it up nor in the way he sits in his car. If we use our bodies as Nature intended and as animals use theirs, every act is an exercise working in our favour so that artificial and contrived movements become unnecessary. Many people find housework a bore, but if done with the ease and fluency that arise out of good habits of use it can become much less tiring and boring.

Another conclusion that follows from untrustworthy feeling is that it is unwise to correct faults purely by verbal instruction. To exhort a child to stand up properly is likely to induce an over-tense stance which is briefly maintained until the inevitable reversion to normal occurs. The child's idea of a good stance may be based on what he has seen of the military posture which at its worst combines the over-stiffened neck, the raised chest and shoulders, the hollowed back often with breath partly held and knees pressed back. The conscientious child will suffer most because he will try harder and longer, while the contra-suggestible one will sag even further out of pure cussedness!

Because verbal instructions did not produce good results Alexander developed a method of using his hands to guide and persuade (rather than to manipulate) his pupils. He could then give the verbal direction with the knowledge that his pupil would receive the sensory experience that he intended to give with much less danger of misinterpretaion. The use of mirrors, so essential when he was re-educating himself, became less important when he was teaching others. The accurate use of the teacher's hands is perhaps the most important part of his training. For unless he has acquired this he will constantly be giving his pupils bad sensory experiences instead of good ones.

Alexander began his lessons by observing by eye and touch the condition the pupil was in; then with his hands, starting with the head, neck and back, he would gently undo the false tensions and misdirection of energy that he found. After this he told the pupil to do some simple movement. The pupil had to inhibit his immediate reaction to comply and, instead, to project directions to his head, neck and back which would prevent him from falling back into his old misuse. This was usually followed by the pupil being allowed to do the movement, but sometimes Alexander would vary it without warning to make sure that the pupil had effectively inhibited his response. Contact by touch was maintained throughout the movement so that Alexander could feel faults that might occur, while all the time he would be using his hands to guide and direct. He did this with the ordinary basic movements of life that he could control manually. The emphasis was not so much on *doing* the movement as on allowing it to happen. This was only possible if the pupil had adequately inhibited his automatic response and had projected the preventive verbal directions. If the pupil co-operated properly he would be rewarded by a feeling of unusual lightness and ease. But very often, especially in the early stages, he would try too hard to do the movement (as he thought) well, with the result that he failed to receive the new sensory experience that Alexander was trying to give him. This giving of the sensory experience in simple movements repeated many times in a series of lessons is unique and basic to the Alexander technique. From this it naturally follows that all teaching apart from instruction in the general principles has to be done individually rather than in groups.

One of the dangers in teaching people to be more relaxed is that relaxation may become a task which the pupil tries to do excessively well. A pupil of mine, a rather dynamic lady, told me she had been to see a specialist for a medical examination. As he helped her on with her coat at the end of the interview he said reassuringly there was nothing she need worry about except that she must relax more. Her comment to me was, 'I tried it for a week and it nearly killed me!' The Alexander approach makes this kind of reaction unlikely since all the emphasis is put on undoing and unlearning, on indirect rather than on direct means, never on trying to be right but always on awareness on what has to be undone. Thus the more relaxed state is encouraged to emerge in its own time rather than be anxiously striven for.

One of the criteria for judging whether a person is using his body well or badly is how much margin of safety his pattern of muscular use allows. A well-aligned flexible back will obviously be less accident-prone than a stiff back with exaggerated dorsal and lumbar curves. The latter will have no reserves. It will be like a hinge working at the extreme end of its range of movement and hence highly vulnerable to careless use. In the same way some slight false move like stepping unguardedly off the pavement in the dark may cause serious trouble. This is only an aspect of the wider truth that any well-balanced person will be much better able to survive crises and emergencies than someone basically less stable. Actors become extremely nervous at first nights but those who are fundamentally secure and well balanced in themselves are more likely to rise to the occasion. In other words, the prevailing mood is a more potent determinant of reaction than the nature of the external event.

The Alexander technique not only increases the body's natural margin of safety by establishing a better muscular balance, but also, owing to the fact that muscular tone is inseparably bound up with mental states, tends to lead to greater tolerance, calmness and open-mindedness, with a corresponding improvement in personal relations. Increased self-confidence is often remarked upon by pupils. Especially is this so when their chief problem has been a weak, unstable back. It is almost as if the technique has given them more backbone.

Alexander always worked on the principle that mind and body are a unity and preferred the term psychophysical to describe his technique. A good example of the influence improvement in bodily use can have on mental states was the case of an actor whose main problem was backache. After I had given him a few lessons he remarked how he had always been very liable to depression. He had felt this beginning to come over him the previous weekend, but by refusing to let his muscular system collaborate with the depressive tendency he had succeeded in fighting it off. It should be admitted that not all depressions are so easily dealt with because there is not always a strong enough conscious urge *not* to be depressed. But there is no doubt that the Alexander technique can at least help to make people less depression prone.

The way asthma can be dealt with is a good example. Most asthmatics misuse their bodies even when they are not particularly short of breath. There is usually abnormal tension in the neck and shoulders, often a retraction of the head and a breathing habit of quick, shallow breaths using the small lung capacity at the top of the chest rather than the lower thoracic area and the diaphragm. This involves raising the shoulders at every intake of breath. Moreover the breath is often, even during periods when there is no asthmatic spasm, sucked in noisily and gaspingly, rather than, as happens in normal breathing, allowed to enter the lungs silently and effortlessly. The asthmatic spasm therefore is only an intensification of a permanently abnormal state. It follows that the most appropriate form of therapy is to increase the margin of safety by teaching the sufferer how to behave habitually in a non-asthmatic way. If this can be done – and it can be even with children of eight or nine – spasms become less frequent and less severe. Any success will build up confidence and reduce anxiety which, by a virtuous circle, will make the sufferer less asthma prone.

Take an actual case history. A little girl of nine to whom I had given ten lessons came to me in a state of great excitement and triumph.

She had woken up in the early hours of the morning feeling, as she called it, 'puffy'. When this happened the routine was to call her mother who gave her pills which helped her to go to sleep again. But this time she decided to be independent by trying to apply what I had taught her. She was so successful that she went off to sleep again and did not wake until her usual time for getting up. But then again she had a feeling of breathlessness and again got rid of it in the way I had shown her. The rise in this child's morale was wonderful. No longer was she a helpless victim of a hostile force that came to suffocate her. She had confidence in her ability to defend herself. I was in touch with her the whole of the following year. She only had asthma (and then mildly) for half a day.

There have been many other cases, from different teachers, of asthmatics, not only children, being much helped by the Alexander technique. It must be emphasized however that, more than in almost any other condition, a great deal of co-operation and perseverance is needed from the pupil. The improvement, the result of re-education and not of some drug, has to be worked for.

In this approach no change of habit is being attempted independently of other changes. If the overall muscular tension has been reduced it will make the change in breathing easier. Muscular habits interlock with other habit systems throughout the body. That is why dealing with one habit by itself is often unsuccessful.

A question asked but not easy to answer is: how many lessons are necessary? The answer depends so much upon what the pupil is looking for. If all he is concerned with is relief from headache or backache he may easily go away cured, perhaps permanently, after about six lessons. One of my own cases is typical. A young woman who had ridden since childhood came to me complaining of backache. She had been X-rayed but no abnormality was found and no treatment given. She was puzzled about her symptoms because some horses gave her backache and others did not. After five lessons she discovered the answer herself. When she was riding a lively horse she gripped it more tightly with her knees and in so doing she tensed and bent her spine in the dorsal area. It was at this exact spot that the ache occurred. Having become aware of this habit she was able to deal with it and was not interested in continuing further lessons.

To prevent pupils from having too few lessons some teachers offer courses of not less than twenty or thirty lessons. This is to enable them to put over the Alexander ideas not merely as a form of therapy but as a way of life – as an aid to helping their pupils to become more aware of themselves and their reactions, rather less end-gaining, less of a slave to sheer habit, rather more able to adapt appropriately to new situations and new tasks, and a little less prone to hold on to fixed positions mentally as well as muscularly. It must be admitted that all these desirable ends are only rarely attained and there is a good deal to be said for leaving it to the pupil to decide whether, after his special problem has been solved or his symptoms relieved, he wishes to continue lessons. Pupils should be entitled to take as much or as little from the technique as they feel they need. Equally, teachers, are not compelled to teach those who are only interested in a quick cure. The best solution is the one most teachers adopt: not to fix the number of lessons but sufficient to arouse interest in pupils for them to want to spend the extra time and money to gain a deeper understanding of the full implications of Alexander's work.

Though not a panacea, the scope of the technique is extremely wide. Dr Peter Macdonald writing in 1926 said,

There seems to be a distinct betterment in cases of angina pectoris, asthma, epilepsy, tremor, spinal curvature, difficulty in walking from locomotor ataxia, and from infantile paralysis. In short I have seen, during the application of an educative process not directed to cure disease, manifestations of disease disappear so that I personally am convinced that Alexander is largely right when he says that disease is the result of wrong functioning. . . .'

It is regrettable that despite the fifty years since this was written the medical profession has with very few honourable exceptions ignored his work. Dr Wilfred Barlow, one of the few qualified Alexander teachers who is also a doctor, has contributed most to converting members of his profession to Alexander's ideas. In his book, *The Alexander Principle*, published in 1973 he details a great many conditions for which the Alexander technique is extremely valuable. He writes: 'In all the types of situation mentioned above in which physiotherapy is given – the rheumatic disorders, the spinal disorders, neurological disorders, breathing disorders, ante-natal and post-natal care, general ward care and rehabilitation, the Alexander Principle has much to offer.' He also has found it very useful in dealing with a wide variety of stress conditions, such as hypertension, gastric and duodenal disorders, spastic colon, ulcerative colitis, rectal spasm, and anorexia nervosa in the young. About migraine sufferers he writes: 'It is rare to find one who cannot be helped by learning to release faulty tensions around the head, neck and face.' He also adds that gynaecological conditions 'can be helped by the Use approach'. To quote him again: 'The most obvious field of application is in the therapy of the various muscular tics and cramps, which can vary from the occupational palsies such as writer's and telephonist's cramp, to severe conditions like spasmodic torticollis and persistent spasm of the shoulders and trunk.'

Alexander considered himself more of an educator than a therapist and so did not bother much about keeping detailed case histories. He regarded his job as being to teach people to use themselves better. If symptoms disappeared in the process, well and good; if not, at least there was a general improvement in functioning. But in *The Universal Constant in Living*, his last book, he does list several outstanding therapeutic successes such as cases of spasmodic torticollis, tic douleureux, asthma and others. Another case, one of osteoarthritis in the neck, is of particular interest because the pupil produced a photograph of himself in a school group taken thirty years previously. It showed how the disease process was already beginning with a marked muscular pull of the head to one side, and it is difficult to suppose that if the boy had then been given Alexander lessons the arthritis would have developed at all. Misuse of this kind lowers resistance locally by interference with normal movement and free circulation, and so opens the door to disease.

It is arguable that the technique can best be used as a contribution to positive health and in the sphere of prevention rather than as therapy. A certain amount of work has been done in schools by a few teachers. But there is always the problem of how to apply what is essentially a form of individual teaching to groups. There is, too, the fact that the technique needs a lot of co-operation from the pupil and to obtain this there needs to be quite strong motivation. For this reason pupils in discomfort or pain which they find is being relieved naturally work more conscientiously than healthy young people with no feeling of need.

The technique has the priceless virtue of combining prevention and therapy. The sufferer from disc trouble whose symptoms it relieves will also find that learning to use his body better makes it unlikely that he will have recurrence. In this way it works like a cure produced by a change of diet or some other basic modification in the way of life. This approach to the problems of health and disease is probably the only way of achieving a real advance in human well-being. Drugs, though sometimes necessary, should be regarded as a last resort. The really important and fundamental question is: what habits of life have made the use of drugs necessary? And this question is hardly ever asked.

Eric De Peyer

APPLIED KINESIOLOGY

Kinesiology is the science of muscle testing to determine the inter-relationship of the physiological processes of the body with respect to movement. In practice, kinesiology (pronounced 'kin-easy-ology') is used to determine the range of movement of the various muscles, and their opposing partners, and to obtain an analysis of the relative muscle tone.

Applied kinesiology on the other hand is an extension of this science which has been developed over the last few years principally in the United States by leading members of the →chiropractic profession. Applied kinesiology uses the application of muscle testing to diagnose physiological conditions, and anatomical problems of the human body. Foremost in this work is Dr George Goodheart, who has developed the science to a much greater degree than ever before by identifying the links between the energy pathways known to the Chinese as meridians and specific sets of muscles.

Further, his research led to discoveries that there are also more links which relate not only the muscles to the meridians, but also to what we call neuro-vascular reflexes, neuro-lymphatic nodes, and the organs of the body. The effects of stress on the human organism may be accurately monitored by this method of simple muscle-testing procedures, which may be used by practitioners in health care as an extremely useful adjunct to other forms of diagnosis.

Another group of chiropractors in the United States have produced a synopsis of the basic understanding necessary to apply both the tests and the various corrective therapies which are advanced to rectify energy imbalances designed especially for the lay public to use. Courses are available to all interested in learning more about health and how to maintain it, rather than disease and how to cure it. This information is called Touch for Health, and there are instructors being trained in their dozens across the American continent. They are then able to teach the principles to anyone who is willing to take the time to learn some basic anatomy and physiology, the techniques of muscle testing, and the methods of systematic balancing which are simple to do, and have proved to be completely safe for lay people to use.

In no sense does this qualify or license people to become any sort of 'doctor', nor does it enable the diagnosis of disease or provide 'cures'. It does enable them to take a more informal interest in the active care and maintenance of the health of their families, to detect energy imbalance in the body, and to apply massage and touch to bring relief to the person concerned. It is a reason to touch others for purposes other than sex or violence. Many chiropractors and osteopaths (→osteopathy) are utilizing this information, and many are now employing qualified Touch for Health instructors to assist them in their practices. Since 1975, there are also qualified instructors in Britain from whom this training may be received on several levels – basic courses, advanced courses, and seminars for professional practitioners.

For thousands of years, oriental medical practitioners have been aware of the energy patterns that relate to the various body functions. Research into applied kinesiology has drawn from this knowledge, and combined it with the fruits of western work on anatomy, human biology, and biochemistry.

The body is run by energy, which in a healthy person is perfectly distributed within all of the systems of the body, whether it be concerned with the maintenance of correct posture, or the proper function of the organs, or the motor reflexes of the musculature. When this energy is in balance and a state of homeostasis exists, the body reflects perfect health. Whenever these energies are disturbed, diminished or increased through any form of stress, whether it be physical, chemical, or psychological, the functions of the whole organism are thrown out of balance.

If this situation is allowed to continue, impairment of function begins to manifest itself in the form of mild symptoms at first, but as time progresses the onset of disease begins. Uncorrected, this may lead to acute problems, the disease may become chronic, and inevitably leads to the health of the individual deteriorating further. Unfortunately this happens all too frequently, as most people feel unwilling to bother anyone when the initial mild warning signals are felt. The further the disease process progresses unchecked, the harder it becomes to rectify.

Applied kinesiology provides a means whereby these energy imbalances may be detected long before many other tests, whether by observation, biochemical analysis, or even X-ray, would reveal the impending problem. Once the problem is pinpointed by muscle testing, energy-rebalancing therapies can be given which will begin to reverse the process, and allow vital body energies to flow normally again within the distressed system. This brings energy to the organ, strength to the related muscles, and relief from symptoms.

In our present-day society, we are constantly under stress every moment of our day. The physical stresses of gravity, and normal human activities involved with our daily working, eating, and sleeping, should be easily and automatically taken care of by a healthy person. Stress in our age has developed into a scourge for vast numbers of people. The human frame can cope with a given amount of emotional stress without causing the onset of any disease process. The problem comes when these pressures are incessant.

It is becoming more apparent that all disease begins with a lack of energy in a muscle, organ, or system. When undue emotional stress drains the energies necessary to achieve the physical and mental work away from those centres, health begins to suffer. Ideally we should be able to grow up in an environment free from emotional trauma. Instead, we live in a society where television, films, books, magazines and all the media seem intent upon whipping up our emotions to fever pitch. Is it any wonder that the health and productivity of a country go down when its greatest national resource, its energy, is being squandered upon negative expressions like anger, worry, irritability, greed, jealousy, impatience, anxiety, boredom, fear?

Too often, small children learn wrong emotional habit patterns within the confines of the family, express them at school, then suppress them during business and social life, only to find these inner pent-up pressures explode in outbursts of relationship-destroying proportions. Or worse, they develop in the prime of life the illnesses which inevitably result from energy imbalances initiated, maintained, and aggravated by habit patterns over the years.

Fortunately, applied kinesiology is available to a better educated public, so that each family or unit may make itself a committee of one to exemplify and epitomize good health and how to maintain it. Touch for Health emphasizes the need for proper emotional direction, and shows how postural, dietary and physical information can help to relieve the effects of the inevitable stress, and also gradually bring about the ability to become immune to the internal and external pressures which would otherwise distress the body. This surely expresses the fond hope of all mankind, to live happy, healthy lives.

Applied kinesiology has revealed that virtually all muscles have a common relationship with an internal organ. That is to say that they might share the same spinal nerve pathways, or the same lymphatic drainage system, or the same blood vessels, as well as being linked to the same →acupuncture meridians.

Whenever subjected to stresses beyond what the body can handle, it actually shuts down, or turns off certain parts in an attempt to protect the system, just as fuses blow in an electrical system. The systems that shut down can involve nerves, blood vessels, lymphatic drainage, muscles and organs. So it can be seen that if these portions of the body are left open circuit, or shut off for an extended period, malfunction and disease can eventually occur in the tissues involved.

Emotional problems have a direct effect on the alimentary canal. Stomach ulcers, duodenal ulcers, indigestion, constipation or diarrhoea, and a host of other ailments can arise as a result of stress. No portion of the frame escapes, and so heart disease, kidney malfunction, neck and shoulder pains, lumbar and low back pain, migraines, headaches, and hundreds of other diseases can result from excessive stress.

The treatment is preceded by analysis. The relative energy level of each system is first tested, and the results recorded. There are fourteen major systems to check, with over thirty-five muscles in groups which help to pinpoint problem areas of energy imbalance.

Then one or several techniques are tried to see which is most effective in achieving a proper balance. A test applied after each therapy shows how effective it has been, and whether or not the system requires further activation. Finally, when balance has been restored, a final muscle check of all the weak systems is made to indicate whether homeostasis has been restored for the time being. How long this lasts depends upon the degree to which the original stress which caused the problem has been brought under control. It is usual for the activation to be progressively more effective for longer periods, until tests show that there is no longer any need for help in that particular area.

This may be after a single treatment in some cases, but others require several over a fairly short period, gradually tapering off with longer intervals between each occasion. To a greater extent, this also depends upon the state of health and mental approach of the individual, but essentially too upon the control of causal stress factors. The different therapies used to activate energy balance are now listed in order of probable use.

Neuro-vascular points, mainly situated on the cranium, appear to be electrically or energy-controlled switch points for the flow of energy to all the main systems of the body. The lightest touch on these points for a short period results in a gradual realignment of energy levels. This is apparent to the one using the technique, as pulses which are apparently unrelated to the heart beat begin to be felt under the fingertips after only a few seconds. After a further few seconds, these pulses begin to synchronize with each other, indicating that a strengthening effect has taken place. When the muscles associated with that system are

31

re-tested, they are found to have gained in tone.

Neuro-lymphatic reflexes, nodes, and switch points, some of which do not necessarily appear to have a physiological origin, but merely exist as a force field, are treated next. Pressure is applied to these in a circular motion in a fairly firm massage, friction being similar to that used on the scalp when washing the hair. The human body contains approximately twice the volume of lymph as it does blood, about two gallons depending upon the size of the individual. The function of lymph is to drain the by-products of metabolism and other débris in the body back to the blood vessels for filtering and disposal. It follows that any blockage or impedance of the flow of lymph will result in the gradual accumulation of undesirable waste products which initially leads to local discomfort, then pain, and finally infection and disease. When these reflexes are reactivated, flow is normalized and strength returns to the related muscles and organs.

The third possible approach is the holding of acupressure points. On many occasions these are the same points which an acupuncturist may use in the course of his treatment, but in Touch for Health no needles are used, merely the lightest touch of the fingertips. Surprisingly this brings about the needed balance in many cases. It is also very effective in pain control, especially in cases of muscle spasm which can cause agonizing pain. As the energy flow is restored again in the meridian, the hypertonus of the muscle relaxes and the pain eases. This assists any misalignment of the bone structure to correct itself, as the pressure is taken off any nerves which have been affected.

The fourth possible method of activation is to brush lightly the meridian pathways. This has a relaxing and soothing effect upon anyone in distress, and again is useful in pain control.

The next possibility lies in the treating of the origin and insertion of the muscles. When a muscle is passively stretched, that is the origin or fixed portion of the muscle is drawn away from the insertion or moving end of the muscle, the strength or tone diminishes. This is necessary in the case of a spasm. When the origin and insertion of muscles are drawn towards each other the energy in the muscle increases, rectifying the weakness.

In addition to all these, there are many dietary considerations, which can help towards alleviating symptoms. Each system in the body needs the benefit of specific vitamins or supplements where any deficiency has developed. It is even possible to determine the relative extent to which a person is allergic to any given substance.

It is necessary to pay attention to postural defects which have been habitually adopted and might be aggravating the situation. The approach is toward the whole person, as work, food, posture, environment, and especially emotional outlook all affect the degree to which the individual may be affected by undue stress.

Applied kinesiology may be used even on small babies. Parents can help children with tummy upsets, colds, and other minor problems, and bring about an amazing amount of prompt relief for those conditions which would not normally require the attention of a doctor, or until contact with one can be made. Sportsmen find they are able to perform to higher standards of excellence after muscle balancing, as many of the athletes at the last Olympics would testify. There is almost no one who will not benefit in some way from the application of these gentle techniques.

None of these therapies is set forth as a cure for pathological conditions, but they act powerfully to stimulate the body to bring into play its own ability to restore proper balanced function to all the organs, energy pathways, musculature, and lymphatic systems. Sometimes, following the release of toxins, a person may at first feel some slight adverse effects, although these pass off very quickly leaving the individual to feel the full benefit of what has been done.

Chiropractors, osteopaths, acupuncturists, and other therapists are finding applied kinesiology a very useful adjunct to their knowledge, and of value in diagnosing and treating many of the problems their patients have. Many claims for the remarkable results achieved could be given, but essentially the only effective way to evaluate how good these principles are, is to give them a proper trial.

Brian H. Butler B.A.

CONTRIBUTORS, p. 220

AROMATHÉRAPIE

Recent research has enabled the renaissance of an ancient therapeutic method based on the use of essential oils and essences extracted from flowers (→**flower healing**), plants, resins and other substances.

The use of essential oils in cosmetology and as an aid to good health formed a major part of traditional medicine in Tibet, India, China and the Middle East. Ancient Egyptian medicine, dating back as far as 4500 B.C., was almost entirely based on the use of aromatic substances which are the key to modern aromathérapie.

Modern aromathérapie was developed in Europe by the late Marguerite Maury. Working in France with her husband – a →**homoeopathic** doctor – she was able to translate the traditional methods into a modern form more suitable to the pressures and life-style of today. In 1962 she published *The Secret of Life and Youth* in which she described the evolution of her new method. Also in 1962 she was awarded the Prix International d'Esthètique et Cosmetologie for her work in the field of aromathérapie which had achieved a major break-through in the modern use of essential oils. In 1967 she was awarded the C.I.D.E.S.C.O. prize for the development of aromathérapie preparations enabling widespread use of the method. Though much of her work was carried out in France, she lived and worked for several years in England. As a result her influence is strongly felt in Britain.

The initial work of Mme and Dr Maury was aimed at 'rejuvenation' – as indicated by the title of her book. They had found that aromethérapie encouraged the reproduction of skin cells and restored the elasticity of muscle tissue. In this way the skin remained clear and healthy, and wrinkles could be limited.

But it is evident and was recognized by Mme Maury that aromathérapie offers much wider potential. Because essential oils can be absorbed by the body through the skin, which is effectively the body's largest organ (weighing approximately twice that of the liver in a normally healthy person), it was found that the application of essential oils and essences to the skin provided a very efficient means of treatment. By their nature essential oils penetrate the skin (through osmosis) and are rapidly distributed around the body with a direct stimulating or healing effect on the internal organs and muscles.

Essential oils do not act by a chemical process alone, but rather through the odoriferous molecules which are composed of free electrons. Whereas every organic molecule possesses a certain number of free electrons the odoriferous molecule possesses them in even greater number. The Maurys found that this was crucial to the concept of aromathérapie and that it was possible to influence physiological functions by means of the free electrons possessed by aromatic substances.

The natural essential oils used are derived from flowers, plants, trees, resins and other biological substances, for example:

Flowers: carnation, rose, neroli, jasmin, lotus, lilac.
Aromatic plants: cinnamon, cardamom, camomile, angelica, tonka beans, violet leaves.
Resins: rosewood, galbanum, styrax, sandalwood.

In order to retain the properties of the essential oil the method of extraction employed is very important. If the essential oils have been obtained by distilling, their effect is not as remarkable as those obtained by *enfleurage*. This is a method of extracting by the following process. Flowers or plants are spread out on filters which are then placed in a bowl of oil. The oil, after a period of time, absorbs the odoriferous molecules of the plants, which have to be replaced frequently until the oil is completely saturated. The oil is then separated from the essence by volatile processes. The essences are then dissolved in cold pressed vegetable oils. Alcohol is never used as it destroys the valuable properties of the plant. It is obvious from the description of this method of extracting the essences that very small amounts of essential oil are obtained from huge quantities of plants and this results in the essences being very expensive and precious. For example, a tonne of rose petals is required to make 1 kg of essence.

The reason for the success in the use of essential oils is easy to understand. Highly concentrated natural substances are used. These extracts contain the quintessence of the plant, energy in its purest form, which enters the human body, carrying with it very considerable revitalizing properties. The famous physicist, Romanet, said, 'The odoriferous molecule is the only living hormone.'

Each essence possesses different properties which act on the body and mind, influencing the emotions. They work in a different way from the herbal extracts used by herbalists. To name a few examples:

Angelica: stomachic, stimulant and tonic of the digestive system; general tonic; good for affections of the respiratory system.

Benzoic: expectorant, pectoral pulmonary antiseptic; helps cicatrize wounds; cures skin trouble.

Bergamot: strong antiseptic and bactericide; helps heal wounds, helps pigmentation of skin in the sun.

Cinnamon: stimulant of the circulatory, respiratory and cardiac systems; general tonic; aphrodisiac; eupeptic, antiseptic.

Cypress: haemostatic; astringent; diuretic; pectoral; sudorific.

Lavender: stimulant of the nervous system; tonic cholagogue; antispasmodic; carminative; diuretic.

Myrrh: antiseptic; vulnerary; skin disease; pectoral.

Neroli: nervous stimulant; anxiety cure; antitoxic, anti-virus; sedative; paraticide; hypnotic; cardiotonic.

Ageing, both of the tissues and of the appearance of a human being, comes when the new cells are biologically too weak to enable these processes to take place, but if the rhythm of the regeneration is maintained there is no reason why anyone should fall victim to premature old age or degeneration. The life-long use of essential oils will help prevent debilitating, ageing illnesses and malfunction of the body.

Aromathérapie at a salon is recommended and patients are advised to take a course of from six to ten treatments, two or three times a year as required. An initial consultation is usually given before recommending treatment.

At the consultation a sample of the patient's blood is taken and analysed to discover the essential oil needed for one's organism. Radiesthesia is sometimes used for this analysis. An individual oil based on the result of the analysis is prepared for the patient. Each composition is unique and consists of a combination of essential oils selected from the 250 available. The patient uses her individual oil and creams at home and follows the instructions given at the clinic.

When a particular treatment has been decided for a client at a clinic, a massage is given, concentrating on the back and along the spine, using the method of German soft tissue massage and acupressure points. Depending on the treatment required, other parts of the body are massaged, in particular the feet, hands, arms and neck, using the patient's individual oil. The treatment concludes with a facial massage.

Amongst those cases treated with success are acne, wrinkles, skin troubles, seborrhoea, broken capillaries, poor circulation, obesity, muscular asthenia, rheumatism, sinusitis and depression.

Danièle Ryman

ASTROLOGICAL DIAGNOSIS

The association of astrology and medicine goes back to the remotest times. In Egypt and Chaldea, and in European and Arabic cultures a long tradition of great physicians upheld in precept and in practice the value of astrology as an adjunct to medical art and science.

From the time of Hippocrates a considerable science of planetary cycles, climacteric periods and critical days was developed and enlarged by such men as Galen, Avicenna and Paracelsus. Of these, the first two were both known as 'the prince of physicians' in their own day and for centuries afterwards. Whatever their shortcomings of medical knowledge they were undoubtedly powerful and original intellects whose teachings dominated medicine for fully fifteen hundred years.

Many of these astro-medical teachings (especially as developed by the Arabs) were, for example, preserved by the English herbalist–astrologer, Nicholas Culpepper, in his *Semeiotica Uranica*. In his later years Rudyard Kipling who was interested in medicine (and who, incidentally, has a short story, 'Unprofessional', about a doctor who went in for healing by cosmic radiations), was invited to address the Royal Society of Medicine. On that occasion he told the members of that illustrious body the following anecdote:

Nearly three hundred years ago Nicholas Culpepper, an astrologer physician, was in practice in Spitalfields, and it happened that a friend's maid-servant fell sick, which the local practitioner diagnosed as plague. Culpepper was called in as a second opinion. When he arrived the family were packing up their beds, preparatory to going away and leaving the girl to die. He took charge. There was no silly nonsense about taking the pulse or looking for the characteristic plague tongue. He only asked what hour the young woman had taken to her bed. He then erected a horoscope and enquired of the face of the heavens how the malady might prove. The face of the heavens indicated that it was not plague, but just smallpox, which our ancestors treated as lightly as we do. And smallpox it turned out to be. So the family came back with their bedding and lived happily

ever after, the girl recovered, and Culpepper said what he thought of his misguided fellow practitioner. Among other things he called him a man of forlorn fortunes with sore eyes.[1]

With the Renaissance men conceived a new interest in the world about them. They observed the world in a way that was, at first, not only a refreshing change but also a much-needed corrective to the excesses of rationalism in the middle ages. It was not long before this impulse to pay attention to the *outsides* of things, regardless of what the theologians and philosophers said about their *insides*, was, in its turn, carried to excess and became a new dogmatism. Science and religion split apart to become the basis of 'the two cultures': heaven and earth were separated from each other; the protagonists turned their backs not only upon one another but also upon astrology – which had been from time immemorial (as it will be again) one of the great forces which kept earth and heaven, man and the cosmos, together.

Since the beginning of this century a steady revival has been taking place in the study of astrology. Although at first this took the form chiefly of an attempt to recover the traditional teachings, in the past twenty years great strides have been made in re-examining and reformulating (or at least in laying the foundation of a reformulation) of astrology on a sound scientific basis.

The few practitioners today (and they are *very* few) who are able to make good use of astrological knowledge are obliged to look back to the old traditional teachings for their insights. They have not yet been able to make use of the new discoveries which are only now beginning to take coherent shape.

Unfortunately, although astrological tradition contains so much that is valuable, it also contains much dross. Therefore it is better at this stage to concentrate upon laying sound foundations for the future using the old ideas as a guide, re-testing and rebuilding astrological knowledge step by step upon demonstrably secure findings. So, this article is not intended to show the applicability of *traditional* astrology to medical science *today*, for that would be like trying to put old wine into new bottles. Rather it is to show the potentialities of the new astrology in its emerging applicability to the medical science of tomorrow.

One of the most important contributions which astrology makes to medicine is its capacity to indicate from the nativity the *kind* of diseases to which the native will be susceptible. A simple, generalized example is in the four temperaments which correspond to the four elements, fire, earth, air and water, which are woven into astrological symbolism and correspond to the four 'humours' beloved by earlier generations of physicians, each of them having its characteristic diseases.

But in recent times much more precise correspondence between planetary patterns and specific diseases have been found. A good example is demonstrated in a brilliant study by Charles Harvey (President of the Astrological Association) in which he traced the occurrence of haemophilia in all those descendants of Queen Victoria whose birth dates are available, showing that in all those who suffered from haemophilia the precise astrological positions in her horoscope were repeated.

Haemophilia is an hereditary disease of the blood in which bleeding even from a slight cut is difficult to control because the blood does not clot normally. The exact causes of this condition are not fully understood, but they seem to relate to a deficiency of two components in the blood, known as Factors VIII and IX.[2] Those who suffer from haemophilia – haemophiliacs – are almost invariably males, yet the disease is always transmitted through the female line; that is, the disease is due to a sex-linked recessive gene. A haemophiliac may have an apparently normal daughter who may none the less transmit the condition to her sons, or through her daughters to her grandsons. These female links are known as 'carriers'.

Queen Victoria would have been a carrier but it is usually considered by geneticists that she was the person in whom the mutation responsible for the disease took place since there is no clear evidence that she herself inherited it.

One of the important discoveries in modern astrology is the outstanding significance in the horoscope of mid-points between pairs of planets. These mid-points carry precise values appropriate to the combination of the planets involved. Therefore, for this study, a detailed comparison, including computerized mid-point analysis, was made of the birth charts of all the haemophiliac and haemophilia-carrier descendants from Queen Victoria whose birth data were available. Non-haemophiliac siblings were also included in the study and these showed a negative relationship in terms of the factors involved.

Highly significant astrological correlates emerge very clearly and are all the more striking because of their extreme simplicity. There are two sensitive points in Queen Victoria's chart which are repeated again and again in the charts of those of her descendants who suffered from or were carriers of haemophilia. These are Queen Victoria's Saturn at 28°46′ Pisces and her Mars/Saturn mid-point at 8°10′ Aries. These points are exactly duplicated in the haemophilia-affected descendants by 45° aspects. (That is to say, the afflicted descendants showed appropriate planetary or mid-point positions either exactly in conjunction with Queen Victoria's Saturn or Mars/Saturn mid-point, or at exact 45° intervals round the zodiacal circle.)

In the highly simplified pedigree diagram (*Figure 1*) the contacts with Queen Victoria's Saturn are shown *on the left* underneath each case name, and the contacts with her Mars/Saturn mid-point are shown *on the right*. The *orb* of the contact (i.e. the distance in degrees and minutes from the exact point) is given in brackets in each case and, as can be seen, there is only one case out of twenty-four where the orb is more than 1°!

Figure 2 shows the eight points at 45° intervals round the Zodiac starting from Queen Victoria's Saturn at 28.46 Pisces. A similar diagram could be shown for the eight points involving her Mars/Saturn mid-point. *These are the points which are exactly occupied by appropriate planets or planetary mid-points in the charts of the affected descendants.*

Fig. 1 Simplified pedigree of heredity haemophillia with cosmic correlates

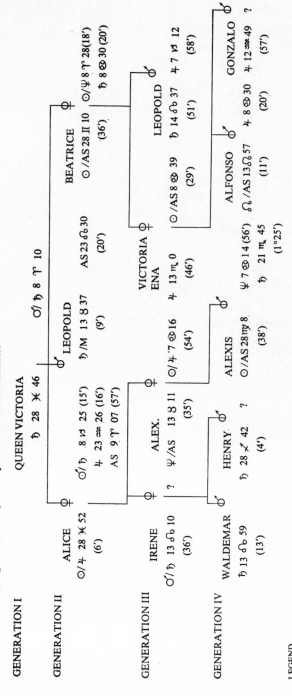

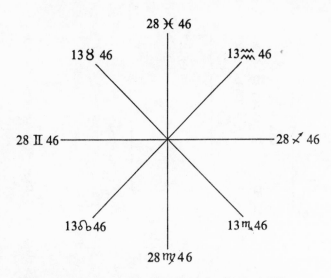

28 ♓ 46

13 ♉ 46   13 ♒ 46

28 ♊ 46 ──────────────── 28 ♐ 46

13 ♌ 46   13 ♏ 46

28 ♍ 46

Fig. 2   Queen Victoria's Saturn and points at 45°

It is not necessary to understand all the symbols and signs of the Zodiac to appreciate the significance of the pedigree. A mid-point between two planets is shown by an oblique stroke between two symbols. Thus Queen Victoria's daughter, Alice, has the mid-point of Sun/Jupiter at 28.56 of Pisces, that is within 6′ of her mother's Saturn; her ascendant is at 9.07 Aries, almost exactly on her mother's Mars/Saturn mid-point, and her own Mars/Saturn mid-point is just 90° away at 8.25 Capricorn.

Saturn and Mars/Saturn mid-point symbolize the hereditary deficiency. The planets and mid-points which are involved in the charts of descendants are also thoroughly appropriate for a disease of the blood. Jupiter has traditional rulerships of the blood while Sun/Jupiter is related by Ebertin[3] to the ability of regeneration in the blood. The carrier Princess Beatrice has Sun/Neptune = Saturn. This is interpreted by Witte[4] as 'blood disease'. However, no record of Princess Beatrice having suffered from a blood disease has come to our attention. The condition was only latent but came out in her son and was passed on to her grandsons through her daughter.

The 'cosmic pedigree' described above[5] characterizes the transmission of haemophilia with a minimum of astrological factors and a precision of zodiacal location. If this type of finding is corroborated by other studies it opens up the possibility of a science based on 'one-to-one' correspondence between cosmic factors and genetic structure. Perhaps we are close to the discovery of a chromosomal 'zodiac' as hinted at by Russell.[6]

It may surprise some readers, accustomed only to the shallow trivialities of newspaper astrology, to learn that the hereditary link between parents and children is clearly shown in a properly calculated horoscope for the exact time and place of birth. Yet this link has been scientifically demonstrated by the French researcher Michel Ganquelin.[7] In his first experiment Ganquelin used the dates and times of birth of 25 000 parents and children (all these birth data have been published) and he showed that where certain planetary positions were present in the charts of one of the parents there was a statistically significant tendency for the same position to be present in the nativities of offspring. Where the same position is present in the horoscopes of *both* parents the tendency for it to be present in the child's horoscope is twice as strong. This is in conformity with genetic principles. Recently Dr Ganquelin has repeated this study with the dates and times of birth of 36 000 *new* parents and children with identical results. The astrological reflection of the hereditary link must now be recognized as scientifically established. The discovery that genetic factors can be expressed in astrological terms is of immense importance to medicine and to other fields of study. This relationship is certain to be a focus of intense interest and inquiry in the coming decades.

The writer's contribution to modern astrological researches has been to show that all astrological forces (and therefore all the traditional lore of astrology handed down through centuries of tradition) are based upon the harmonics – that is the rhythms and subrhythms of cosmic periods.[8] The signs of the Zodiac, the 'houses' of the horoscope, the 'aspects' between planets, are all derived from this concept of regular rhythms within cosmic periods. 'Cosmic periods', or periodicities, mean any regularly recurring cyclic phenomenon in the astronomical field. The turning of the earth in its axis the various lunar, solar and planetary cycles, of which there are many, are all examples.

As an example of how these rhythmic forces manifest astrologically in relation to disease the writer has made a study of the nativities of 1024 children suffering from paralytic poliomyelitis.[9] From these it was possible to show that there are distinct and regular rhythms in time according to which polio-prone nativities occur in greater or fewer

numbers. A follow-up study of 257 polio sufferers with timed births confirmed the findings.

There are a number of implications of these and similar studies. First, the discovery that all astrology is based on cosmic rhythms immediately places astrology in the same, or a similar, category to that of circadian and other biological rhythms. Despite difference in philosophies, the astrologer and the biologist who study rhythmic phenomena in nature and man are now looking at the same kind of thing. The difference is that the biologist is not yet aware that his field of study is related to cosmic cycles of an all-various nature. He knows that many physiological rhythms are circadian, that is 'about one day' or a fraction of a day in length, and even that some of the creatures of nature, for example the crab, follow lunar rather than diurnal rhythms; but he does not yet realize that other cosmic rhythms are abundantly present in biological phenomena.

Another important consequence of the discovery that identifiable rhythms are at work in the manifestation of various diseases, together with the fact that the degree of susceptibility to them is potentially distinguishable from the nativity, is the relevance of this to medical research.

Most medical research proceeds on the assumption that everyone starts life with an equal chance of contracting various ailments and that the causative factors are to be found in the environment. The truth is that environmental factors are usually triggers which may set off the disease in those who were born with a susceptibility to it.

Thus, much has been made of the association between cigarette smoking and lung cancer. Yet it can easily be shown that the generation born about 1900–10 was the most susceptible to lung cancer and that since then successive generations have been less and less susceptible to it.[10] This largely unrecognized fact has invalidated many of the conclusions drawn about the relationship. When about 1970 the government started its campaign to discourage smoking among young people the incidence of lung cancer had already been falling at all ages below thirty for over twenty years and was by then in a state of run-away decline, those being born having an ever-decreasing tendency to lung cancer. 'Lung cancer deaths up again,' said a government poster. 'This will continue as long as cigarette smoking continues to increase.' Yet this was entirely untrue. The death rate from lung cancer among the heaviest smokers, say those at age fifty-five and under, has now been falling for a good fifteen years, and the only reason that lung cancer deaths have, even now, scarcely begun to decline is because the high death rate from this disease in the generation born in the first two decades of the century (now reaching its allotted three score years and ten) is still offsetting a falling death-rate at all ages below sixty-five.

In short it is the inborn tendency rather than the environmental hazard which is the primary regulating factor in this, as in most diseases, and which needs to be studied.

Although the immediate contribution which astrology can make to medicine is limited, it is now certain that new approaches to this age-old belief are beginning to produce results that will restore astrology to a key position in the physician's armoury of knowledge.

John Addey M.A., A.F.A.S.

ASSOCIATIONS, p. 212
BIBLIOGRAPHY, p. 244
PRODUCTS, p. 224

Notes

1. *Daily Express*, 16 November 1928.
2. R. G. MacFarlane, 'The clotting of the blood', *Science Journal*, December 1966, pp. 58–63.
3. Reinhold Eberton, *The Combination of Stellar Influences*, 1960.
4. A. Witte, *Rules for Planetary Pictures*, Hans Niggermann, New York, 1959.
5. J. B. S. Haldane, 'Blood royal', an essay in his collection *Keeping Cool*; and additional details most kindly given by James Russell, Director of the Astrological Association Genetics Research Group.
6. James Russell, 'Astrology and heredity',

Astrological Journal, Autumn 1966.
7. M. Ganquelin, *Cosmic Influences on Human Behaviour*, Garnstone Press, 1975.
8. John Addey, *Harmonics in Astrology*, L. N. Fowler, 1976.
9. John Addey, *The Discrimination of Birthtype*, L. N. Fowler, 1974.
10. T. W. Lees M.D., *Smoking and Lung Cancer* and *The Wave Theory of Cancer Mortality*, published by the author.

AUTISM

The word is derived from the Greek *auto* – self. The syndrome was first described by the American psychiatrist, Leo Kanner, in 1943. In Britain four to five children in every 10 000 suffer from the illness, with a larger percentage of boys than girls. Considerable controversy has surrounded its causes. Is it a purely behavioural abnormality arising from environmental factors and/or due to genetic or intra-uterine events? It is worthy of note that a number of mothers of autistic children have particularly stressful experiences either during pregnancy or at the child's birth.

From babyhood the typical autistic child resists physical affection and is inconsolable in what appears to be its grief and isolation. Usually there is good physical health, features are often beautiful with fine penetrating eyes – that is, if eye contact can be made, as avoidance of gaze is characteristic of the autistic child. There is often over-alertness in the body posture, giving the impression of readiness for flight, or a fixed position in which a rocking movement may continue for hours. There may be twiddling with string, the spinning of objects (with considerable skill), dribbling of sand through the fingers, pouring water without any obvious purpose and similar stereotyped activities. If these actions are interrupted, the reactions may be loud screaming, attack on people near by, even attempts at self-mutilation.

At times autistic children insist on carrying sharp objects – pins, a piece of broken glass – as other children would carry a soft toy. They appear not to notice extremes of cold or heat and will sometimes remain in front of a fire until they are burned, with serious injury resulting. Two examples of idiosyncratic behaviour were of one child who refused to allow its parents to remain together in the same room. The father had to feed him and stay with him all evening, while the mother, to avoid the inevitable tantrums, remained in another part of the house. Another child insisted that every person entering his home brought in a blown-up balloon.

An autistic child will note where objects are placed and if these are moved may show resentment or fear and in their agitation scratch, bite, bang their head, poke at their eyes or tear their clothes. In other circumstances some children will threaten to run away or jump out of a window. They may have to be kept in a locked room with barred windows. Speech is normally absent or used in a repetitive manner. Occasionally a sentence may be spoken, but will rarely be repeated. A high level of ability is not unusual, notably in mathematics or music, but practical application is lacking.

The effect on the family is traumatic. The parents become exhausted and distraught, other children are constantly interfered with, their possessions damaged, homework interrupted and their schoolfriends frightened away.

Generally the orthodox approach interprets autistic behaviour as arising from children who lack the necessary speech receptors in the brain, cannot understand the spoken word, are confused and unable to make sense of their environment. To help overcome this confused state the education method works to make connection between words and objects and groups of objects. Simple language, clearly spoken, combined with reading and writing exercises, where applicable, are used. Obsessional behaviour is, as far as possible, curbed. Drugs are sometimes used to quieten the child. In cases where there are recurrent attempts at self-mutilation, splints are used on the arms to prevent the child reaching his face or other sensitive parts of his body.

Despite the comprehensive time-table of activities which are normally provided, little time is allowed to promote self-motivated activity. Signs of latent intellectual ability tend to be seen as symptomatic of the autistic phenomena and are left undeveloped in favour of practical routine tasks. The results of this approach are generally disappointing. After leaving school some children go to adult training centres but more end up in psychiatric or mental subnormality hospitals. A small minority find places at a residential home for autistic adults, while a few continue to live at home and are able to take light employment.

An alternative approach to the problem began in 1967 at an autistic unit in London. It continued in this setting and later developed on an individual teaching/therapy basis. Positive results indicate that re-motivation can often occur in unpromising situations. The method is based on the hypothesis postulated by the ethologist and Nobel Laureate Nikolaas Tinbergen, who has stated:

The primary cause of the deviation [childhood autism] must, in most cases, be sought in the fact that genetically or otherwise, over-timid children live in a state of severe motivational conflict between hypertrophied fear of unfamiliar physical and social surroundings and frustrated sociality; a conflict aggravated by over-intrusion by frightening, though often well-meaning adults, including in many cases parents, who themselves live under considerable stress. All the evidence so far available suggests strongly that many of the well-known autistic symptoms – incapacity to 'relate', perceptual malfunctioning of many kinds, stereotopies, withdrawal or hyperkinetic behaviour, lack of exploratory behaviour, non-development or regression of speech and, in general, unteachability, are secondary, invetable consequences of the excessively fear-slanted, motivational conflict. This hypothesis fits with modern and experimentally tested ethological interpretations of conflict behaviour.

Professor Tinbergen noted that autists show an electroencephalogram that indicates a high over-all arousal.

The alternative approach to the treatment of autism employs the following precepts:

1. Presume the child can understand. Talk quietly and normally. Do not ask questions

unless the child speaks and uses language to communicate.

2. Never discuss the child in his or her hearing.

3. Be prepared to interest yourself in some creative activity in the presence of the child without expecting participation. (The child is expert at resisting conformity.) Eventually he may attempt the activity when you have left the room. He may need to do so secretively in order to make progress. Here a two-way mirror is valuable to observe his activity.

4. Where intelligence exists it can be further developed by finding someone to share it and teach the child at an advanced level. Such sessions will enable the child to fulfil himself, dispel his isolation and, later, work at mastering everyday chores which have previously been a problem for him.

5. Take non-verbal communication seriously.

6. The child is in an extreme state of distress and can unload some of it through emotional discharge if sympathetically supported. This discharge can take the form of laughter, tears, trembling, yawning, stretching or perspiration. When any of these occur, the child needs support in a quiet setting to enable the discharge to continue. Later it is likely he will want physical comforting and this should be given. (As an example, I know of a child who was integrated into a primary school. In the middle of work there would be a build-up of tension, whereupon he would leave the room, close the door, scream loudly and return to finish his work without further fuss. This child went on to complete a grammar school education and has become a skilled musician.) In most cases distressed behaviour is beyond the child's control and little reference should be made to it. Moralizing is totally inappropriate. Basically the child wants to receive and give love.

7. Any self-motivated behaviour of a positive nature should be accepted and encouraged.

These suggestions for a new approach to childhood autism are in keeping with the teaching methods of the educationalists Froebel and Montessori and have proved, in my experience, to benefit the children nurtured in this way. If there is any single recommendation to make it is that autistic children should be treated as human beings who have within them the potential for normality and happiness.

Barbara Roberts s.r.n., a.f.phys.

BIBLIOGRAPHY, p. 244
CONTRIBUTORS, p. 220

BALDNESS

Most so-called baldness cures tend to be more profitable for their vendors than those in need of them, but two which arose in unexpected circumstances appear to have led to hope for balding men.

One concerned an almost totally bald man in Stockholm who, in addition to his lack of hair, suffered from hardening of the arteries. It was for the latter ailment that he began receiving treatment at a Swedish hospital with nicotinic acid, one of the B vitamins which doctors were testing as a treatment for arterial disease. After three years he was delighted to find he was the owner of a full head of hair. Apparently the dilating effect the nicotinic acid had on the blood vessels had increased the blood supply in his scalp and brought about a vigorous growth of hair.

Another unintended cure was reported in the *British Medical Journal* by a doctor who had been treating patients suffering from a disease of the blood vessels with the drug betapyridylkarbinol, derivative of a vitamin substance pyridin-3-carbonic acid. As an unexpected bonus of the treatment the doctor noticed that some of his bald patients were growing new hair. One of them who had been completely bald arrived in his surgery with a 'beautiful and well-combed head of hair'. Following results such as these, preparations have been marketed with ingredients including nicotinic acid and other of the vitamins of the B-complex, together with iron, iodine and other trace-elements. There have been some favourable testimonies from users.

John Newton

BIBLIOGRAPHY, p. 246
CONTRIBUTORS, p. 220

BATES METHOD

Dr William H. Bates practised as one of the foremost eye physicians in New York. Born in 1860 he held posts at five hospitals and taught in the New York Post Graduate Medical School and Hospital. By the time he died in 1931 he had revolutionized the knowledge about and treatment of the eye. For in the course of examining more than 30 000 pairs of eyes, he made one startling observation: many defective cases recovered spontaneously, or changed the nature of their defect.

This was so startling because it ran completely counter to the theory of vision defects held universally then, and still widely today – that all defective vision was due to irreversible damage or deterioration of the eye's lens.

So Bates began to investigate further. He carried out some of the most far-reaching studies yet undertaken of the function of both human and animal eyes and came to this revolutionary conclusion:

Accommodation which is the process that governs near vision, like reading, and distant vision, like spotting the lightning conductor on top of the church spire, is not a function of the lens, as hitherto believed, but of the two oblique extrinsic muscles which encircle the whole of the eyeball.

That discovery had one practical and epoch-making consequence. It meant that visual defects were no longer incurable. For eye muscles, like all other muscles, can be trained and retrained. And the beginning of all retraining is relaxation.

That is the basis of the Bates method. It makes spectacles as irrelevant as are crutches to the cure of a sprained tendon.

It corrects, totally or partially, depending on the stage reached, the following defects:

Myopia or short sight where distant vision is difficult.

Presbyopia or old-age sight, where near sight is defective.

Hypermetropia, where both far and near vision are impaired.

Astigmatism where sight is blurred or distorted and the eye is abnormally sensitive to light.

Strabismus, or squint.

All can be eased or corrected by a treatment based on relaxation. Bates set up a number of ways in which relaxation can be induced in the eye muscles. These form the core of his treatment.

They start with *palming*. Dr Bates said that most patients are benefited merely by closing the eyes. But since some light comes through the closed eyelids, an even greater degree of relaxation is obtained by excluding it. This is done by covering the closed eyes with the palms of the hands – the fingers being crossed upon the forehead – in such a way as to avoid pressure on the eyeballs. That is all there is to palming – one of the most efficacious ways of relaxing the eyes and obtaining better vision.

Of no less importance as an aid to relaxation and better vision is swinging. It particularly counteracts the damage done by the strain of *staring*.

It is impossible, said Bates, for the eye to fix a point longer than a fraction of a second. If it tries to do so, it begins to strain and the vision is lowered. This is staring, a common fault among most people with vision defects.

Dr Bates found that by swinging the body from side to side, you not only relax but you consciously establish a new pattern of movement for the eyes. The reason is that the rhythm of the swing is gradually transmitted to the nerves which control the extrinsic muscles. And this new rhythm re-establishes shifting as the dominant pattern of eye behaviour.

Here is one of the most effective ways of swinging. Stand with the feet about one foot apart. Turn the body to the right while rotating the left foot. Then move in the opposite direction, rotating the right foot. Keep head and shoulders aligned. It is important not to move the eyes while you shift, nor to pay any attention to the apparent movement of stationary objects. The illusion of stationary objects moving indicates that you are swinging correctly. Continue the long swing for a minimum of five minutes.

Another way of creating the effect of movement by stationary objects is the *variable swing*. Hold the forefinger of one hand six inches from the right eye and about the same distance to the right. Look straight ahead, and move the head a short distance from side to side. The finger will appear to move.

The next essential element in the Bates system is *blinking*. This is not so much an exercise as a habit. The normal eye blinks *gently* and frequently. The defective eye blinks too rarely. So get back into the habit. Blinking always clarifies vision, if only momentarily.

Those are the basic essentials for restoring normal vision. Among the chief auxiliary factors is *sunlight*. This, Bates taught, is as necessary to the normal eye as relaxation. But here is a word of warning. *Never* look into the sun with the naked eye. Instead, close your eyes, and let the sun shine on your closed lids. Move the head from side to side while sunning so that no single part of the eyes get the full force of the sun for long. Do this for only two or three minutes. And always palm after sunning.

One of the most powerful aids to normal vision is imagination. Bates insisted that persons with normal vision use their memory, or imagination, as an auxiliary to sight. When the sight is imperfect, he said, it can be demonstrated that not only is the eye itself at fault, but the memory and imagination are impaired, so that the mind adds imperfections to the imperfect retinal image. He therefore devised a number of exercises to retrain memory and imagination.

The Bates system has never failed to correct or improve the defects listed above, given a chance by diligent application.

Tense and nervous types need more time for re-education than the more placid. But people who are looking for instant success,

had better think again. The essential ingredient of re-education is time.

One of the most spectacular successes of the Bates method was personified by the writer Aldous Huxley. He wrote a book about it, *The Art of Seeing*, which is still in print. Because of a teenage illness, reading to him was a constant problem, overcome only by powerful glasses and a constant administration of atrophine to dilate the pupils, until the day, when in spite of greatly strengthened glasses, reading became increasingly difficult. 'My capacity to see was steadily and quite rapidly failing,' he reported. That was the crisis point at which he heard of the Bates method. He gave it a try. 'Within a couple of months,' he wrote, 'I was reading without spectacles [something he had not been able to do for more than a quarter of a century]. And what was better still, I was reading without strain and fatigue. The chronic tensions, and the occasional spells of complete exhaustion, were things of the past.'

Finally, here is Dr Bates's own advice to doubters who wish to test the principle of his method:

Close your eyes and rest them, remembering some colour, like black or white, that you can remember perfectly. Keep them closed until they feel rested. . . . Now open them and look at the first word or letter of a sentence for a fraction of a second.

If you have been able to relax, partially or completely, you will have a flash of improved or clear vision. . . .

Continue this alternate resting of the eyes and flashing of the letters for a time, and you may soon find that you can keep your eyes open longer than a fraction of a second without losing the improved vision.

Evelyn B. Sage

BIBLIOGRAPHY, p. 244
CONTRIBUTORS, p. 220

BELLY DANCING

This ancient and erotic art has few competitors as both a slimming method for its devotees and a particularly pleasant source of entertainment for the men in their lives. Referred to somewhat clinically as the 'abdominal dance' by Curt Sachs in his major work *World History of Dance*, and of which the poet Martial wrote, 'Tirelessly the lustful move in gentle tremor eager limbs,' belly dancing incorporates in its classic form a trembling and undulatory trunk motion, movements of the breasts and back muscles and gyrations of the rectus abdominis.

A modern advocate of belly dancing as an aid to slimming is 'Soraya', herself a talented belly dancer and author of *Slimming: An Oriental Approach*. She says that her method of exercises, if properly performed, will help to improve health, remove fat, promote a better sex life and do so in a way far more gentle than the hard work involved in many other types of exercise. The movements of the belly dance are smooth and lithe, each performed with a flowing grace. Some of the rhythmic movements for the stomach muscles can even be performed while washing or cooking the dinner. 'Soraya' points out that the original purpose of the belly dance was sexual and it is possible through her method to train the muscles that come into play during lovemaking. By this means women can enhance the quality of their sex lives and that of their husbands or lovers. The muscles controlling the pelvis, important in love-making, can, when properly controlled, considerably aid sexual satisfaction. Equally the 'internal muscles' of a woman can, through appropriate exercise, be made to tighten and relax at will, providing no little pleasure for the male partner.

John Newton

BIBLIOGRAPHY, p. 244
CONTRIBUTORS, p. 220

BIOENERGY AND BIODYNAMICS

Bioenergy is life-energy of cosmic origin in man. It was discovered and used in psychotherapy by Wilhelm Reich (→**Reichian therapy**), who was a pupil of Sigmund Freud. This energy is known in eastern philosophy as 'prana' in yoga, and 'ch'i' in →**acupuncture**. The flow of bioenergy in the organism promotes well-being and good health, while its blockage causes nervous tension and muscular pain. Bioenergetic treatment is used in psychotherapy and for treating psychosomatic illness in both individual and group therapy, as in Reich's orgonomy and Alexander Lowen's bioenergetics. Biodynamic psychology employs all these methods and owes much of its development to them. In bioenergy and biodynamic psychology one works with both body and mind, with the focus on the body's psychological defences, which are anchored in muscle tension (muscle armour). Massage and breathing techniques are employed in order to help patients to get in touch with their own feelings.

Biodynamic psychology is a science of somatic-oriented psychotherapy I have developed during more than twenty-five years of clinical experience in psychology, vegetotherapy and dynamic physiotherapy. My discoveries, through research in psychosomatic disturbances and mental illness, revealed complementary hypotheses to Wilhelm Reich's orgonomic science and his theory that pathology is a disturbance of the bioenergy metabolism. In particular the dynamic behind repression is amplified by my focus on visceral tension and its regulation mechanism: 'psycho-peristalsis'. This discovery explains the rôle of the digestive organs in relation to emotions, namely the capacity to regulate and dissolve nervous tension and stress, and its effects, via *metabolic* discharge.

Since this particular intestinal function is related to nervous tensions and not the digestive processes, it is called *psycho*-peristalsis (in general physiology, the contractive movements of the intestines brought on by the digestive juices are called peristalsis). During my extensive work with psychosis and other mental illness, I noted particularly positive results when attention to the intestinal response was directing the treatment.

The underlying theory is that psycho-peristaltic activity is a natural function in the healthy organism, preventing nervous tension and stress from becoming chronic disabilities. Neurosis, as such, is the gradual inhibition of this organismic self-regulation. The restoration of function of psycho-peristalsis will detoxify tissue and aid in the release of muscular and respiratory tension.

Whilst highlighting the importance of visceral tension in the formation of neurosis, the biodynamic method works on all aspects of the personality, including the muscular, vegetative, psychic and spiritual levels. By this approach one can influence cellular functioning in any part of the body, so that life-energy (bioenergy) can flow freely and vitalize every cell. Underlying the biodynamic approach is a methodology based on a wide range of therapeutic concepts drawn from Freudian and Jungian analysis, the Reichian vegetotherapy of Ola Raknes and the dynamic physiotherapy of Dr Braatoy and Bulow-Hansen and other related methods.

In the biodynamic context there is a consistent goal to integrate the new methods and findings with those of Wilhelm Reich.

'Psycho-peristaltic regulation' is the main somatic method applied in biodynamic therapy. It is divided into three groups of visceral treatment:

1. *Harmonization* techniques which provide emotional vitalization by generating visceral energy.
2. *Distribution* techniques which provide emotional relaxation by drainage of excessive visceral energy.
3. *Mobilization* techniques which provide emotional excitation by activating repressed visceral energy.

(All approaches stimulate self-regulative functioning of the viscera almost from the very start of the treatment.)

For this purpose a stethoscope is placed on the navel region of the patient in order to pick up psycho-peristaltic responses during treatment, which consists of various massage and touch stimuli on the peripheral nervous system (the skin and muscle membranes).

Other Reichian and neo-Reichian methods are synthesized into the biodynamic therapy, although the psycho-peristaltic principle remains the guiding line throughout. These methods are applied according to the patient's needs and alternate between somatic and psychoanalytic techniques. The bodywork of vegetative massage, deep draining and breathing exercises, for example, has a mainly biological function in loosening muscular tension and establishing bodily harmony by encouraging the flow of pleasurable and relaxing feelings. Parallel with it is the psychological approach, referred to as 'dynamic relaxation', which is used to bring repressed emotions, such as memories, dreams and libidinal feelings into consciousness.

What is essentially presented in biodynamic psychology is a physiological basis for psychotherapy, with the consistent linkage of body and mind. The unique principle expressed in the therapy is the confidence in the individual's vital and creative self – the primary personality – the body itself wants to rid itself of the neurosis. This is an (often unconscious) biological drive which impinges from within. And it is just a matter of penetrating the first layer of resistance to contact this drive.

Gerda Boyesen

CONTRIBUTORS, p. 220
TRAINING, p. 232

BIOFEEDBACK

The biofeedback principle is this: if one can become aware of some body function of which one is not normally aware, then one can learn to control that function. The bathroom scales give feedback on the success or failure of one's attempts to control weight. Similarly biofeedback instruments are an aid in reducing, for example, tension and the effects of stress.

In one sense, though, biofeedback cannot be effective. If one has an electrical skin resistance meter and a book of instructions, then the act of trying to understand the use of the instrument will cause arousal; if one has E.E.G. (electroencephalogram) to aid in the detection of alpha brain rhythm, then involvement with the machine will cause the opposite response – alpha-blocking.

A guide is therefore needed so that the beginner's attention may be given to the desired result rather than the process until sufficient proficiency has been attained. We prefer to call this guidance biomonitoring rather than biofeedback where the instructor indicates to the subject the usual difficulties of the first encounter with the biofeedback instrument. Later the subject can open his eyes and read the meter, or even walk around the room without losing his alpha-rhythm. Later still, he has learned the feel of these altered states of consciousness and dispenses altogether with instrumental aid.

The use of biofeedback divides into two categories: it is being used in hospitals to supplement or replace other forms of treatment. For example it is effective in the treatment of →**migraine and tension headaches**, epilepsy, tachycardia, Reynaud's disease, high blood pressure, gastric and duodenal ulcers, re-training of muscles, and a wide range of nervous disorders, and biofeedback achieves this without the side-effects which are often found when using drugs.

The layman asks, 'How does all this help me?' The answer is that biofeedback is far more effective in the prevention of disease than it is in treating it. The implications of prevention, though, are wide-ranging. Stress, for example, may be caused by maladaption to tension at work, or it might be due to dissatisfaction with what we are achieving with our life, so that the border-line is very nebulous between prevention of disease and positive expansion of our total capacity.

Indeed prevention of disease is a rather boring subject; think of how many people continue to smoke even when they know of the likely damage to their bodies. Fortunately, expanding our total ability is far more interesting and does achieve a dramatic reduction in our susceptibility to all the stress-related disorders. This is confirmed by subjects attending biofeedback courses who have made the following typical comments afterwards: 'I

used to have migraine headaches', 'I used to suffer continuously from colds', 'I used to have mild epilepsy', etc.

The inference from this seems to be: if we trained our mental muscles, increase our mental fluency, i.e. become what Maslow calls a self-actualizing person, then we will be more healthy. The courses given by C. Maxwell Cade combine the ancient technique of →**yoga** with modern biofeedback technology, the aim being to increase self-control through self-awareness.

What physiological changes can be measured? How may we use this information to improve our health and creativity? One of the ways in which we measure our state of awareness and also of relaxation is by monitoring electrical skin resistance (E.S.R.) using a meter such as the Omega 1 connected to contacts at the palm of the hand. Skin resistance provides a number of clues as to how we, as mind, interact with the world. This electrical measurement is possible because the meter-readings are related directly to the behaviour of the autonomic nervous system. The rate of blood-flow varies with body tone and this causes changes of polarization at the sweat gland membranes. The changes of meter-reading are not caused by the apparent wetness or dryness of the hand but by this polarization which varies according to how tense or relaxed we are. The reactions which actually make us tense or relaxed are the 'fight or flight' response and its mirror image the 'relaxation' response – the response from the sympathetic and parasympathetic nervous system respectively. Our ability to cope with stress depends on whether these responses are free-ranging so that we can react appropriately to a situation or whether habitual reactions have caused them to stick somewhere on the scale.

The systems can best be understood with an example. If a tiger is on your tail panic is the correct response, but if you survive the first few seconds it is not. The fight or flight response mobilizes the body's systems to face danger: heart rate is increased, blood pressure goes up and blood is forced from the skin and organs into the muscles, muscle tension is increased, the digestive system closes down, and the cortisone level in the blood increases.

Immediately, the slower parasympathetic branch of the autonomic nervous system (the relaxation response) is energized to reverse these reactions so that rational thought and action take over. Reaction to stress in everyday life can arouse our bodies in a similar way. In this situation the arousal is followed by action and the relaxation response eventually returns the body systems to normal. However, often the modern reaction to stress leaves us in a state of partial tension causing, it is increasingly believed, many psychosomatic disorders. High blood pressure causes extra straining on the heart. Unused cortisone is not easily reabsorbed and reduces the body's immune response to disease. An inefficient digestive system results in ulcers, and continuously tensed muscles may be the cause of fibrositis.

The relaxation response is the very opposite of stress (fight or flight response) and can be learned through the biofeedback principle of monitoring these inner changes and learning how to relax by invoking the parasympathetic system and helping it to work as it should.

The effect of E.S.R. biofeedback training is to normalize the readings. Under-aroused people become more alert and active; those who are over-aroused become more calm and relaxed, while the normal person can change his range both up or down.

Having measured the physical arousal with the electrical skin resistance meter, we can estimate mental arousal and relaxation by studying the electrical rhythms generated by the brain. Briefly these are as follows. Beta 13–30 Hz (Hz is the measure of frequency in cycles per second) is the normal waking-rhythm of the brain. Alpha B–13 Hz is the most prominent rhythm of brain activity but is the one with least apparent meaning unless the associated rhythms are also known – an empty mind rather than a relaxed one. Theta 4–7 Hz is associated with creative inspiration and deep meditation. Delta $\frac{1}{2}$–4 Hz is primarily associated with deep sleep.

The left- and right-hand sides of the brain are physically identical but in fact share the work load. In most people the left-hand side of the brain deals with logical thinking, and because it is also concerned with speech the left-hand side acts as spokesman for the right-hand intuitive side of the brain. The left-hand logical side also tends to be the most developed and used half of the brain because we live within a technologically orientated society. The two halves of the brain, though, are joined by a massive nerve connection so that theoretically we do have all the brain's ability waiting to be used if we know how to activate it.

There are exercises to aid this development which begin with deep physical relaxation. Experience with meditation groups suggests that in a matter of a few hours the right-hand intuitive side of the brain may be encouraged to express itself so that the measured alpha and theta brain rhythms from the two halves of the brain become identical. When this relaxation can be maintained with the eyes open, then the beta rhythm will be found added. We call this tri-state rhythm 'state five' in the list of increasing levels of awareness.

These brain rhythms may be measured by a simple E.E.G. instrument such as the Monitor–M, though complex rhythms are more easily seen with a multi-channel E.E.G. such as the Mind Mirror made by Audio Ltd.

We hope by this training to increase our creativity using more of the brain's capability but at the same time to be more physically relaxed so that our vulnerability to the stress-related diseases is decreased.

There are other physiological measurements to give further aid in biofeedback training. The temperature meter used with visualization training assists muscular relaxation. A more sensitive electrical skin resistance meter (Omega 2) may be used in desensitization exercises. The E.E.G. Monitor–M also has a myograph facility which gives a direct response to the activity of a muscle.

The preliminary goals of biofeedback may well be concerned with physical well-being, but we believe that the potential is much greater. To quote Professor Ernest Woods, 'Our modern scientists now know that the age of natural selection has gone, and men must look to themselves not to their material environment, for the direction and impulse needed for their future progress.'

Geoffrey Blundell

BIORHYTHMS

I must consider more closely this cycle of good and bad days which I find coursing within myself. Passion, attachment, the urge to action, inventiveness, performance, order all alternate and keep their orbit; cheerfulness, vigor, energy, flexibility and fatigue, serenity as well as desire. Nothing disturbs the cycle for I lead a simple life, but I must still find the time and order in which I rotate.

GOETHE 26 March 1780

Everyone is conscious of the fact that their performance varies. It is possible to perform exactly the same task day after day and to finish in the evening feeling completely different. Sometimes you feel as fresh as when you commenced in the morning, but on other occasions you have just sufficient energy to get home and watch television. Sometimes you feel benevolent and capable of handling all the pressures at work and home – on other occasions you feel raw and all your nerve endings are exposed.

This is what biorhythms are about. They are about your variations in mood and performance – about your patterns of behaviour.

You have a number of self-recognizable moods and patterns of behaviour. So does everyone else. If you play sport, for instance, there is the recognizable state of being 'late' for every shot; of not being able to 'get it together', of total frustration because you know you can beat the other guy – and here you are losing.

All of these, and more, of your individual reactions can be related to your biorhythmic pattern.

What then are biorhythms?

Biorhythms, in this context, are the variations in performance and mood that have been measured, and to a great extent can be explained and predicted by assuming that we all have three basic energy cycles.

The *intellectual* cycle which has a rhythm of thirty-three days and affects, amongst other things, your concentration, judgement and learning abilities.

The *emotional* cycle which has a rhythm of twenty-eight days and controls moods, creativity and emotional life.

The *physical* cycle which has a twenty-three-day rhythm and governs your energy, co-ordination and stamina.

Each cycle has an active phase, with a good supply of energy; a passive phase during which there is a less plentiful supply and changeover periods where the energy supply is unstable and can switch backwards and forwards between the two phases.

All these cycles commence at birth.

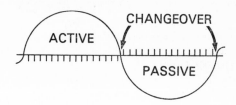

For a concept which at the moment is in the realm of 'fringe' medicine, biorhythms have remarkably respectable origins.

The original discovery, or observation, that behaviour varied as though there were two cycles, was made simultaneously and independently by two doctors. One, Wilhelm Fliess, a German, was working in Berlin, and eventually became President of the German Academy of Sciences, and the other, Herman Swoboda, an Austrian, worked in Vienna and became Professor of Psychology at the University of Vienna, a post he held until the mid 1950s.

Both doctors observed that their patients had symptoms, emotional and physical, which seemed to recur regularly. On investigation they found that the physical symptoms of pain, inflammation and fever seemed to recur as if the body followed a twenty-three-day cycle. The emotional symptoms, on the other hand, recurred as if the body had a twenty-eight-day cycle.

On working these cycles back to their points of origin the doctors discovered that both appeared to commence on the date of birth. This study was undertaken around 1900 and the first book was published in 1904.

Later, Alfred Tetschler, a Swiss, discovered that there was a thirty-three-day cycle which affected the learning ability and academic performance of his pupils at a high school in Switzerland. This cycle too appeared to originate at birth.

The Swiss maintained their interest in the subject of biorhythms, as these cycles were called, and produced the first calculator for plotting them in about 1927.

Since then very little serious academic work has been done. The Japanese and later the Americans in the 1960s have taken up the theory and made practical application of some of its aspects in industrial safety work. The Swiss have continued to use biorhythms, not only for industrial safety, but also, it is claimed, in their hospitals for determining the most suitable time for surgical operations, and in sport for the selection of their national gymnastic teams.

It is only recently in 1974 and 1975 that the theory has once again been put to the acid test of academic examination. This occurred in the United States Navy Postgraduate School at Monterey in California, and the programme arose out of an intention to disprove the theory.

I quote from the *United States Navy Times*, 25 June 1975:

In an effort to disprove the old theory, Professor Neil and Naval Postgraduate School students conducted a series of experiments which included monitoring the physiological, emotional and intellectual responses of volunteers by having them perform a series of tasks over a period of time.

Professor Douglas Neil of the Department of Operations Research and Administrative Sciences said, 'Frankly, it sounded like a lot of bunk. We started out with the intention of disproving it. But . . . our laboratory results took us by surprise.

'The figures showed human performance does vary according to biorhythms. They showed that the rhythms did indeed last for twenty-three, twenty-eight and thirty-three days cycles as the old theories had claimed.'

Let us now consider the implications and applications of biorhythms in the areas of health and self-help and stress reduction.

Firstly, biorhythms are not 'things that cause events to happen to you'. No dark handsome strangers are going to enter your life because of biorhythms.

Biorhythms are connected with energy. If you think of physical energy only, you get a useful picture of the action of biorhythms.

The energy you have available at any time is like a storage tank of water with two taps; one is always emptying the tank – this is you deciding how to spend your energy, by sitting still, or jogging, or perhaps playing tennis. The other tap, which is filling the tank, is controlled by your biorhythms. Sometimes it releases a plentiful supply (the active phase), and sometimes a less plentiful supply (the passive phase). Sometimes it vacillates. It can be active or passive (the changeover periods).

This model enables us to understand how biorhythmic variations can influence our behaviour and mood. If we try to spend a constant amount of energy while the supply varies, there are going to be times when we still have a good reserve of energy (the active phase) and times when our energy is depleted, or exhausted (the passive phase), depending on our level of expenditure.

The English language is full of phrases which describe our reaction to these conditions: 'I was mentally exhausted'; 'I had no reserves of physical energy left'; 'I was emotionally drained'; 'I was bubbling over with ideas'; 'I was full of energy'.

The point of knowing about one's biorhythms, seeing the pattern of the ebb and flow of energies laid out, is that it is then possible to come into harmony with the natural rhythms. If one continually over-rides the cycle of supply, one pays the price. The latest work on heart attacks being done in America by Rosemann and Freidman suggests that compulsive deadline-meeting and competitiveness are a major factor in the incidence of heart attacks.

It has to be remembered that biorhythms reveal only the pattern of variations in your energy supplies. The absolute level, if you can call it that, and your reaction to it, are depen-dent on your genes, your background, your situation and your natural make-up. Because of their nature and life style many people do not respond well to the times when they are active (i.e. have a good energy supply) in all three cycles. They feel edgy, irritable, tense and can even end up depressed, because they are just not spending sufficient energy to use up their supply. It is as if the storage tank were overflowing.

An everyday example and a suggestion as to the cure, is to consider what might happen to a little boy locked up in a room on a rainy day. He would tend to become destructive, because his latent energy has to go somewhere. The solution, which wise adults know, is to get him to go for a run and get rid of that surplus energy.

When you have your pattern of energies, your biorhythms laid out in front of you, you can then begin to see how it relates to your own pattern of behaviour. You will gradually find that when a particular pattern of energy repeats (for example active on all three cycles), then so does your pattern of behaviour (all things being equal, no broken legs for example).

Changeover days, when your energy supply is unstable, are often the easiest days to cor-relate with your behaviour. What seems to happen is that one is going along, spending energy as if it were a normal period, and suddenly the supply seems to dry up. The result is that one's reactions suddenly change to those associated with over-spending one's reserves; the sudden onset of physical tired-ness; the inability to find the correct word; the sudden irritability. All these symptoms appear to relate to changeover days. There are, of course, the reverse symptoms, when suddenly there is a plentiful supply of energy; sudden euphoria; a great upsurge of activity. Altogether changeovers produce an unstable period of energy and are therefore generally quite noticeable.

A knowledge of one's biorhythmic cycles can be regarded as a tool which will enable you to succeed in getting the best out of yourself in many fields.

Family life can be more harmonious where people use their knowledge of each other's biorhythms to help understanding. In some way the knowledge that another person is going through, say, an emotional changeover depersonalizes the irritating aspects of their behaviour. The behaviour is no longer directed at you, but is the result of their dealing with their energy supply situation.

Large families have found knowledge of biorhythms a great help in reducing tension. To be able to relate the children's behaviour to their energy patterns explains a great deal. Gone are many of the worries like, 'How have I failed as a parent?' The knowledge of bio-rhythms can change situations from a potential family trauma to a shared family memory.

Business colleagues have reported a great easing of tension arising from a knowledge of each others' biorhythms. The percentage of arguments, as opposed to disagreements, that have a biorhythmic basis varies, of course. Some people have discovered that 80 per cent of their conflicts had their roots in the bio-rhythmic state of one or the other participants.

Athletes have found that they can use a knowledge of biorhythms to organize training schedules. Dr Peter Burrows, the England soccer squad doctor, has drawn up a training schedule for his local club, Luton Town Foot-ball Club, based on biorhythmic information.

The idea is basically that when you are in the active phase of the physical cycle you can extend or push yourself to build up your stamina or strength. During the passive phase of the physical cycle you can just run a maintenance schedule rather than push yourself with the consequent excessive tiredness and risk of injury.

Winning or losing are much more complex subjects than training and the combinations of energy that suit one person may not suit another because of their personal temperament. Even the sport you are playing makes a difference. For example, the intellectual cycle, as it affects concentration, plays a significant role in golf.

Failure to slim or even maintain your healthy weight arises from eating too much. The points on which one 'breaks down' can be divided into two categories, both of which tie in with a particular energy cycle.

Firstly, there is the compulsive sweet-eating – cakes, sweets, buns, all the 'treats' that one has given up. These outbreaks are tied into the emotional changeover days.

Secondly, there are the days when one just feels incredibly hungry. A desire for 'bulk' foods, potatoes and bread for instance. The correlation here is with the physical change-over days.

A recognition of these correlations and a little forward planning has led people to a simple and reliable method of weight maintenance after years of fluctuating 'feast-and-starve' behaviour.

The area of application grows continuously as we receive more information from users of biocalendars. Investigations are going on in conjunction with a driving school, long-distance runners, teachers of remedial reading and migraine sufferers. A useful correlation seems to be emerging between all these areas and biorhythms.

There exists a relationship between the repeating patterns of a person's moods and performance and the pattern of their biorhythms. One can learn to observe and use this relationship. The benefits of this additional knowledge lie in the reduction of tension and the increased opportunity to make the best of one's abilities.

Michael McDonald B.SC., M.I.E.E.

CONTRIBUTORS, p. 220
PRODUCTS, p. 224

BREATHING – KNOWLES THERAPY

How to breathe healthfully is an art to be learned. The purpose of the Knowles system, which can be by personal consultation or by post, is to outline a method of daily exercise whereby better breathing can become a habit; so that whether you are awake or asleep you can be sure of a better supply of oxygen.

How you breathe matters supremely to your health and ability to combat disease and fatigue. Better breathing may help sufferers of asthma and nervous debility. Too many people imagine that they breathe rightly by instinct. Experience shows that wrong breathing habits have become almost universal. A greater supply of oxygen will purify and enrich your blood, renewing the structure and vitality of your mind and body.

No one is too old to breathe correctly. Everyone derives benefit from it. No one needs fear overstrain or inability to carry out the simple yet scientific exercises which, in a short time, establish for life correct and healthful breathing habits.

The key to breathing lies in the action of the diaphragm, a large muscle which separates the lungs from the abdominal cavity. When you inhale and make the lungs larger, it flattens out. When you exhale and make the lungs smaller, it rises. Most people take in only a limited supply of air. This means the diaphragm is not as active as it might be. If this inadequate breathing becomes a habit – and may be further curtailed through over-indulgence, such as smoking – then when any sudden stress or prolonged tension takes place the heart may suffer.

Such conditions as thrombosis (or stroke) are brought about by continued tension in the sympathetic nervous system caused by worry overtaxing one's energy. This condition appears more frequently in middle age. If attention to breathing were to become common practice, as common as shaving or attention to one's hair, there would be a remarkable reduction of this suffering.

It is an extraordinary fact that here is something given in abundance by nature – the breath of life – free for all to use, and yet in many ways it is not only neglected but actually impeded by bad habits and over-indulgence. In our cars we do not tolerate choked petrol lines, faulty carburettors, or anything that leads to poor engine performance. Yet we accept poor body performance caused by an inadequacy in the oxygen supply that is essential to the health and well-being of our trillions of cells. We *can* breathe our way to better health and better living if we bother to learn.

The object of the Knowles course is not primarily that of curing disease. Rather it is a means of strengthening the nervous system by an all-round toning up of physical and mental powers. It supplies the perfect means whereby the healing power of air and exercise can be brought to the aid of all who suffer from physical disabilities or whose occupations are sedentary.

Breathing exercises are prescribed by medical practitioners and hospital doctors for the relief of asthma, neurosis and emphysema. Asthma in particular yields to air treatment. Its cause is tension in the autonomic nervous system due to shock or prolonged strain. Although this nervous system cannot be consciously controlled it can be restored to more normal functioning by better oxygenation, which is induced by breathing exercises. Records show that a very large proportion of asthmatic patients have obtained permanent good results.

Here is something you can try for yourself.

Take a full easy breath and start to read a paragraph from a newspaper. Without causing the slightest strain, see how much of the paragraph you can read on one outgoing breath. Then after a slight pause – be careful not to gasp for breath – repeat the process. A few days' practice, just a few minutes at a time, will prove that by learning to breathe out slowly and steadily you have learned to relax. You will also find you have increased the amount of air that you can inhale.

Take for example the end of the day when you feel depleted and possibly out of sorts; the remedy is simple and only requires a few minutes. Sit in an easy chair and gently draw the shoulders slightly back, relax the arms and hands, then breathe out a long gentle sigh. Then slowly and gently, as though smelling a flower, breathe in, pause a second to allow the breath to remain in the lungs and then slowly and gently breathe out, pausing a second to allow the excess of carbon dioxide in the blood to be exhaled. Repeat twelve times and you will be surprised how different you feel. Why? Because you have given nature the chance she needs to recharge your system.

I use the rhythm of seven which is the basic rhythm of life. This rhythm adequately fills and empties the lungs. Consequently I have made this rhythm the first basic exercise and this has been proved by students to stimulate both body and mind to better health. In short, if you practise this exercise of seven in and seven out for twelve times at each session, at least three times a day, nature will have shown you a simple way to establish better health.

Captain William P. Knowles M.C.

BIBLIOGRAPHY, p. 245
CONTRIBUTORS, p. 220
PRODUCTS, pp. 226, 229

CANCER

The history of unorthodox methods for the treatment of cancer is long and controversial but there is increasing evidence that a number of them have produced successful results. It is conceivable that among them are some that will become the established therapies of the future.

Dr Josef Issels

Perhaps more controversy has surrounded Dr Josef Issels and his approach to the treatment of cancer than any other doctor this century. Born in 1907 in the German Rhineland, Josef Issels graduated in medicine in 1932 and soon developed skills as a surgeon.

His experience in cancer surgery made him realize that removing a tumour did not remove the cause of the growth and it was the cause he sought. For a time Issels became a ship's doctor and later became absorbed in the principles of homoeopathy and the associated methods of fasting and diet control. It was in the years after the war that he developed his philosophy of *Ganzheitstherapie*, the belief that the only rational approach to the cancer problem is 'whole-body treatment'. In 1951, with the help of a grateful cancer patient, Issels opened the Ringberg-Klinik in Bavaria. There he set out to treat the so-called incurable patients who had been given up by other doctors after all conventional methods of therapy had failed. His treatment included the elimination of focal infections such as septic teeth and tonsils, the administration of oxygen and ozone to help cellular regeneration, and the injection of a drug which irritated the fever control mechanism in the brain. This raised the patient's temperature to a peak of 105°F (40·5°C) which was maintained as long as possible. The effect of the fever was to stimulate the natural resistance of the body so that toxicity could be more easily removed. Issels also corrected nutrition, emphasizing the importance of keeping the blood slightly alkaline, eating raw foods and excluding flesh-foods. He also fortified and increased the bacterial flow of the intestine with special bacterial and enzyme preparations.

In 1959 independent statistical evidence was produced by Dr Arie Audier of the University of Leiden, after investigating 252 case-histories of Issels's patients. He found that on his sampling of the cases, all with a diagnosis of cancer no longer treatable by conventional means, forty-two of them, all 'terminal cases' with a life-expectancy of less than one year, had survived for five years living a normal life. This gave a statistical survival rate of 16·6 per cent – and this for patients who were regarded as beyond further treatment by some of the leading hospitals of Europe.

According to the figures of the World Health Organization less than 2 per cent of such patients could statistically have expected to experience 'spontaneous regression'. With his treatment Issels had achieved eight times better results.

Despite his achievements Issels continued to meet with opposition from medical circles and in 1973 the Ringberg-Klinik closed. Issels claimed that its closure was the result of a systematic campaign in West Germany to stop his whole-body system of cancer treatment. Nevertheless, three years later he was back, this time to continue his work at a private hospital in the Bavarian town of Bad Wiesse.

Orgone therapy

Dr Walter Hoppé, a Reichian orgone-therapist in Tel Aviv, Israel, was trained in psychiatry at the University of Berlin and has been in private practice in Israel for the past forty years. In November 1969 he was nominated a member of the Sybaris Magna Graecia Accademia, in Sibari, Italy, in recognition of his work in cancer research. He was one of the first physicians to confirm the effectiveness of Wilhelm Reich's (→**Reichianism**) orgone-accumulator, which made possible the accumulation of orgone-energy that Reich had discovered existed in the atmosphere. For the past thirty years Dr Hoppé has used the accumulator to treat a wide range of physical illnesses, including cancer. In his work on cancer Hoppé has applied and extended the results which he learned from his studies with Reich. A detailed article of his treatment of a malignant melanoma appears in the book *In the Wake of Reich*, edited by David Boadella, published by Coventure, London. In the article, originally a paper delivered by Hoppé at the Second International Seminar on Cancer Prophylaxis and Prevention held in Rome in October 1968, he states:

The accumulator can and will have a great prophylactic significance against cancer. For this purpose, everyone who wishes to protect himself in this manner against the cancer sickness should try to use the accumulator regularly and over a very long period of time. Not a single case of cancer has been registered, as far as I know, among those who have done this for years.

Relaxation healing and mind training

A new form of therapy for terminal cancer sufferers was introduced in May 1974 by Dr Ann Woolley-Hart and Gilbert Anderson L.N.C.P. after consultation with Dr Carl Simonton, an American cancer specialist and radiologist. The therapy took the approach that stress is largely responsible for many diseases, in particular stress involving suppressed emotion for which there is no outlet; therefore, removing these factors and creating within the individual the will to live and the feeling that there was something to fight for might result in a reversal of the stress situation. Both Dr Simonton and Dr Woolley-Hart had suffered from cancer and were convinced that they had been helped to overcome the disease by other agencies in addition to medical science – either by spiritual healing, a changed attitude and determination to live – or a combination of both.

In a first pilot study, seven advanced terminal cancer patients, with various forms of cancer, including leukaemia, bone cancer, breast cancer, lung cancer and uterine malignancy, were invited to take part. Two of them died, however, before it was possible to start therapy. In June 1974, after a thorough investigation into their past histories to discover their hidden stresses and release them, group-therapy began with the five terminal patients.

It was first necessary to eliminate the fear that their terminal verdict had created and to replace it with hope. It was felt that in many instances the patients themselves had brought the disease into being by their negative attitudes, due to the suppression of fear, hate, envy, resentment or other forms of worry, that had gained control of their thoughts. The purpose of the group-therapy was to teach relaxation, meditation and thought directive, so making the group-members more receptive to spiritual healing, which was given during their relaxation by the laying on of hands. Before long there was an encouraging reaction within the group. Increasingly members began to display a happier state of mind and over

the months their medical reports, too, became more encouraging: 'My drugs have been reduced'; 'The consultant can't understand the change; it's quite contrary to the normal pattern'; 'I'm so thrilled, my blood is normal'; 'The last X-ray shows the shadow much less and I feel fine'; 'I've been able to do some gardening without any ill-effect and the specialist said I'd never be able to do anything like that again.'

After two years, three of the terminal patients who survived showed no trace of cancer on medical examination. Of the two deaths, one patient suffered from the side-effects of radiation treatment; the other succumbed to severe shock when the specialist she idolized was killed in a bomb incident.

Following the encouraging response to the pilot study, further groups are being set up in various parts of the country. In a booklet produced by the founders of the relaxation healing and mind training therapy, they emphasize that their approach does not imply that the advice of medical practitioners should be ignored in favour of the therapy, and that it does not represent the whole picture; but it is intended to deal with the person as a whole and to explain how emotional problems and attitudes can affect health.

The lactic acid fermentation diet

Professor Johannes Kuhl M.D., PH.D. of Westphalia, West Germany, was the originator of the lactic acid fermentation diet for the treatment of cancer. He took the view that cancer is caused by impaired cell-respiration, where the cells have become choked with an excess of pathologically increased lactic acid. This can be removed, he said, and cell-respiration regenerated by the intake of certain fermented foods, rich in *nutritional* lactic acid. 50 to 70 per cent of the daily diet should consist of these lactic acid fermented foods which include fermented wheat-grains, fermented milk products (buttermilk, curd, yoghourt) and fermented vegetable juices. Unleavened bread (bread-dough without yeast) is also a part of the diet.

Red beet therapy

Two leading European physicians, Dr Sigemund Schmidt of West Germany and the Hungarian Nobel prize-winner, Dr A. Ferenczi, advocate the use of red beet (*Beta vulgaris*) as a supplementary treatment for cancer and leukaemia. Dr Schmidt has stated that in cases of tumorous diseases and leukaemia the juice from red beet has produced favourable results. Daily doses have also reduced the toxic effects of ionizing radiation.

In a speech given at the 21st Conference of the International Vegetarian Union in 1972, Dr Ferenczi reported that he had been treating cancer with red beet since 1950. In its application to thirty-eight of his cancer patients, thirty-six showed signs of recovery; of the thirty-eight, eight recovered to such an extent that clinically no symptoms remained. In all cases their general health improved. However, the recovery lasted only as long as the patients continued with the treatment.

Another researcher in this field, Dr Seeger of Berlin, has found that beetroot juice increases the respiration of cells with oxygen up to 400 per cent, thus destroying toxins through oxidization. Because of its high iron content the juice regenerates and activates red blood corpuscles, increasing oxygen in the corpuscles and cancer cells as well as activating respiratory ferments. That the main cause of cancer is the lack of oxygen in the body was the view of Dr Otto Warburg, Nobel prize-winner and head of the Max Planck Institute of Cell Physiology in Berlin.

Robert Bell M.D.

The story of alternative therapies for the treatment of cancer includes its quota of rebels against medical orthodoxy. One of the most eminent of these was the surgeon Robert Bell. Dr Bell, who was elected a Fellow in the Royal Faculty of Physicians and Surgeons in 1872, was in charge of cancer research at the Battersea Hospital in London. He abandoned the use of surgery for the treatment of cancer in 1894 and until his death in 1928 conducted a militant campaign for a non-surgical approach to the disease. His major work, *Cancer – Its Cause and Treatment without Operation*, was published in 1903 and was later followed by *Cancer and Its Remedy* in which he wrote: 'It is of no more avail to excise the local manifestation of blood contamination – which cancer undoubtedly is – and thus expect to eradicate the constitutional affection, than it is to cut out a piece of dry rot in a beam without adopting means to remove the cause of the mischief.'

Having given up surgery for the treatment of cancer, Dr Bell advocated in its place the adoption of a vegetarian diet consisting of raw vegetables, salads, fresh fruit, wholemeal bread and honey. He considered that intestinal stasis was one of the chief causes of cancer and recommended that each morning before breakfast a pint of hot water should be drunk to help bowel movement and assist elimination through the kidneys. He also emphasized the importance of deep breathing and exercise in the open air. Having observed the large proportion of myxoedema – low-functioning thyroid conditions – in cases of cancer, he argued that as the thyroid gland has a powerful influence upon the metabolism of epithelial cells, the development of cancer might be due to inefficiency of this gland. This led him to employ thyroid extract in cancer treatment and after four years of research he was able to demonstrate that his conclusions were in the main correct. Dr Bell advanced his dietary approach to cancer, citing a number of cases he had cured, in a paper read to the British Gynaecological Society. His views led to bitter controversy with medical colleagues and he became involved in several law suits. In 1912, following an attack in the *British Medical Journal* by the general superintendant of the Imperial Cancer Fund, who called him a quack, he instituted a suit for libel which he won and was awarded £2000.

F. W. Forbes Ross M.D.

A pioneer of the nutritional approach to the treatment of cancer, Dr Forbes Ross was a physician who practised in London during the early part of the century. He rapidly lost faith in the orthodox cancer treatment of surgery and irradiation and began his own researches into the physiology, anatomy and chemistry of the cancer cell. Arriving at the conclusion that the cause of cancer was the deficiency of a vital biochemical element which enabled the healthy cell to maintain its proper function, he finally identified the missing element as potassium salts. Forbes Ross believed that these salts were being processed out of foods, that deficiency existed because the soil was being depleted of essential minerals and that even more of these salts were lost in the process of cooking meat and vegetables. To correct the deficiency he prescribed potassium citrate and phosphate together with a weekly dose of potassium iodide. His treatment also included a radical dietary re-education of his patients, many of whom he noticed regularly ate rich spicy foods, disliked vegetables and rarely drank the water in which their vegetables were cooked. They also had a preference for distilled liquors to beer and wine, products which generally retain their potassium.

In his studies of healthy, primitive races, Forbes Ross found that their diets included raw and fresh foods which retained all their nutrients. He noted:

The Negroes of the West Indies on sugar plantations, who have in the past shown a singular immunity from cancer, have always been prodigious consumers of crude sugar. Crude sugar contains a large proportion of potassium salts (and also iron) which for the most part is removed from the white or refined article.

Many of the cancer patients he treated were either inoperable, or had rejected surgery or irradiation and in numbers of these cases he was remarkably successful. A tribute to the work of Forbes Ross, after his death, came from Mr Barton Scammel M.S.C.I., President of the Radium Institute in Dover, who wrote in the journal *Truth*:

The radioactive alkali, potash, is the great oxygen-attracting element in the body. It forms over 70 per cent of the mineral ash of the red corpuscles in the blood. Owing to certain defects in diet and the preparation of food, the modern civilised human being suffers from 'potassium starvation' and the increase of cancer is a corollary in this state of affairs. The great work of the late Dr Forbes Ross finds an explanation in this discovery, also it explains the success secured in the treatment of cancer with the administration of attenuated solutions of citrate and radio-phosphate of potash – which restore the recuperative power of the blood, thus causing the cancer to retrograde and disappear.

Johanna Brandt and the grape cure

Few practitioners in the field of unorthodox cancer therapy have followed the dictum 'Physician, heal thyself' with as much fortitude and ultimate success as Johanna Brandt. A South African naturopath with a practice in Cape Town, Mrs Brandt came from a family many of whose members had suffered from cancer, her mother having died of the disease in 1916. After suffering herself from severe stomach pains, Johanna Brandt went into the General Hospital in Johannesburg for an X-ray examination which revealed a large malignant growth. Despite the advice of a leading surgeon that only surgery would prolong her life, she refused, convinced that an alternative solution could be found.

At this time she came across the book *The Fasting Cure* by the American writer Upton Sinclair. As a result she began a period of fasting in the belief that even if it did not provide a cure, it would at least keep the growth under control. Of this period she wrote:

I fasted myself to a skeleton. I fasted beyond starvation point, consuming my own life tissues in the effort to destroy the growth. With every fast the growth was unmistakably checked. But it was not destroyed. On the contrary it seemed to take a new hold whenever I broke the fast – because I took the wrong foods afterwards.

Finally she discovered the food she had been seeking, one that would 'destroy the growth effectively, eliminate the poison and build new tissue'. It was the grape. She lived on grapes alone for six weeks and was completely and permanently cured. Johanna Brandt claimed that grapes are a perfect food, rich in potassium, iron and other essential salts. 'Apart from their rich organic sugar,' she wrote, 'the fact that they contain proteins, the great body builders, partially explains why new tissue is built with such extraordinary rapidity on an exclusively grape diet. But science has not yet discovered what elements in the grape break down the malignant growths.' After the publication of her book *The Grape Cure* she received thousands of unsolicited testimonials to the effectiveness of her cure from every part of South Africa, Australia, the United States, Canada, England and Ireland. Still vigorous and fit in her mid eighties she continued to visit and treat patients with the cure she had discovered through her own experience.

John Newton

BIBLIOGRAPHY, p. 245
CONTRIBUTORS, p. 220
(See also **Gerson therapy**)

CHIROPRACTIC

Chiropractic was discovered in 1895 by Daniel David Palmer in Davenport, Iowa, U.S.A. He was born of English and German ancestry in the little Canadian town of Port Perry, near Toronto. Palmer was an extraordinary man, intelligent and with wide interests chiefly concerned with healing which in those days centred on medical practices of blood-letting, use of chemicals, necromancy and potions. Amongst this confusion and lack of any real principle or system, Palmer directed his researches. He investigated the infant science of →**osteopathy** founded in 1874 by Andrew Still but believed that its principles of manipulation of joints to restore normal circulations of the blood were inadequate, though he felt that the theories were a big advance on the then current medical ideas and practices.

Previous to Palmer's discovery of chiropractic, he treated patients by mesmerism and magnetic healing at Burlington and later in Davenport, Iowa, where he performed an experiment on Harvey Lillard, a Negro janitor who claimed he became deaf after a strain in his back whilst doing some strenuous work. Palmer located a very painful and prominent vertebra which coincided with the region of sprain Lillard experienced in his back injury. Palmer then proceeded to manipulate forcibly this prominent lump where a vertebra seemed to be displaced. A short time later Lillard said he could hear somewhat better than before. This was most encouraging and Palmer followed up the case with further repeated hand treatments until Lillard's hearing became completely normal. Today it is verified that certain →**acupuncture** points even in a remote part of the spinal regions can cause hyper-sensitivity which can lead to deafness, though neurologically this cannot be proved.

Since Daniel D. Palmer experimented, observed and recorded his results, he thus complied with the first requirement of science. He further studied anatomy and physiology to find the explanations for his results and reasoned that they were based on 'bones, nerves and the manifestation of nerve impulses'.

After a time Palmer achieved better results in his patients by these 'hand treatments' than by his magnetic healing, so he gave up the latter and became well reputed for his successful treatments of a wide variety of conditions after many other therapies had failed.

Daniel Palmer did not pretend he was the first person to discover spinal derangements or displacements (subluxations) – manipulation of joints had been practised for thousands of years – but he did claim that he was the first to do so by special and specific lever techniques for the particular purpose of removing irritation to the nervous systems.

One of Palmer's patients, a Reverend Samuel Weed, a famous Greek scholar, christened his work by combining two Greek words, 'cheiro' and 'praktikos', literally meaning 'done by hand', and so coined the word 'Chiropractic'.

Palmer stressed that disease was not only an 'entity' invading the body but was also due to alterations of body functions caused by neuro-irritations resulting from abnormal muscles and joint physiology. This principle was entirely new and very advanced for his time. Some quotations from his writings make interesting reading:

Inordinate excitement of the moral and malevolent emotions indirectly irritate the nervous systems both voluntary and involuntary. . . .

Spasms, muscular contraction, nerve tension is caused by autosuggestion, poison or nerve impingement. I was the first to promulgate that the above mentioned caused vertebrae to be drawn out of alignment and by their correction tension was relieved.

A modern definition of chiropractic is: a method and system of manipulation of the joints of the body by hand, especially those of the spinal column, to restore normal function of them and the nervous system and thus regain health.

During life the body is prone to various traumas both muscular and skeletal, caused by accidents, falls, sprains and strains, postural and occupational distortions, mental and physical stresses. These incidents induce abnormalities of joints, muscle tonus and distortion, resulting in pain, neurological disturbances, vascular congestion, malfunction, disease and illness, both physical and even in some instances psychological. In fact in the most modern schools of learning it is now being scientifically established that man is much more than matter, mud and clay, for he is a being motivated by mind. Thus it is in no way surprising to find that both health and disease are psychosomatic states. In other words one can say, 'The body disposes what the mind supposes and vice versa.' This is not far removed from what Daniel David Palmer stated in his day; with this concept as a basic principle chiropractic can claim to be perhaps the foremost therapy in understanding the nature of man and his problems. In the medical world today this notion is now being well considered and accepted at long last.

The skeletal and muscular formation of the body is important in the chiropractic profession since it is here physically and in the engineering sense too that 'structure can be said to govern function'. How else can performance, in the bodily sense physiology, be otherwise determined, both in health and disease? It is not surprising the two associate; rather would it be alarming if they did not. Hence the purpose of the chiropractor is to improve both these states by corrective manipulation of joint and muscle aided by complementary and auxiliary treatments, exercise, relaxation, diet and rest. These may take the form of remedial exercises, posture correction, surgical corsets, massage, physiotherapy, water, heat, light and sound, acupressure, some →yoga practices of relaxation, respiration and →biofeedback. Correct dietetics, vitamins and behaviour play their part, as do other practices, but fundamental to all these is the basic chiropractic adjustment to the joints. There is no exclusive claim to help all conditions; in fact referrals to medical and other forms of treatment are frequently made but for certain types of condition associated with the basic principle mentioned there is as yet nothing superior.

The prognosis of any suitable condition depends very much on the extent of pathology, age and vitality of patient, duration of condition, recuperative powers, co-operation of patient and desire to get well; hence recovery, and to what degree, depends to a large extent on all these factors. In consequence there is never any claim to 'miracle cures', though there have been innumerable instances of remarkable and inexplicable results through chiropractic treatment.

The usual chiropractic procedure is firstly to consult the patient for the history of the condition and all relevant matters in the normal medical way, then to examine the patient physically not only with the appropriate standard medical, clinical and neurological tests but also with additional emphasis on a precise examination of the spinal column, pelvis, posture and muscle tissues relating to the pain pattern; palpation, range of mobility, muscle tensions, areas of pain and tenderness, distortions of skeletal and organic structures, neurological disturbances, etc. In addition and where necessary, the help provided by all other special medical tests and procedures such as blood pressure, cardiac and respiratory auscultation, reflexes, blood and urine samples, allergy tests and any other procedures carried out in hospitals or medical laboratories is welcomed. The use of radiography is especially necessary and most practitioners have such equipment of their own or access to it. Chiropractors are specially trained to use X-ray equipment for diagnostic purposes both for the protection of their patients and themselves from malpractice; in consequence some cases are refused and referred to other more suitable practices. There is no opposition to conventional medicine or other forms of therapy, but in some ways there are contradictory opinions to orthodox methods.

It is difficult to say how often and how much treatment is necessary because so much depends on the correct assessment of the patient, the degrees of pathology, the duration and type of case and last but by no means least, the cooperation of the patient. Generally in suitable acute cases the response is swift and good depending on age and successful application. In chronic situations with pronounced pathologies or complications, results may vary from slow to tedious or none at all. All too commonly one is confronted with the problem of chronic life-long neuro-muscular habit patterns of distortion which take a lot of repetitive manipulative treatment coupled with remedial exercise and posture correction over a long or permanent period; in this respect our work is no different from that of any other therapy. However, as a means of prophylaxis chiropractic plays a vital rôle, since health depends very much on good transmission of neuro-energy and impulses throughout the body to the glands, tissues and organs, all of which reflect on the state of the mind.

What ailments does the chiropractor treat? Unfortunately one can only speak in general terms. Even within the range of conditions which respond extremely well to chiropractic treatment there are always certain reservations due to pathologies, age, chronicity and so on. Be that as it may, the following categories respond favourably and well:

Spinal disc lesions, spondylosis of spinal vertebrae with associated and resultant neuritis, sciatica, neuralgias, articular and muscular pains.

Rheumatic and arthritic conditions of neuro-muscular or vascular origins affecting spinal and extremity joints.

Limited traumatic joint and muscle states where pathology is not too advanced, such as peri-articular damage to extremity joints like the elbow, wrist, hip, knee, ankle, etc. Bad postural states, sprained joints, strained muscles and ligaments.

Psychosomatic dysfunctions of high or low blood pressures, migraine and other types of headaches, some asthmas, neurasthenias, emotional neurosis and factors due to stress.

Visceral dysfunctions have also been cured where the aetiology has been associated with irritation of the autonomic nervous system.

The list cannot be totally embracing as sometimes without any good reason unexpected results occur. However, the above categories are responsive.

The present minimum requirements for practitioners are a full-time four-year attendance at a recognized chiropractic college. The preliminary years are concerned with the study of anatomy, physiology, chemistry, micro-biology and pathology with particular studies in radiology and physics. The next two years cover the more specialized chiropractic studies with emphasis on the spinal column, neurology, psychology, body mechanics, diagnosis and adjusting (manipulative) procedures. In Britain there is only one college, the Anglo-European College of Chiropractic, situated in Bournemouth, which provides a recognized four-year course with entrance qualifications of five O-level G.C.E. passes and two A-level passes in science subjects.

Since 1925 the British Chiropractors' Association has maintained a Register of all qualified practitioners in membership, limited exclusively to graduates from approved chiropractic colleges. As a registered association it has upheld the principles, aims, practices and research on a sound professional basis.

The growth of this profession throughout the world has been rapid. Today there are over 35000 practitioners alone in the United States and Canada where it is recognized by State and Provincial Law; so also in Switzerland, Western Australia and New Zealand. Legislation is pending in Europe for Denmark and Norway, and in the near future we hope for Britain too.

R. Gerald Cooper D.C.

CO-COUNSELLING

Co-counselling is a method of personal development through mutual support for persons of all ages and both sexes including, with suitable modifications, children. It is not for those who are too emotionally distressed to give attention to a fellow human on a reciprocal basis. It is a tool for living for those who are already managing their lives acceptably by conventional standards, but wish significantly to enhance their sense of personal identity and personal effectiveness. It is part of a continuing education for living which affirms the peer (equal) principle.

All persons are differently stressed by virtue of their immersion in the human condition which has at least the following sources of stress: the separation trauma of birth and death; the tension between physical survival and personal development: the relative inscrutability or apparent meaninglessness of many phenomena; the intractability of matter; the inherent instability of unprogrammed and probably unlimited human potential; the presence of other stressed humans. On the one hand such stressors can be enabling, providing the shock of awakening that promotes personal development and cultural achievement. On the other hand they can be overwhelming

and disabling so that personal and interpersonal behaviour become distorted and persons interfere with each other, either unawarely or deliberately and maliciously. There are thus two sources of distress: the primary source in the human condition, the secondary and derivative source in the interference of other people. The latter is what co-counselling is most obviously and immediately concerned with.

Human infants have remarkable though undeveloped capacities for love, understanding and choice, but lack the information, skill and experience with which to actualize them. They await wise and loving education, but are also highly vulnerable to interference by others – the blocking, frustration, rejection or neglect of their deep human potential. The result of such interference is a line of distress in the mind-body, the emotional pain of grief, fear, anger, shame and embarrassment, together with correlated physical, often muscular, tension. The effect of such distress is to suspend the effective response of human capacities – of love, understanding and choice – so that the child is left with an undiscriminating recording of the traumatic interfering interaction, including the child's own maladaptive response. These distress recordings can become ingrained and extensive through cumulative repetition of interference from parental and other sources. There is invariably a double interference, firstly with the deep human potential, and secondly with the child's attempt to find a way of dealing with the pain of this through catharsis: hence the double negative message – 'Your human capacities are no good, and the pain that you feel at their interference is no good.'

In our emotionally repressive society, distress recordings acquire a dynamic functional autonomy, often unidentified and unacknowledged. They are the source of unaware, compulsive, maladaptive and rigid behaviour patterns. Some of these patterns are periodic, triggered by particular types of situation that significantly resemble the early interference situations: for example, when rational behaviour breaks down in the presence of someone seen as an authority figure. Others are endemic or chronic, a persistent distorted way of feeling and thinking and doing that infects behaviour in a wide range of situations: for example, a chronic self-deprecatory attitude. Here the trigger is being in the world at all – which has become associated with a deeply ingrained distress recording.

When triggered in later life, the distress recording unawarely plays itself out, either the child's end or the parent's end of the recording being reproduced in behaviour and attitude, depending upon the situation. Or both may be reproduced at the same time as in a chronic internal pattern of self-condemnation. Typical composite recordings are those of: the victim and the oppressor – the compulsion to oppress, to manipulate, to denigrate and despise; the helpless and the rescuer – the compulsion to depend on, to lean on, to seek help from, and at other times the compulsion to be responsible for, to look after, rescue and care for. Such patterns may be acted out, in interactions with other people; or they may be acted in, in internal transactions within the self. In either case they are, for the adult, maladaptive. For the child they have some survival value – the trauma and pain become encoded as a ritual distortion that at least enables the person to continue without total breakdown and disruption. But they restrict and constrain mature, flexible and innovative response to changing circumstances in the adult.

Co-counselling theory also holds that catharsis is a way of releasing distress from the mind-body. Keeping some attention in the place of the aware adult in present time, the client in co-counselling reaches down into the hidden place of the hurt child, honours and experiences the pain, and releases it – grief in tears and sobbing, fear in trembling, anger in loud sound and storming movement, certain core or primal pains in screaming, false shame and embarrassment in laughter. This is a healing of the hidden memories, a reintegration of the occluded past. The effects of sustained catharsis are: (1) spontaneous insight – the traumatic past is seen in a new light, re-evaluated, perceived with a truly discriminating awareness for the first time, and its connection with the current distortions is understood in a way that illuminates; (2) the break-up of patterns, of rigid distorted behaviour and attitude – the tension of contained distress that sustains them has been released; (3) the liberation of frozen needs and capacities – love is freed from its distorted childhood fixation, intelligence can function flexibly instead of in a stereotypic and dogmatic way, choice is released from the illusion of powerlessness. The person can thus live more creatively and awarely in response to what is going on now.

Finally, the way of regression, catharsis and reintegration of the distressed past is complemented and indeed consummated by the way of celebration – the joyful affirmation of felt strength, of experiences and projects that are worthwhile, enjoyable and creatively rewarding.

Co-counselling is a two-way process among peers, each taking a turn as client and counsellor – typically a two-hour session with each person taking an hour in each rôle. Client and counsellor exercise appropriate skills, acquired on a basic training course of at least forty hours – with on-going groups, intensive workshops and advanced workshops for systematic follow-up. Co-counselling is not simply client-centred – it is client-directed. The client is the person who is taking his or her turn, working on the way of regression and catharsis, and the way of celebration and affirmation. The basic techniques are primarily for the client to work with on herself, with the aware supportive attention of the counsellor. This is particularly important in the early stages so that the client does not become strongly dependent on counsellor interventions. The counsellor does not interpret, analyse, criticize or advise on problems, but only acts within a contract indicated by the client. This contract may ask for non-verbal attention only; for occasional interventions when it seems to the counsellor that the client is missing her own cues, is getting lost in her own defences; or, at a later stage when the counsellor has acquired the requisite skill, for intensive interventions which work with every cue evident in the client and which hone in on areas of primary material. The counsellor's interventions are always in the form of a practical suggestion about what the client may say or do. The rationale of the suggestion is not verbalized; and the client is in principle free to reject the intervention.

On the way of regression and catharsis, the client is trained to take charge of the discharge process by always keeping a focus of attention in the place of the aware, mature adult outside the distress of the child within, and to work with accessible and available distress, with what is on top. This ensures that the healing of the memories occurs in a relatively un-disruptive way, in a sequence and at a pace which the client can readily handle. The client works not only upon childhood experiences but also on more recent and present relation-ships both personal and professional and also on future expectations and on political and institutional tensions. Some of the introduc-tory techniques the client uses – and which the counsellor recommends when she inter-venes – are those of: literal, evocative descrip-tion of early events, rather than analytic talk about them; repetition of words and phrases that carry an emotional charge or loading; association – catching emergent thoughts, images, memories, insights that occur spon-taneously; rôle play – becoming oneself in the early scene and expressing directly the negative or positive feelings that were suppressed at the time; contradiction – verbally and non-verbally putting energy in the opposite direc-tion to the constraints of the negative self image. Many other techniques are used, and co-counselling at its various stages of develop-ment can accommodate the four primary ways of managing catharsis: active imagination, passive imagination, active body work, and passive body work. Transpersonal co-counsel-ling is an important development for working on the repression of the sublime and arche-typal. Fundamental throughout is the valida-tion, affirmation and celebration of the inali-enable worth of humans and their capacities.

Co-counselling was developed out of other influences by Harvey Jackins in Seattle, U.S.A., in the 1950s and 1960s. Under his auspices it spread through the U.S.A. and to Europe in the late sixties and early seventies, and networks of co-counsellors were organized under the title Re-evaluation Counselling Communities. This organization became theo-retically rigid and internally authoritarian. Co-counselling International is an alternative network, that federates entirely independent communities or co-counsellors in several countries: these communities develop their own decision-making procedures consonant with the peer principle and their own approach to the training, assessment and accreditation of teachers of the method. Co-counselling as a practice primarily occurs in people's own homes on the basis of one-to-one informal arrangements. The purpose of a network or community is to provide up-to-date address lists of trained co-counsellors, and to provide a continuous programme of groups and work-shops for follow-up, group support, intensive co-counselling, refresher courses, advanced training, teacher training and social change activity.

John Heron

ASSOCIATIONS, p. 214
CONTRIBUTORS, p. 220
TRAINING, p. 232

COLOUR THERAPY

The use of light for therapeutic purposes is not new. The area seems new to us today, but ancient cultures have used it extensively. The great difference between the past and today is that we can actually measure the effects of light on living substances. It was Gerrard and Hessey, two Californian psychologists, who in 1932 made the discovery that blue light has a calming, and red a stimulating effect on human beings.

Colour is only a very fine way of controlling light. Each colour has a specific density and a certain order of these make up the spectrum. The natural spectrum consists of three primary and three secondary colours.

In a quite different order, but appearing in optics, we find that colour appears on the edges where darkness meets light. Light is denser than darkness and out of the darkness that plays with light arise the colours. There are two halves of the natural spectrum: red, orange and yellow on the one hand, and violet, blue and turquoise on the other. By way of a prism (a piece of glass with a triangular profile) the edge of darkness and light gets enlarged and the eye can see more easily this emergence of colour.

By shifting two black fields so close together that only a narrow strip of white remains the yellow and the turquoise of the two edges merge and produce green. Conversely, if two white fields are shifted together with only a narrow strip of black remaining, the colour of magenta is produced from the merging of violet and red.

Red is the densest colour and violet is the least dense colour. Green holds the balance and the human eye reacts to it least of all. Dark blue objects are focussed in front of the retina and red behind.

These are just a few basic facts in optics. To go deeper into the effect of colour, new, sensitive instruments can register the lowering of blood pressure by the use of blue light and the raising of blood pressure under red light. It is in this area that colour therapy begins to be an effective method to support medical work.

Like all areas of the manifest world around us, colour is never just 'colour' – it has to be linked to form, intensity of light source, pigment and many materials which are either opaque or translucent. Pure colour is not so easy to produce, in fact almost impossible, as there must be a medium by which colour becomes visible to the eye. Colour is a very subjective experience and its effect on the individual has to do with a complicated nervous reaction.

It is in the linking of light, colour and form we can create a harmony experience or a tension experience. In colour therapy it is important to use colour and form together with a rhythmic timing that produces a response which, by way of the movement of the living organism, can achieve a realignment. Such a realignment can introduce a healthy molecular structure in the cells of plants, animals and humans. The colour therapist can introduce a therapy to the body of a sick person. The effect of the eight colours, and many of the shades in between them, is beginning to become an integral part of all medical work – the colour of hospital wards, furnishings, windows, artificial light, etc.

Colour therapy helps both to prevent and to cure disease. There are conditions when colour therapy offers a good, quick and easily available aid. For instance during an attack of asthma normal daylight is dimmed and a blue light is switched on. Research shows that general tension is greatly reduced under blue light, which in asthma can sufficiently relax muscles and tissue to relieve the attack. Conversely, the switching on of a red light under such conditions can lead to the death of the patient.

However, much better and specialized therapy needs to be given through an instrument called the Colour-Form-Rhythm Beamer. In this instrument are combined the colour, made available through an aperture (window) specially chosen for one of the eight colours, and a timing computer which increases the specific colour chosen for the therapy of a patient, and the complementary colour on a rhythmically decreasing scale. There are only a dozen or so colour therapy centres in Europe. One treatment session lasts for $24\frac{1}{4}$ minutes; between one to four treatments per week should be sufficient. The patient is asked to wear only white clothes whilst attending the therapy. The whole or part of a body can be treated. This therapy is an auxiliary to 'straight' medicine and in no way eliminates the help of a doctor. Nevertheless, it has been found that whilst all other channels have been explored, this therapy has produced results which have not been possible with any of the other methods tried before.

Theo Gimbel D.C.E.

BIBLIOGRAPHY, p. 245
CONTRIBUTORS, p. 220
TRAINING, pp. 231, 233

CONSTIPATION

Some years ago a consumer survey revealed that one in three children on a British housing estate were dosed with aperients every day. The laxative industry is flushed with success.

We are obsessed with the need for regularity. If you do not 'go' punctually as a cuckoo clock your mother will not love you, the boss will pass you over, even Rover may snarl.

For my first thirty-five years I was a non-daily goer. Twice a week, with luck, saw my allotted span of the gracious throne. The straining sessions were time-taking and painful. Still, I had been told life was a vale of tears, so what should I expect – violets? Thankfully a quaintly isolated childhood had kept me innocent of the daily doings of the rest of humankind. Only through a chance remark heard at the age of twenty-two did the awful truth dawn – I was *different*! After that I was not only a young man with stomach-ache – I was a man with a secret shame.

I took pills and I did not take pills. I drank five pints of water every day and did not drink anything at all. I ate uncooked vegetables, morning cereals, starved, did exercises. For thirteen years my insides were subjected to every known cure. Nothing worked.

At thirty-five I revealed my secret to a doctor. 'Is there,' I asked, 'something physically wrong with me? Could I be fixed with surgery?'

He said, 'If that were the case you'd have died thirty-five years ago.' He then proposed the most stupid cure of all: 'Come and talk to me about it for an hour once a month.'

Twelve months later I reported, 'Everything works. It just happens right after getting up.' We continued six more months to consolidate our joint success.

What did we talk about? Rarely my bowels. We talked about my relationships, my work, my love-life. From his position of authority he gave me permission to let go, to feel free to be fond of people, to love. I have not taken a pill since.

There is rarely a physical reason for constipation. The sufferer is far more likely to find permanent relief through psychology than laxatives.

When they were emotionally moved the Anglo-Saxons would say, 'It goes to my bowels.' In their simple way they thought the heart was down in that department. Maybe they were right.

Malcolm Hulke

COPPER

The use of copper to ease rheumatic pains has been known for centuries, as it seems to relieve pain in nearly all types of rheumatism, lumbago, sciatica and even arthritis. It does not always work and cannot effect a permanent cure, but it is remarkable how often it helps and how quickly it takes effect. Treatment is extraordinarily simple: you simply wear copper next to the skin – a bangle, a special inner lining to an otherwise normal leather wrist-watch strap, or as an attractive bracelet or necklace.

In modern times, however, its use in western culture originated in South Africa where it was found that tribesmen wearing copper were free from aches and pains. Alastair Cooke has estimated that 5 million Americans wear copper.

Why does it work? American researchers found that most rheumatic subjects have in their system an element causing a copper deficiency. Dr Donald A. Gerber of the State University of New York Downstate Medical Center, Brooklyn, perfected a new laboratory technique for diagnosing rheumatoid arthritis. It was based on the increase of copper ligand excreted in the urine. He studied a group of 78 patients with rheumatoid arthritis and another of 183 patients suffering from un-unrelated illnesses. In 51 per cent of the patients in the first group, compared to 2 per cent in the second, the copper-binding capacity of the urine was greater than that of a 90 mg per cent solution of hydralazine used as the basis of comparison. Steroid therapy was not, of course, used in any of the patients examined.

Dr Gerber also tested more than 200 substances to discover which caused this singular copper-binding activity of the urine of patients with rheumatoid arthritis. Evidence pointed to the following compounds: histidyl-histidine, 3-methylhistidine, histidinol, histidine, and hydralazine. It was pointed out that administration of the latter sometimes causes clinical patterns similar to rheumatoid arthritis and he thus drew the conclusion that an increase in copper-binding substances may be responsible for some of the symptoms of this disease.

Dogs, cats, horses, and all kinds of animals may benefit from wearing copper. The racing horse Black Prince went lame and neither trainer nor veterinary surgeon could pinpoint the trouble. Copper insets were introduced into his straps and he went on to come second in the 1965 Epsom Derby. Perhaps the most curious case was that of a much-loved old Aylesbury drake who was able to resume his normal waddling life after small copper rings had been fitted on each leg.

Lt Col. A. Forbes

COSMETICS

A blooming and delicate complexion can be discovered by turning to simple home-made preparations. Many ingredients are already present in your kitchen. Making your own preparation is satisfying. The improvement to one's skin makes the effort worthwhile. We can easily make many lotions and creams by combining plants with other natural ingredients.

Home-made creams and lotions can cleanse, moisturize, tone and soothe; and they can heal and feed your skin depending upon the ingredients. Herbs, oils, nuts, seeds and flowers can be made into preparations that can improve even the clearest of skins as they are gently absorbed and uncover your natural beauty. Cosmetics based on natural ingredients must be complemented by a proper diet. Both health and beauty increase when one follows the natural path.

To maintain a healthy complexion you need foods rich in natural vitamins A, E, C and B complex. Some of these foods are whole grains, green and yellow vegetables, citrus, watercress, brewer's yeast, natural vegetable oils and yoghourt. Foods with few carbohydrates will help free an oily complexion of its enlarged and dirt-trapped pores, whilst the addition of vegetable oils, nuts and green vegetables bring great benefit to those with dry skin.

A healthy complexion is a clean complexion. It is through our skin that we eliminate toxic wastes. We need not depend upon soap and water alone to accomplish this task. Vegetable oils, used for centuries, smooth away dirt when wiped with cotton wool. Any natural polyunsaturated vegetable oil will serve the purpose, but the best are almond, wheatgerm, olive, sunflower, avocado and soya. Acid-based natural oils will not remove the protective acid mantle surrounding our bodies. When massaging with the oil, rotate your hands in an upward motion. Lemon juice cleans away surface impurities and dead skin. It is also very effective in removing dry patches from knees, elbows and heels. An oily complexion greatly benefits from tomato slices. The juice inhibits the sebaceous glands from producing too much oil.

Cold drying winds and burning sun play havoc with unprotected skin. We can smooth away lines and maintain healthy skin texture by utilizing the plants which surround us. Moisturizing becomes necessary as skin ages and the natural sebum decreases. Left unattended, those thin lines will become deep wrinkles and the skin will sag. Vegetable oils lightly massaged into the skin will help moisturize a dry complexion, the best being avocado, almond and wheatgerm oils. One replaces much-needed oil which has been lost, improving skin texture and transforming a dry, blotchy complexion into one of shining supple radiance.

Honey is recognized as a cosmetic as well as a healing food. Over the ages women learned that honey alone or combined with other natural products helped to keep their complexion and hands soft and wrinkle-free. Honey will also ease a rash and help moisturize a dry complexion. Having the ability to attract water from the lower layers of skin and from the air, honey helps the moisture balance necessary for dry skin. Mix a tablespoon of honey with a little oil and spread the mixture thickly onto your skin. After twenty minutes rinse off with warm water.

To remember that the skin is the regulator of the body and indicator of its general state of health is to understand it. By discovering the use of natural ingredients in caring for the skin, we can improve and enhance our complexions, thereby giving a glimpse of the natural beauty within.

Rona Batson

CONTRIBUTORS, p. 221
PRODUCTS, p. 225

'CRANIAL' OSTEOPATHY

Most people are now familiar with the terms osteopath and →osteopathy, although their meanings are not immediately obvious. Osteopaths do not, on the whole, treat bone diseases as one might infer from the Greek roots of the word. Similarly, practitioners experienced in 'cranial' osteopathy might refute the obvious conclusion that their work is confined to the head, or cranium. However, in both cases the terms have been imported from the U.S.A. and are now in relatively common usage.

'Cranial' osteopathy is a more specific approach to diagnosis and treatment which fully conforms to the basic principles of osteopathy. These were developed by Dr A. T. Still in the late nineteenth century and incorporate the inter-relationship of the body's structure and function.

A further premise is that the body has an inherent capacity to maintain itself in a state of 'health' or stable equilibrium. Where this is not possible, or is prevented, a state of 'dis-ease' ensues and osteopathic diagnosis and treatment will be directed to discovering and dealing with any malalignment of structure and function. The osteopath thus attempts to assist the body, usually by the use of his hands, in its efforts to help itself. This self-stabilizing mechanism, when all aspects of it are considered collectively, is very potent indeed and further reference will be made to it.

In 1899, during his training as an osteopathic student in Kirksville, Missouri, in the U.S.A., William G. Sutherland found himself contemplating the bones of a skull which had been separated and mounted in a display cabinet. He was struck by the fact that the edges of the bones were bevelled, notched and angled where they had originally fitted together. He became convinced that there had to be a reason why such a large variety of joint types and shapes should be developed and maintained well into late adult life. Further, the overall pattern, allowing for small individual differences, could be identified in every skull that he examined. He then asked himself whether there could be a *functional* reason for the consistent pattern and orientation of these joints.

Such a notion appeared at first preposterous when viewed from the standpoint of classical anatomy, based as it is on the study of the rigid, dried bones. However, he was intrigued and began an intense study of all twenty-two components of the skull and its internal membranes which support the brain. Only after many years was he able to convince himself that every single detail of the cranial anatomy reinforced his hypothesis that the cranial bones were indeed designed to accommodate *very slight* motion. The next question, of course, was – what was causing this movement? There were, after all, no appropriate muscles within the cranium. Eventually he concluded that the brain tissue or grey matter itself goes through a rhythmical and continuous cycle of very slight expansion and contraction – quite independently of the movements of breathing or heart beat. This was naturally another hard-to-accept idea until, to his astonishment and delight, he found that he could detect this motion on his own head and later also on the heads of his family and patients. He found the motion conformed to a distinct pattern which was precisely in keeping with his painstaking studies of the individual cranial bones.

Later he found that it was possible to detect variations in the frequency, amount and even 'quality' of this cyclical motion between different patients – and even in the same patient – depending on the age, state of general health, emotional state, and history of specific injury – especially injuries involving the head. It was found that effective treatment of any kind produced changes in the characteristics of cranial motion and thus the findings became useful in diagnosis itself.

With a detailed knowledge of the mechanics of the cranium and its contents, it became possible to get an idea of the dynamic state of the mechanism as a whole. All this requires a sense of touch, or rather an ability to detect movement (not at all the same thing) which may be difficult to appreciate. In fact, remarkably little research has been conducted into the tactile and proprioceptive senses as compared for instance to sight and hearing. However, it has been accepted that the joints of the hand are capable of detecting extremely small increments of movement and that they are also able to detect quite complex patterns of motion. Both these capabilities were developed consciously by Dr Sutherland who was by this time a highly trained osteopath of many years' experience.

Further development of Sutherland's concept has led to the question as to whether the cranium alone is endowed with the ability to move involuntarily and rhythmically. If this is a basic property of living tissue, as postulated by Sutherland, what about the rest of the body? In fact, it has been found that this same pattern of involuntary movement is indeed detectable throughout the body and that, as in the cranium, it can be a sensitive indicator of the state of health of the tissues.

The concept of 'cranial' osteopathy thus lends itself to the application of diagnostic and therapeutic techniques throughout the whole body, in perfect accordance with the basic principles of osteopathy as taught by its founder, Dr A. T. Still.

In treatment the main aim is to refine as far as possible the body's own recuperative abilities. These are mirrored by the 'quality', degree of symmetry and regularity of the involuntary body motion. The experienced practitioner, through his hands, can be aware of the dynamic state of the tissues, cranial or otherwise. Using his detailed knowledge of the underlying anatomy and physiology, he may assess the degree to which the pattern and quality of motion detected differs from what might be expected as 'normal' in that individual. Such an assessment is often itself of therapeutic value.

The patient is occasionally quite unaware, apart from the contact itself, that anything at all is happening. However, more usually, a patient may feel that the osteopath's hands are moving very slowly or are 'undulating'. This is a subjective sensation as there is rarely relative motion between the hands and the underlying tissue, the hands being moved passively by the motile tissues. Perhaps most notably the patient is aware of a distinct reduction of tension physically and perhaps even emotionally. It is not unknown for a patient to fall asleep during treatment. In other cases where a change in the pattern of motion is detected, sensations of localized warmth at the area of contact may be accompanied by a feeling of slight light-headedness. This usually dissipates within a few minutes of the end of treatment.

As with other aspects of manual therapy and diagnosis, the findings and results are extremely difficult to quantify and correlate, the problems being multiplied alarmingly when the findings in several cases are brought together. Many of the subjective impressions gained by the hand are very hard to describe in comparative terms, let alone scientifically. However, in the U.S.A. much work has been done in an effort to provide a factual and scientific basis for Sutherland's concept of 'cranial' osteopathy. This has ranged from direct measurement of the extent of motion of the cranium by sensitive electro-mechanical apparatus to the evaluation of the results of treatment given to a large number of hospitalized patients over a prolonged period. Much work is still going on, sponsored mainly by the Cranial Academy, a component society of the American Academy of Osteopathy, and also by members of the Sutherland Cranial Teaching Foundation.

Hard as they may be to evaluate on a statistical basis, clinical results are undoubtedly obtained in a large number of cases and the practical value of the approach in daily practice is evidenced by the ever-growing interest in this field of study and an increasing number of trained osteopaths in the U.S.A. and Registered Osteopaths in the U.K. who are attending postgraduate study courses under the auspices of the S.C.T.F.

The 'cranial' approach to osteopathic treatment has perhaps special relevance to the problems of children and young people as, of course, any improvement achieved is of proportionately greater significance. In addition, results are often easier to obtain as the whole structure of the body is more pliable and more amenable to change as the patient grows and develops. In the very young, most of the bony structures, including those of the cranium, are separated by soft connective tissues for this reason. Conversely, this very plasticity also increases the vulnerability of the tissues to injury which may therefore have far-reaching effects on the structure and function of the body. Under the term 'injury' one may also include the results of a difficult delivery at birth, especially where the process has been unduly prolonged. As a point of interest, in a few osteopathic hospitals in the U.S.A., babies are examined 'cranially' as soon as possible after birth.

Due to the process by which Sutherland developed his 'cranial' concept, treatment in this field has rightly become most well known for the results of its application to problems mainly concerning the head. These have included conditions such as certain types of migraine headache, vertigo, the after-effects of whiplash injuries to the neck, etc. However, as already intimated, the approach is poten-tially more widely applicable; some practitioners for example, especially in the U.S.A., work closely with dental surgeons in an attempt to mitigate the possible after-effects of dental surgery in susceptible cases. In other patients, treatment has been found to be very effective in some forms of spinal or limb pain, where alternative methods have proved of only temporary or no avail.

The osteopath trained in the 'cranial' approach may, according to his experience, use it more or less in any case. Often he will use it almost exclusively in a very acute case where direct manual methods may be contra-indicated or undesirable, for instance where the patient is in a great deal of pain or in an emotionally reactive state following an accident or injury. Sometimes he will use the technique simply to gain information about the patient's general dynamic state, or to gauge the patient's response to more orthodox treatment. More often, perhaps, he will use the 'cranial' approach to supplement the manipulative techniques more commonly used. The main overall effect here allows him, with experience, to be much more gentle and specific in his application of manual treatment generally.

In the U.K., because of the very detailed postgraduate study and intensive practical coaching required, the number of qualified osteopaths experienced in the 'cranial' field unfortunately is very small. Probably little more than two dozen practitioners use this approach to any significant extent at present. However, the number is steadily growing as successfully treated patients begin to stimulate a demand for this form of osteopathy.

D. E. Gilhooley D.O., M.R.O.

CUPPING

Cupping was used 5000 years ago by the ancient Egyptians to treat disease. Hippocrates appreciated its benefits and Alexander Trallianus, a contemporary of the Emperor Justinian and writer of an extensive textbook on medicine, employed it for treating certain forms of arthritis and rheumatism. The cupping method, which uses suction to draw blood to the surface of the body in treating conditions of deep-seated congestion, has been used to relieve breathing difficulties associated with asthma, bronchitis and pleurisy and in the treatment of lumbago and various forms of rheumatism.

There are two types of cupping, dry and wet. In dry-cupping, a cupping-glass (these used to be available at some chemists) or a thick glass tumbler can be used. First a few drops of methylated spirit are placed upon a small piece of cotton-wool or a fragment of blotting-paper, which is then ignited and while still burning put in the glass, the mouth of which is placed firmly on the appropriate area of the patient's body. A vacuum is produced and the skin swells into the glass as blood rushes into the small blood vessels. The process is repeated four, six or eight times on different parts of the body.

An effective 'massage' treatment can be given by using a cup in its vacuum state and dragging it along the body, chest or abdominal muscles with sufficient firmness to ensure the vacuum is not broken. Cupping has been used to treat →multiple sclerosis by improving the circulation to and through the spinal cord and to relieve congestion. It has also been used on recently healed scars, the alternate suction and release loosening the scar tissue.

Wet-cupping, now rarely used, first employs the dry-cupping procedure; then the swollen skin is scarified – shallow cuts are made in the skin with a lancet or special instrument; the cupping-glass is again applied and blood drawn into it. The vacuum effect achieved in cupping can also be produced with the use of a suction-bulb. In his book *Some Unusual Healing Methods* Leslie Korth devotes a chapter to cupping.

John Newton

CONTRIBUTORS, p. 221

DIANETICS

Dianetics was the fore-runner of scientology and was discovered by L. Ron Hubbard. Those who are trained in the use of the technology of dianetics state that they can understand and handle psychosomatic illness.

This technology is new and cannot be compared to other techniques in this field. Dianetics can readily demonstrate that man is not just an animal. He is a spiritual being and has a mind and a body. His mind is not his brain. The mind is created by the person himself, i.e. the spiritual being. Hence it cannot be reached via the body. However, the mind is real and although not physically solid like the brain, it can be detected just as radio waves can be detected, by using suitable electronic equipment.

The mind is senior to the brain and can be demonstrated to be separate from the body. It contains the recorded experiences of the individual in full 3D technicolour with sight and sound and the other perceptions (although these may be occluded and not readily visible to the person himself). These are mental image pictures and one can experience this simply by closing one's eyes and imagining a picture.

The individual, i.e. the spiritual being, records these pictures in his mind and can recall them at will. Hence these pictures, and indeed the mind itself, are created by the person himself. The person being senior to his mind has the potential ability to correct anything wrong with what he himself has created.

As Buddhists believe, there are levels of awareness. One need only observe the awareness of different individuals walking down the street to find this to be true. A person's awareness can be increased. In dianetics awareness is increased – without the use of drugs, hypnosis or any physical method – to the point at which the person can become aware of the source of his troubles. Interestingly enough the source of the problem will be found in the mind. Therefore any trouble in a person's mind was originally put there by himself. He then proceeded to forget that he had done so. When he regains awareness of what he put in his mind, he can deal with it.

Pictures in the mind include pain and painful emotion from moments of pain and unconsciousness and emotional stress. Such pictures below one's awareness can cause one to act irrationally, such as does a hypnotized subject who has been given a command of which he is not aware.

Such pictures and the stress and pain they contain are not accessible to any form of physical treatment for they are separate from the body. Their ability to cause irrational conduct or psychosomatic illness, however, can be erased. This is done by taking the person through the experience (reviewing the 'picture') in a precise and scientific form. In this manner treatment for psychosomatic conditions is possible, and significant when the Royal College of General Practitioners states that psychosomatic illness constitutes 70 per cent of the general practitioner's workload.

While dianetics is the study and science of the mind, scientology is a religion which deals with the spiritual nature of man. It also contains processes by which one can assist others who are suffering physically. It is done by addressing the person himself, i.e. the spiritual being, i.e. you. The following passages come from a recently published book by L. Ron Hubbard, *The Volunteer Minister's Handbook*. They give you some practical ways in which you could help someone else. It should be noted that religion exists in no small part to handle the upsets and anguish of life and ministers long before the Apostles had, as part of their duties, the ministering to the spiritual anguish of their congregation.

An assist is an action undertaken by a minister to assist the spirit to confront physical difficulties and deal with them. One of the easiest forms of assist is called locational processing.[1] When a person has an injured hand and you tell the person, 'Look at that chair. Look at the floor. Look at that hand,' with you pointing to the objects, the pain will diminish. Another form of assist is a contact assist. In a contact assist you take the person to the exact spot where the accident occurred. (Of course first aid rules apply and any bleeding or immediate first aid must be dealt with first.) Then have the person duplicate exactly what happened at the time of the accident. For instance,

if he hits his head on a pipe, have him go through the action of putting his head against the exact spot on the pipe, having the pipe also touch the exact spot on his head. The rest of his body should be in the position it was at the time of the accident. If the object is hot, you let it cool first; if current was on, you turn it off before the assist. If the person had a tool in his hand, or was using one, he should be going through the same motions with it. Have the person repeat this several times, until the somatic[2] occurs again. It will occur and 'blow off' when he exactly duplicates it. While doing it ask him occasionally how it is going and if the somatic occurred. End off when you get the phenomenon of it turning on and 'blowing off'.

If a contact assist is not possible you can do a touch assist. Just use a simple command like, 'Feel my finger, thank you', run repetitively. This is done up and down the body – around the injury and especially below the injury, i.e. further from the head than the injury. It is a good idea to have the person shut his eyes so that he is definitely looking 'through' the area of injury in order to tell that you are touching him.

Note: Medical examination, diagnosis and treatment should be sought where needed. An assist is not a substitute for medical treatment but is complementary to it.

Injury and illness are predisposed by the spiritual state of the person. They are precipitated by the spiritual being himself as a manifestation of his current spiritual condition. And they are prolonged by any failure to fully handle the spiritual factors associated with them.

An assist is not engaging in healing. It is certainly not engaging in treatment. What it is doing is assisting the individual to heal himself or be healed by another agency by removing his reasons for precipitating and prolonging his condition and lessening his predisposition to further injure himself or remain in an intolerable condition.

Tom Shuster B.A.

1. Location processing – the principle of

making an individual look at his own existence and improve his ability to contact what he is and where he is.

2. Somatic – this is essentially body sensation, illness, pain or discomfort. Soma means body; hence psychosomatic or pains stemming from the mind; a pain or ache, sensation and also misemotion or even unconsciousness.

ENCOUNTER

Encounter groups originated in America in the 1950s and have been in this country since the late 1960s. Most sources agree they originated with the work of an American psychologist named Kurt Lewin, who, in the early 1940s, became concerned at the lack of training in inter-personal relations. Lewin and his associates devised ways of facilitating inter-personal interaction and the first training groups (called T groups) took place in 1947. The participants were mainly managers and executives sent by their employers for training. The results, in terms of increased awareness, honesty and contact were encouraging enough for the work to continue and the National Training Laboratories were set up.

In the 1950s groups started to emerge emphasizing personal growth rather than training. The work spread and by 1962 the demand was strong enough for the first growth centre, Esalen, to be opened in California. By now, groups specializing in inter-personal work were called 'encounter' groups. They became a regular feature at Esalen and the other growth centres which were to open. The first encounter groups in this country occurred in the late 1960s and the first growth centre, Quaesitor, opened in 1969.

Another main influence on the formation and popularity of the encounter group movement was the American educationist and psychologist, Carl Rogers. In 1970, Rogers, the originator of client-centred therapy, became intensely interested in encounter and worth. In order to achieve what is often groups. Such was his prestige and standing within the field of humanistic psychology that many people were attracted to group work. Will Schutz has done much to clarify encounter and to popularize the movement with his books *Elements of Encounter* and *Joy*, and the film *Here Comes Everybody*.

The reason for the emergence of encounter groups seems to be the readiness of people to take the risks which lead to personal freedom. Theologians, psychologists, writers and artists have examined in depth the ends to which man will go to avoid taking responsibility for himself. A good encounter group provides a place where you can learn to take responsibility for yourself and so achieve more personal freedom.

Entering a group you leave the so-called normal world where strangers do not speak and, greatest taboo of all, never touch. A typical opening for an encounter session is for everyone in the room to close their eyes and to wander about very slowly, hands raised and held slightly out. Every time your hand collides with another's you pause and the two hands caress and fondle one another before slowly moving on. For first-timers, raised in our up-tight society, this is a breathtaking experience. When the group leader tells everyone to open their eyes you do so with the knowledge that you are now looking at friends. Whatever shell society made you build around yourself is at last falling away.

The size of a group varies from eight to eighteen, and the age of participants from seventeen to sixty, although I would welcome anyone over sixty in my groups. You will be encouraged by the group leader to express your feelings in relation to yourself and the other people in the room so that you experience your feelings with and in your body. Much has been written about the body, feelings and energy, most notably by Wilhelm Reich (→**Reichian therapy**). Suffice to say that we all have our own body-energy. The more we are connected with our body and the freer our energy, the more alive we feel. From conception we have been receiving messages from our parents and society as to our acceptability only a minimal acceptance, we 'sell out'. We learn to suppress our feelings and stop trusting ourselves. We are afraid to be honest. The physical and emotional symptoms which are the result of this process are varied, but include depression, anxiety, fear of your own and other people's aggression, body pains, excessive shyness, feelings of 'not being here' and not knowing how you feel. If you feel physically sick in any way it is important to be examined by a doctor. If he says, 'There is nothing wrong with you', it is most likely that the cause is emotional. You may find that a good encounter group with a trained group leader can help you. If you feel that you can cope quite well with life but want something more, then an encounter group can provide you with the opportunity to find out what it is you need. Whichever category you belong to, the important thing is to integrate what you learn in the group into your daily life.

Besides work with feelings, encounter can help with building ego-strength, making choices and building self-esteem. Many people, especially those interested in a spiritual approach to life, disapprove of any work designed to build a strong ego. But you need a strong ego before you can 'let go' of it or 'lose' it. It is necessary to have a strong ego to allow the integration of the unconscious and not be overwhelmed by it.

You can experiment in an encounter group with going forward with both positive and negative feelings for other people. Most people turn their negative feelings such as anger against themselves. We grow up afraid of sharing negativity because of fear of rejection. But the clearing of negativity leads to closeness and contact and not to the disaster so many of us fear. The ability to go forward with positive feelings means that you are free to share the deeper and more vulnerable parts of yourself: to have a meaningful and satisfying relationship with another human being, to express yourself creatively: to allow yourself to love and be loved.

There are as many different encounter groups as there are group leaders. There is no

'right' place to start with group work. You should go to a growth centre or to people with a good reputation, training and experience. Training is important. Group leading looks easy, but it is not. A group leader needs to have done at least one and a half to two years' work on her/himself before beginning training and then needs to train for a minimum of one and a half years before she/he is ready to begin leading groups. A good encounter group leader will also be trained in →gestalt, →bioenergetics and regression work. The more techniques she/he is familiar with the better. The work on her/himself is important as no group leader can take someone into feelings that she/he is not comfortable with.

Which type of group would be most suitable for you? Here are some guidelines:

A *one day* newcomer's group. An ideal place to begin as all the people will be new to group work. The group will be geared to introducing you via experience and explanation to the principles of encounter.

A *week-end* group. There will probably not be so much introductory work. There will most likely be more time for people to work on individual problems. Still, a good way to begin.

A *weekly* on-going group. An excellent way to get maximum value from groups, particularly if you feel you have a lot to work on. Also very good for making friends as people commit themselves for a four- or six-week period. A good way to get support while you are changing and integrating what you learn from groups into your everyday life.

A *48-hour* marathon. Marathons were brought to this country by Denny Yuson (Veeresh). The technique derives from Synanon, a drug-free therapeutic community for ex-drug addicts in America. The accent is on honest inter-personal confrontation. Very good for building ego-strength and getting beneath a person's image to their feelings, attitudes and needs. A good marathon is a very special experience. There are interviews before marathons to ensure that no one is psychotic or too disturbed for the group. There is a follow-up group to tie up the experience intellectually and to give feedback. A very good group to do if you do not know how you feel.

5-day groups or longer. These are often in the country so it can be a holiday as well. In a 5-day group you may find it difficult to hang on to your defences and play the games you usually play.

Intensives. An intensive group usually meets one or two evenings per week and one weekend per month for a period of three to nine months. You will be with the same group of people enabling support, friendship and trust to develop. The group leader can get to know you and your emotional history and thus be better equipped to help you. You will also get experience of other techniques as most intensives have visiting group leaders from other disciplines.

In this country group work is gradually becoming accepted as an essential part of training in such professions as social work and management. The treatment of mental illness within the National Health Service is still mainly drug-oriented. However, group work is gradually being introduced and, more important, the concept of self-responsibility is gradually being accepted in many parts of our society.

In writing about encounter groups I have tried to explain what needs first to be experienced. You will get as much out of a group as you are prepared to put in. Merely attending a group will not guarantee any change. If you participate and share your feelings and yourself with the group, you can become more aware of the possibilities of choice in your life and your power to create your own experience.

Margi Robinson

CONTRIBUTORS, p. 221

ENDOGENOUS
ENDOCRINOTHERAPY

Endogenous endocrinotherapy (E.E.) implies the treatment of the endocrine system by bringing about a normalization of glandular functioning *from within*. This immediately distinguishes it from any form of conventional treatment which involves the administration of glandular extracts derived from external sources. Such a form of treatment is 'exogenous' and constitutes a substitution or replacement therapy which does not in any way improve the basic disorder: rather does it worsen such problems by causing further atrophy of glands that are already underfunctioning. E.E., on the other hand, is entirely consistent with the principles of natural therapy in that it stimulates the vital forces, promotes homoeostasis and is harmless if used properly. Exogenous administrations, on the contrary, have considerable risks attached to them, do not stimulate the vital force, militate against homoeostasis in the long term and depend upon unpleasant animal experimentation for their production and usage.

E.E. may be effected in many ways. →**Acupuncture**, zone therapy (→**reflexology**), →**shiatsu**, →**massage**, →**homoeopathy**, →**herbal medicines**, →**osteopathy**, →**colour therapy**, psychotherapy and →**applied kinesiology** are all able to influence glandular functioning in a favourable direction. Where an osteopathic lesion exists, particularly if in the cervical or cranial region, it would be foolish to attempt to restore endocrine balance without first giving osteopathic treatment to correct it. But, whilst all the above modalities are capable of helping to balance the endocrine system, it is customary to restrict the term E.E. to a form of treatment which might more accurately be described as Samuels's treatment. Dr Jules Samuels, who lived and worked in Amsterdam, devoted his life to the development and teaching of this particular therapy, although he did not discover it. Before examining this treatment in greater detail, it is important to describe briefly some of the underlying physiology.

Most people are aware that the body has an endocrine system. They usually think of hormones as being specifically connected with the sexual apparatus and functioning, and in this they are partly correct. In fact hormones have extremely widespread and profound action throughout the body, and constitute a method of passing messages around in a way that might be compared to a postal system where given information can be distributed to a number of recipients. This contrasts with the nervous system which might be compared to a telephone system through which messages may be transmitted very rapidly, but only to one place at a time. In the body, chemical messengers (hormones) are used when a multiple response is required. Sometimes these chemicals are used to regulate the rate of functioning of various activities. Sometimes they determine whether or not a particular reaction will take place. However, the traditional view of nervous and hormone activity has now been challenged[1] and the rôle of the bio-energy or bio-energetic system suggested as being far more direct than has hitherto been thought.

The endocrine glands are quite numerous and the more important of these are the pituitary, thyroid and gonads. The pituitary is a tiny structure situated at the base of the brain almost in the centre of the head approximately at the level of the eyebrows. It stands in relation to the remainder of the endocrine system in much the same way as a conductor to an orchestra. It influences the rate of activity of the thyroid by a hormone termed thyrotrophic hormone and that of the gonads by the gonadotrophic hormone. These must be in balance for healthy functioning. There is a delicate mechanism of feedback and control which enables this balance to be maintained. But if the pituitary may be considered as the conductor, then the hypothalamus must be considered as the place of origin of the score. What is the use of having a good conductor and a good orchestra if the music is poor? Conversely, good music is ruined by a bad conductor or incompetent orchestra. From this analogy it is possible to see how easily the hormone balance may be upset, and health impaired. Such an imbalance may very well be due to adverse mental activity. The hypothalamus is very sensitive to higher (cortical) areas of mental activity and is itself a strong influence on the pituitary. So if the mind is upset by undue stress or negative thought, then the body will be adversely affected, and this adverse effect is mediated through the endocrine system as well as in other ways. Is it surprising, therefore, that we find a considerable amount of endocrine disturbance in the world today?

Severe endocrine disturbances are easily recognized clinically. Grave's disease, Simmond's disease and diabetes are familiar examples. More subtle disturbances present as a whole variety of clinical symptoms including tiredness, fatigue, headaches, depression, inability to concentrate, skin conditions, etc. Such imbalances may be determined by various forms of diagnostic procedures including acupuncture diagnosis, iris diagnosis and applied kinesiology. The specific method used by Samuels was that of the spectroscopic analysis of the blood. This is a simple test carried out on a small amount of the blood which, incidentally, is not removed from the body. A small area of skin, usually the skin between the thumb and first finger, is pinched off in a special pincette. A light is shone through this piece of skin and then observed through a specially adapted spectroscope. This allows the observer to see the spectrum of the blood. The spectrum first observed is that of oxyhaemoglobin (oxygenated blood). This changes eventually to that of reduced haemoglobin (de-oxygenated blood). The change is not easy to observe but with practice most people become fairly proficient at this task within a few months. The time taken for this change in the spectrum to take place is known as the Reduction Time (R.T.) and is indicative of the rate of metabolism which, in turn, reflects the hormonal balance. The R.T. should be twenty-five seconds. Too fast a rate indicates either an over-activity of the thyroid or an under-activity of the gonads: according to Samuels's theory. Such dysfunction is usually related to a pituitary disorder. Each of the three sets of glands are now treated in order to discover more fully the precise nature of the disturbance. Continued treatment of the offending gland or glands brings about a normalization. If stimulation of the pituitary speeds up an already fast Reduction Time, we conclude that the patient is thyrotropic. In other words, the pituitary is over-stimulating the thyroid. Continued treatment of the pituitary brings about a normalization of activity. Conversely, when the treatment slows down the Reduction Time, it is assumed that the patient is gonadotropic, i.e. that the pituitary hormone responsible for gonadic activity is in excess. However, if this were the case the initial reading should, in theory, have been *slow*, since excess gonadic hormone should have the opposite effect to that of the thyroid. In point of fact, slow initial readings are very rare and this is where we reach the point of requiring further knowledge. There seems to be a 'missing link' which has not yet been put into place.

In some cases treatment is required to the thyroid or gonads themselves. This is usually indicated by a change in Reduction Time taking place after an initial treatment of these glands. It has been found in practice that some menopausal and post-menopausal women have benefited from treatment to the ovaries, as well as some cases of infertility.

The treatment given is that of standard short wave as found in any well-equipped hospital physiotherapy department. However, it is applied in a special manner to the glands and the duration of treatment has to be very carefully regulated. Although the treatment would be fairly easy for any qualified physiotherapist to undertake under the direction of a physician, it is not part of the state registered physiotherapist's curriculum; hospital physiotherapists are, therefore, ignorant of it. A patient can be taught to treat himself but this necessitates the purchase or lease of expensive apparatus; so, unless a practitioner who carries out this particular treatment (and very few do) happens to live not too far away, it is difficult to obtain it.

Dr Samuels erroneously thought that his method was a cure for practically every known disease, including cancer, heart disease, multiple sclerosis and other serious, chronic illnesses. Despite the fact that our knowledge of the endocrine system has increased tremendously during the past few years we are still unable to say that this treatment is a cure for these diseases. Samuels was an undoubted genius and was, like many such persons, carried away with the enthusiasm he had for his work. However, he overlooked the important rôle of the pineal gland, the adrenals and that of prostaglandins. He seems to have been unaware of the fact that gonadic secretions vary during the menstrual cycle in the female and he took no cognizance of the profound influence of the mind over the endocrine system. He was so preoccupied with his own theories that he never seemed to relate his findings to any other recognized system. There is still an enormous amount of research to be done by way of monitoring other treatments with the spectroscopic test.

Hormonal balance can be improved by using foot zone therapy (deep massage of the feet with particular emphasis on the big toe and other endocrine reflexes). Several herbal agents are known to normalize the hormonal activity. Bugleweed (*Lycopus virginicus*), for example, works on the pituitary. An infusion of 1 oz. to 1 pt boiling water should be prepared and a glassful taken several times per day. These treatments need to be continued for six months to a year before reaping the full benefit. There are very many herbs which affect the other endocrine glands and the selection of the best ones in any particular case should be done by a qualified herbal medicine practitioner.

The medulla oblongata may be influenced by thumb pressure on Fengfu (sixteenth point on the Governor meridian) which is situated at the centre of the base of the skull where the cranium joins the neck. Deep massage to this point will favourably influence the pituitary, thyroid and adrenals. A deep pressure massage is the optimum form of treatment. Such treatment will ultimately affect the prostaglandin output and, consequently, the life and vitality of every cell in the body.

In this article on E.E. the authors have concentrated mainly on describing the Samuels's treatment which has come to be accepted as almost synonymous with endogenous endocrinotherapy. Whilst the authors agree that the treatment is of value, they firmly believe that it should not be undertaken without full tests and examination of every patient, in addition to the unique spectroscopic test. In many cases individuals can bring about a normalization of their endocrine system through improved mental attitudes and simple physical treatment such as those briefly described. It is felt by one of the authors at least (M.N.) that the use of acupuncture, applied kinesiology and bio-energetic synchronization techniques which balance the energy fields of the whole body are more appropriate in most cases than the short-wave (Samuels's) treatment. It is also realized that normalization of the relationship between the sacrum and occiput or cranium is vital to the restoration of endocrine balance and one of the authors (D.B.) has spent much of his life using techniques designed to bring this about. Whatever techniques are employed to treat any physical illness or imbalance they must be selected with the long-term interests of the patient in view. For this reason, the more that the patient is treated as a complete entity and the more his entire system is brought into harmony and homoeostasis, the better it will be for him. In view of this, endogenous endocrinotherapy, or any other treatment, should never be undertaken unless the practitioner is able to recognize, and put right, any imbalance in any bodily system; particularly that of the energy fields which are the architects of the dense physical body and, therefore, of its health.

Denis Brookes D.O., M.R.O.
Michael Nightingale D.O., M.AC.A.

CONTRIBUTORS, p. 221

Reference

1. M. T. Morter Jr, 'Bio-energetic synchronization technique', *Digest of Chiropractic Economics*, vol. 18, no. 1 (1975), p. 26.

FLOWER HEALING

Flowers are made into teas and ointments, but there is a more subtle and effective way of calling on them for healing: potentizing. By this means the flowers' non-material energies, or radiations, are used as distinct from using their chemical constituents, vitamins, and other material properties. In prehistoric times potentizing was a secret method of healing; it survived as tradition until recently in the many healing wells which were potentized by throwing various nuts or leaves into them before drinking the water. The children of Israel caught none of the plagues of Egypt because Moses potentized the water of Marah (Exodus 15: 23–26). In India, 4000 years ago a system of medicine based on flowers was so successful that it cut out the need for surgery. Modern flower healing using flower potencies can do away with the need for many operations and nearly all painkillers.

A branch of this formerly secret science has been known for two hundred years as →**homoeopathy**, a system of medicine based on the value of 'the hair of the dog that bit you', because a very attenuated dose of the substance which would have made (or did make) one ill often acts as a cure, e.g. homoeopathic remedies and vaccinations, etc.

While homoeopathy and the Bach remedies both see the patient as being composed of body and soul, Dr Edward Bach refined homoeopathy's method of potentizing, cutting out such things as snake venom, chemicals, and the patient's own →**urine**. He used twigs and flowers exclusively. Bach's method of potentizing was less violent than homoeopathy but the twigs or flowers were killed. His method required diagnosis of a difficult type: the remedies were prescribed for psychological dis-ease. Difficult – often impossible – to pinpoint accurately in others, the diagnosis required unhealthy introspection if applied to oneself.

The original work that I did resulted in cutting out the need for diagnosis. I retained one of Bach's ingredients, flowers. But I simplified potentizing still further and in my method the flowers are not killed – they are benefited, i.e. the process is entirely creative. This being so I make potencies of a very different type. I accept the principle that illness is psychogenic, i.e. physical illness arises in the personality as a consequence of inner dis-ease, but I gave inner dis-ease a cause, i.e. failure to resonate with spiritual perfection.

These new-type – 'homoeovitic' – potencies give a lead in activating positive aspects of the personality which are either latent or inactive. They invest the psyche with life and activity in the areas in which, for some reason or other, it does not function properly – or perhaps never functioned at all. To take one instance only: a baby might have acquired the habit of crying for attention. This carries over into the young infant's life so that it will cry for attention no matter if its mother becomes angry as a result. In adult life such persons will automatically expect everyone whose attention they invite to react with anger, and will therefore clam up internally whenever they need attention. This negative and self-defeating reaction to others leads to various physical illnesses in adult life, such as constriction of the arteries, heart troubles, digestive troubles, and skin troubles. All of which have their origin in faulty expectation. But (ripening the fruits of the spirit within the personality) these new homoeovitic potencies gently nudge the personality into open, reasonable, and friendly reactions. The result is that the basic cause of the physical disease disappears, and as a result the heart affliction, skin trouble, digestive upset or arterial congestion have no ground in which to grow. That is, their cause ceases to exist. Now the way is clear for the body's mechanism for maintaining harmony to remove obstructions to harmonious working, malfunction of the heart, skin, digestive tract, etc., disappear.

It has proved possible to blend a large number of these homoeovitic flower potencies (of which the above is only one example) to make a safe, simple and very effective remedy that is useful in almost every type of illness, mental or physical, and in less frequent doses becomes an unrivalled preventative. The blend's universality is amazing and in some cases it cuts out the need for surgery.

It has proved capable of resolving such dissimilar conditions as the horrible aura of depression surrounding thoughts for up to thirty years; lack of vitality and tiredness; it has given a further vitality far beyond that expected even for strong and healthy men and women of seventy and over; sleeplessness; it has resolved leg ulcers even in the very elderly; it has banished symptoms of →migraine without side effects; it has completely freed people of the scourge of colds and sore throats; it has got rid of bunions that had persisted for very many years; and has completely resolved synovial cysts on the finger joints of several years' standing without the operation normally thought essential – and not always successful; painful external haemorrhoids have ceased to exist within three weeks of application; swollen and painful feet have responded, as have tooth abscesses of two and three weeks' standing. In childbirth women report it was as if they had not had a baby, they felt so well afterwards; and it is used with success for strains and sprains; and for arthritic and rheumatic pains and swellings. Inflamed eyes respond after a few drops, and eyesight is often greatly improved. The blend of potencies relieves hay fever and stiffness in the joints. It has dissolved a large growth on the spleen; lumps in breasts, etc., have either dissolved or come to the surface and burst and discharged, relieving the system of all the toxins they contained so that there has been no recurrence. It has got rid of womb polyps and discharge, acne and all skin troubles.

A remarkable feature of the blend is that it can be used for young and old as a tonic, or for ordinary everyday accidents in the home, as well as with absolute safety for the most pronounced illness and for the most severe of accidents.

For all animals the blend is just as effective as it is for people. Given it, plants become strong and healthy, have excellent blooms and crop heavily. The soil's micro-flora and fauna (the true base of soil fertility) thrive on it.

This great contribution to the fertility of the soil is in regular use by premier plant growers and breeders.

This blend of flower potencies is available in various bases: as a water, lotion, or ointment, for people; as a water or salve for animals; for plants as a foliar spray, and as a soil conditioner.

Elizabeth Bellhouse

BIBLIOGRAPHY, p. 244
CONTRIBUTORS, p. 221
PRODUCTS, p. 229, 230

GERSON THERAPY

The Gerson nutritional therapy for the healing and prevention of cancer and other 'incurable' diseases is a total approach to the problem of chronic illness. Dr Max Gerson (1881–1959), of whom his former patient Albert Schweitzer wrote, 'I see in him one of the most eminent geniuses in the history of medicine', developed this dietary method. He found that by 'restoring the body's healing mechanism', that is by correcting the basic metabolic disturbances that allow chronic disease to develop, possibly all body systems may be returned to their proper functioning and the course of the chronic illness including terminal cancer may be reversed. Dr Gerson maintained (and he was borne out by other authors: Fischer-Wasels, Beck, Oberling, Maisin, *et al.*) that it is not the local but the general pathological change which is decisive in cancer. In other words, cancer is non-specific, and the therapy is also non-specific. It is applied to patients of all ages with every type of cancer, and may only be modified in the treatment of the non-malignant chronic diseases such as rheumatoid or osteo-arthritis, diabetes, allergies, asthma, glaucoma, heart disease, arteriosclerosis, mental disease, multiple sclerosis, high or low blood pressure, etc.

As a young physician in Germany, Dr Gerson first developed his therapy to cure his own severe →migraine which for years had kept him in bed for two or three days each week. When no orthodox remedy could offer him relief he attempted a change in his body's chemistry by changing his diet to the fresh fruit and raw food that had nourished man's ancestor, the ape. He soon found that the same diet that cured his migraine was also successful in other chronic 'incurable' diseases.

Dr Max Gerson first received world-wide acclaim in the 1920s for his success in treating tuberculosis with his diet therapy. Internationally renowned physician and surgeon Dr Ferdinand Sauerbruch wrote in *Master Surgeon* (Thomas Crowell, New York) of his Munich experiment with 450 patients with incurable lupus (tuberculosis of the skin). On the Gerson therapy 446 (more than 99 per cent) completely recovered.

During the course of this work with tuberculosis, many of Dr Gerson's patients suffering from other chronic conditions (arthritis, vascular disease, etc.) were cured of these as well. It was at this point that Dr Gerson concluded that in normalizing the body's chemistry, the body reactivates its normal defences and heals itself. His further research and later practical application of his (considerably modified) 'migraine diet' proved him to be correct and he had the same astounding results in reversing the fatal course of cancer. After his arrival in America he continued this dietary treatment of cancer and had such unusual results that in July 1946 he was the first doctor ever to be asked to demonstrate before a Senate Sub-Committee (Foreign Relations relative to appropriations for cancer research) five restored cancer patients who had previously been given up by leading clinics. Unfortunately the medical lobby supporting surgery, radiation and chemotherapy caused the defeat by four votes of the Senate bill which could have supported extensive research into the Gerson therapy.

Dr Gerson felt that chronic disease begins with the loss of potassium from the body cells and the subsequent invasion of sodium – and with it water – to cause oedema (retained water). In this context he stressed the importance of 'our external metabolism' by which he meant the life of the soil and the growth of plants and fruits which we need to live. Plants and vegetables, if naturally fertilized, contain the proportion of these minerals that is required in our bodies, namely an excess of potassium over sodium. Dr Gerson found in the 1920s that when soil was chemically fertilized the potassium content of the fruit and vegetables grown in that soil slowly fell and the sodium content rose.

Food processing (canning, bottling, pickling, smoking, freezing, bleaching, preserving, etc.) further changes the natural mineral balance. The potassium content of the food thus produced is considerably reduced and large quantities of sodium are added at various stages, for preserving as well as flavouring. Even when housewives buy fresh vegetables they often boil them in water, eliminating the natural potassium, and then add salt for flavour. So, slowly but steadily, modern agriculture and food technology cause a cumulative effect of reducing the body's potassium reserve and place great demands on its ability to eliminate the huge excesses of sodium. When this process fails and the potassium level falls too low, sodium invades the cell. Dr Gerson explains that this change in the mineral metabolism is followed by changes in pH content of the cells, which, in turn, affects the building and reactivation of hormones, vitamins and especially of the different oxidizing enzyme systems. It is at this point that he assumes that the weaker 'abnormal' cells that exist in every organism are first hurt and, in their anxiety to survive, change their metabolism from oxidative to fermentative. Thus they leave the harmony of the normal cells and sustain themselves by destroying neighbouring tissue with their toxic metabolic products, eventually killing the host body itself.

Why does the body not defend itself? Dr Gerson answers that in the pre-cancerous stage there is already heavy damage to all essential organs and the body is unable (a) to produce the necessary enzymes to digest the over-heavy load of fat and protein contained in our modern diet; (b) to sustain an immune reaction; (c) to produce inflammation fluid. These are its usual defences.

The treatment of the degenerative disease has to penetrate deeply to correct all the vital processes, writes Dr Gerson. When the general metabolism is restored we can again influence the functioning of all organs, tissues and cells through it. He stresses the importance of the liver as the central organ for maintaining health as well as the central organ for the body's healing mechanism.

The therapy works in three ways simultaneously to restore the chronically deficient liver. The first step is detoxification. This is achieved by giving patients large amounts of freshly pressed fruit and vegetable juices, a special soup which stimulates elimination through the kidneys, and a large number of coffee enemas, where the caffeine helps to open the bile ducts which release large masses of toxic material. The many fresh juices given also contribute to the second part of the therapy: to help the body obtain the essential nutrients, minerals and vitamins in easily digestible form. Other foods are also given: raw and freshly cooked fruits and vegetables (preferably organically grown), fresh green salads, and the soup mentioned above freshly made from specified greens and herbs. For the first six weeks all animal proteins are eliminated in order to allow the pancreas, already greatly reduced in its ability to break down proteins, to attempt to kill and digest the cancerous tumour tissue. The juices also stimulate the liver and kidneys to eliminate and flush out toxic accumulations. The third area of the treatment is the supportive liver-therapy, in the form of crude liver-extract, organic and inorganic iodine (thyroid extract and Lugol's solution), large amounts of a combination of three potassium salts in a 10 per cent solution (potassium acetate, gluconate and phosphate), pancreative enzyme and raw liver juice.

The treatment forbids all processed, canned, salted, pickled, prepared, bottled, frozen, jarred, bleached or refined foods; also stimulants of all kinds such as coffee, tea (black), nicotine, alcohol, spices, salt; also toxic materials such as hair dyes, drugs and pain-relieving agents; all butter or butter fats, oils, fluoridated water or toothpaste. Temporarily forbidden (until the restoration of the liver is completed): cheese, eggs, fish, meat, milk, cream.

In his last book, *A Cancer Therapy – Results of 50 Cases*, under the chapter heading 'Reactions–flare-ups', Dr Gerson describes the healing crises undergone by patients after three to ten days of the treatment, and periodically thereafter, when the body begins to rid itself of some of the vast amounts of toxic material that is blocking its functions. After these flare-ups (nausea, headaches, depression, in some cases vomiting, spasms in the intestines, more gas accumulation than usual, inability to drink the juices and difficulties with coffee enemas) pass, patients feel greatly relieved, normal circulation resumes and they are able to eat and drink again. Dr Gerson supplies full instructions as to how to deal with these reactions. He writes, 'Clinically these "flare-ups" are favourable reactions and should be regarded as part of the healing process.'

Depending on the extent of damage to the patient by radiation, chemotherapy or the inroads of the cancer itself, some patients cannot be totally restored to the extent that they are able to return to a 'normal' diet. They must be warned that they have to restrict their food intake to fresh foods, little meat, no salt or fat, on a permanent basis. But in cases where the liver is able to regenerate itself, Dr Gerson found that this was fully achieved after a year-and-a-half to two years' strict adherence to the diet. Most patients have no desire to return to the way of life that originally caused the onset of cancer.

It is difficult to determine the exact percentage of results obtained by the Gerson therapy because too many factors are involved. With the rarest exceptions, patients came to Dr Gerson after all orthodox methods had failed and they had been given up as hopeless. But in all cases pain was very quickly relieved or disappeared without the administration of any drugs; patients had quiet, restful nights.

One doctor who saw a patient fail after some early response remarked that if it is only for the fact that these patients die peacefully and free from pain the Gerson therapy should be made compulsory in all hospitals. In fact the actual recovery rate of Dr Gerson's patients, almost exclusively terminal cancer cases, all with metastases, was about 40 per cent. This compares with the recovery rate for terminal cases achieved by orthodox methods of less than one in 10000 cases. Dr Gerson's results in healing brain tumours were not duplicated anywhere, with any other approach. (See the first six cases in the book *Cancer Therapy – Results of 50 Cases*.) Early cancers (Cases nos. 33 and 36 are two of these) which had had no other treatment whatsoever were easily returned to normal health.

At the time of his death Dr Gerson was working on the publication of an additional 100 cases which had come to him in terminal condition, then recovered under his treatment and remained well and could be described as 'cures'. Unfortunately the book was not completed and could not be published. This is to note that there were many more than the fifty published cases among the material Dr Gerson collected over the years. (All the published and recorded cases have biopsy reports and diagnoses from hospitals or doctors other than Dr Gerson.)

Dr Gerson's ideas met with well-organized opposition from vested medical interests (cf. S. J. Haught, *Has Dr Max Gerson a True Cancer Cure?*, London Press, 1962) both during his lifetime and after. For this reason the Gerson therapy is not being used by any doctor or in any clinic at the present time. The exact treatment prescribed and used by Dr Gerson was applied only by one other doctor in New York. Dr Lance Vallan used the method with some terminal cancer patients, basing himself entirely on Dr Gerson's book. He was able to duplicate the results Dr Gerson obtained. Unfortunately he died in 1966.

The most complete literature on the Gerson nutritional therapy is available in Dr Max Gerson's book *A Cancer Therapy – Results of 50 Cases*. In it he discusses the theory, background, research and exact practice of the therapy, besides giving documented case histories of fifty cases. All of these cases recovered for at least five years; some are still alive and well more than twenty years later. Since there is now no physician using the method, some patients, in desperation, have actually used the book entirely on their own. Many have been able to follow the directions accurately and have had excellent results.

Dr Gerson's daughter, Charlotte Gerson Straus, lectures extensively on her father's work and both she and the author of this article counsel on the practical problems and application of the therapy.

Dr Gerson wrote that it was impossible for cancer and other chronic diseases to be eliminated in the future unless the entire civilization of our present age were changed and people returned to nature and its eternal laws; unless the soil were made healthy again, mothers nursed their babies again, fed them natural foods (and not canned and jarred baby food), and we eliminated so many of the things which start so early to undermine the health of our children and youths (i.e. canned and bottled drinks, sausages and ice cream, white flour, cakes and sweets, denatured foods of all kinds, cigarettes). But bearing all this in mind, since it seems possible to cure cancer and other chronic illnesses, it is obviously simpler and more painless to prevent it.

Margaret Straus

BIBLIOGRAPHY, p. 245
CONTRIBUTORS, p. 221
PRODUCTS, p. 229

GESTALT THERAPY

Gestalt therapy has developed out of gestalt psychology, Freudian psychoanalysis and the writings of Otto Rank and Wilhelm Reich (→Reichian therapy). Its basic principles are the work of Fritz Perls, author of *Ego, Hunger and Aggression*,[1] *Gestalt Theory Verbatim*,[2] and (with Hefferline and Goodman) *Gestalt Therapy*.[3]

A gestalt is a pattern or configuration. If we look at the sky at night we have difficulty in finding the Pole Star without identifying constellations such as Ursa Major (the Great Bear). Our habit of 'seeing shapes', however arbitrarily, causes us to focus attention on the *figure*, the rest of the sky becoming *background*, and so to orient ourselves and find our way around the sky.

If a bright shooting star comes within our field of vision, our attention is drawn to this moving object, which becomes figural, and the constellations, as well as the rest of the sky, become background.

This process of gestalt formation and destruction is going on in all of us all the time. It follows the perpetual flux of our attention, which, if we are healthy, follows the rhythm of our needs. If need-fulfilment is blocked, however, there is confusion or a lack of awareness. The person does not know what he wants or cannot reach out to get what he wants.

The blocking of need-fulfilment is manifested in repetitive behaviour, lack of interest in the body or a feeling of effort when any task is attempted. The gestalt therapist is more active than the psychoanalyst or the Rogerian. He breaks up the patient's poorly organized field of awareness, heightens each emerging figure, and helps the patient to recognize what he is doing that prevents him from getting what he wants at that moment.

He constantly emphasizes the here-and-now. He invites the patient to change questions, which he sees as an attempt to cling to authority figures and to remain a child, into statements, which represent taking responsibility for one's own feelings.

He keeps bringing the patient or group back to the 'open now' of what is being revealed, and the 'hidden now' of phantasies. He encourages the person to change impersonal statements, such as 'My shoulders are tense', to 'responsible' ones such as, 'I am tensing my shoulders'; and 'why' questions to 'how' questions: 'How am I tensing my shoulders?

He encourages the person to change nouns into verbs, in order to become aware of the constant flux of sensations, feelings and relationships. Instead of *gossiping* about absent people, the person is invited to play both roles, himself and the one he is concerned with. This is part of the process of initiating a dialogue between the person and parts or aspects of himself he has *disowned* or alienated and *projected* into the outside world.

Such projection leaves holes or gaps in the personality, and the gestalt therapist helps the person to fill the holes by taking minor risks in the here-and-now.

Dreams are seen as dramatizations of projection, and the therapist encourages a dialogue, not only between the humans who appear in the dream, but also between animals and objects, all of which are projected and disowned fragments of the personality.

I remember the first session with a new patient in which the whole hour was taken up with a tiny fragment of one dream. A rabbit, chased by a large, growling, barking dog, continued to run although its intestines were falling out and its legs were collapsing from exhaustion. It was too terrified to turn round and look at the dog.

After repeated encouragement, the patient, playing the rôle of the rabbit, eventually turned and faced the dog. In the rôle of the dog, the patient snarled and barked savagely, but each time he changed rôles and faced the dog, the dog became smaller and less terrifying.

At one point, as the rabbit, his terror reached the point of catatonic stupor. His jaw locked, and his breathing was almost imperceptible. Suddenly his energy was released, a dialogue was initiated between rabbit and dog, they became reconciled and friendly, and the dog carried the weak and exhausted rabbit on its back.

The nightmare which provided the material for this session was a dramatization of what Perls calls 'top-dog and under-dog', the two warring parts of the personality which split the body and enfeeble it like a civil war. Until they are reconciled the person's energy is locked in a struggle between impulse and repression. In gestalt theory repression is both unawareness of the impulse and the contrac-tion of antagonistic muscles which inhibits the impulse.

As the false or phoney self is progressively abandoned, the person's individual hierarchy of needs is clarified, and a healthy rhythm of gestalt formation and destruction, in harmony with that hierarchy, can be established.

When the patient was in the rôle of the dog, the sadistic satisfaction he was deriving from terrifying the dying rabbit was manifest in his expression, body movements and voice. In order to escape from the paralysis of civil war, he had to abandon both the sadistic satisfaction of the persecutor and the masochistic submissiveness of the victim. The body can then be unified and function harmoniously.

The gestalt therapist calls the tyrant–victim struggle *game-playing*. The person maintains the *phoney layer* of his personality and plays manipulative games ('I'm doing this for your own good'; 'He wouldn't hurt a fly'; 'You don't want to make Mummy unhappy, do you?') in order to avoid his fear of finding out what and who he is.

If he breaks through this controlling layer and tries to become more honest and genuine, he reaches the *phobic layer*, the resistance against accepting what he is. This resistance takes the form of an elaborate system of *shoulds* and *should nots*. 'I should not have murderous or hurtful impulses. I should be kind and considerate. I should love my neighbour as I love myself. I should love my mother, and so I shouldn't hate her.'

If both the phoney layer and the phobic layer are broken through, we reach the *impasse*. We feel that we are nothing, dead, machines or robots. The phoney self has hitherto attracted so great an energy-charge that the person cannot believe that the suppressed and disowned self can be real, can grow, can have vitality. The terrified rabbit, in my patient's image, is dying because its intestines are falling out, and it dare not even look at the danger.

The acceptance of this despair, when the false self is rejected and there seems to be no self to take its place, brings us to the *implosive layer*. When my patient reached this layer in his first session, he went into a catatonic state, his whole body stiff and rigid as if in *rigor mortis*. He could not utter a sound or move any muscle of his body.

When he realized that the dog and the rabbit, two sub-personalities drawing upon one source of energy, his own body, might be able to cooperate instead of persecuting each other, the catatonic, implosive state was suddenly dissolved, and an *explosion* of energy occurred. Lying on the mattress, he kicked, shouted, breathed strongly and deeply, and expressed his immense relief.

Perls describes four types of explosion: into joy, into grief, into orgasm, into anger. According to my experience he overlooked a very important type: the explosion into the total bodily discharge of fear and physical hurt. Perhaps this omission is due to the extreme cultural taboo on the violent shaking and cold sweating which is the only discharge of fear which brings total bodily relief.

An alternative or a mitigation of the explosion is *melting*, when the implosion or catatonia is dissolved into streamings, a highly pleasurable sensation of the flow of energy through the body.

The strength of gestalt therapy lies in its compatibility with other important developments in humanistic psychology since the publication, in 1951, of *Gestalt Therapy*.[3] It is not so much an alternative to primal therapy, bio-energetics, psychomotor therapy, psychodrama or meditation as a shift of focus from authoritarian treatment or teaching to the encouragement and guiding of the person to discover his own doctor-guru in his own dreams, his own relationships, his own lifestyle and his own body in the here-and-now.

The only important psychotherapy with which it is incompatible is psychoanalysis. The gestalt therapist regards psychoanalysis as an encouragement of the patient's need to remain a child, to remain weak and ill, to accept the authority of an adult, and to have himself and his illness explained to him.

Although, like Perls, I derived my basic understanding of psychodynamics from Freud, Rank, Klein and other psychoanalysts, as well as from pioneer gestaltists such as Kurt Lewin, I have abandoned Freudian dream-interpretation in favour of gestalt dream dialogues and dream extension (letting the patient be the director of his own 'dream-film'), combining the dialogue with bodily expression. Yet the use of Freudian insights in here-and-now group therapy, as illustrated in *Treatment or Torture*,[4] has become well established over the last two decades.

An account of gestalt therapy would not be complete without mention of Perls's own idiosyncratic style of working. *Gestalt Therapy Verbatim*[2] and *Gestalt Therapy Now*[5] give the reader a glimpse of his use of the group as background, with himself and one person in the 'hot seat' as figure.

He would focus on a fragment of a dream until its significance for the person's way of life became evident, and then he would dismiss the person and invite another to take the hot seat. Sometimes members of the group would be called on to participate, but most of them would learn only vicariously.

His method is what I would call 'the limelight method'. Perls pointed out that Freud's phobic symptom, hating to have to look into the patient's eyes or be stared at, led him to the method of putting the patient on a couch and sitting behind him, which has become the standard procedure of psychoanalysis.

There is no reason why Perls's exhibitionistic 'symptom', having the short, dramatic intervention in front of a group who are not effectively relating to each other, should become standard procedure in gestalt therapy.

Gestalt therapy has great survival power because it is flexible enough to be used in conjunction with the great flood of insights flowing from Sigmund Freud, with the body-work derived from Wilhelm Reich, with the group methods of psychodrama and encounter, and with the deep, intensive therapy of primal release and reintegration.

G. Seaborn Jones B.A. (Oxon.), PH.D. (Lond.)

References

1. F. S. Perls, *Ego, Hunger and Aggression*, Allen & Unwin, 1947.

2. F. S. Perls, *Gestalt Theory Verbatim*, Real People Press, Moalo, Utah, 1969.

3. F. S. Perls, R. F. Hefferline, and P. Goodman, *Gestalt Therapy*, Julian Press, New York, 1951, and Dell, New York, 1965.

4. G. Seaborn Jones, *Treatment or Torture*, Tavistock, 1968.

5. J. Fagan and I. L. Shepherd, *Gestalt Therapy Now*, Science and Behaviour Books, 1970.

GINSENG

The root of the ginseng plant, much revered by the Chinese for thousands of years, has recently attracted much attention in the West as a natural tonic and anti-stress agent. One of the reasons is the growing interest in natural substances and preventive medicine. Another is that more research has been done on this oriental herb in the last decade than in the preceding hundred years.

Panax ginseng grows in China, Korea, and eastern U.S.S.R. Related varieties grow in Japan (*Panax japonicus*), the Himalayas of India and Nepal (*Panax pseudoginseng*), and in North America (*Panax quinquefolium*).

Panax ginseng C. A. Meyer is the botanical name of a rare shrub of the family Araliaceae. It grows in secluded and forested areas. The medicinal part of the plant is the root, which is white, branched and fleshy, and covered in tendrils. The shape of the root is often likened to that of a man. Hence its Chinese name, meaning 'man-plant'. The root takes four to seven years to mature and is now extensively cultivated in Korea and China.

Ginseng is said to have been used in China as a medicine as long ago as 3000 B.C. The earliest written record concerning its medicinal use comes from Emperor Shen Nung's *Materia Medica*, which regarded it as the highest, most potent herb among the thousands mentioned. Shen Nung wrote that it was 'a tonic to the five viscera, quieting the animal spirits, strengthening the soul, allaying fear, expelling evil effluvia, brightening the eyes, opening the heart, benefiting the understanding and, if taken over a period of time, will invigorate the body and prolong life'.

There is a rich history and mythology surrounding this 'root of life'. At one time the Chinese and Tartars fought battles over the possession of lands where ginseng grew. It was considered the property of the emperors. A Tartar warrior-king is said to have built a wooden palisade around an entire province in order to protect his precious supply. In 1714 a Jesuit missionary, Father Jartoux, was given a root to suck by a mandarin when he was utterly exhausted and could no longer sit on horseback. Within an hour, after sucking half of it, his fatigue had completely gone. An account of the 'miraculous herb' was read by Father Lafitau, stationed in North America, who then 'discovered' a herb of the same species, five-finger root (*Panax quinquefolium*), known as American ginseng.

Ginseng does not appear to possess any specific, well-defined action, but exhibits a number of pharmacological activities, all of which contribute towards its total therapeutic effects. On the one hand, it acts as a mental stabilizer or depressant of the nervous system; on the other, it reacts as an activator or stimulant, balancing the equilibrium of both mind and body. Modern science is beginning to admit the need for remedies that strengthen the overall resistance of the organism. Ginseng acts to build up the non-specific resistance of the body to stressful conditions, whether social, environmental or pathological.

Ginseng has a stimulatory effect on the cerebral cortex of the central nervous system. Using condition-reflex methods it was found that ginseng simultaneously stimulates the process of excitation and active inhibition in the brain cortex. Thus ginseng, unlike the stimulants known so far, does not disturb the equilibrium in the brain processes.

Many of the activities of ginseng have been positively connected with components called glycosides. A whole series of glycosides have been isolated in Russia, and are called panaxosides. The same series has been isolated in Japan, and are named ginsenosides. Besides glycosides the dried ginseng root contains essential oils, fatty acids, ginsenin, phytosterin, mucilaginous resins, enzymes, vitamins, sugars, certain unknown alkaloids, minerals, silicic acid, and not more than 13 per cent moisture.

The best roots are submitted before being dried to a process of clarification, which renders them a light brown or buff colour, giving them a semi-transparent appearance. Its commercial value is determined by its size, shape and age. Ginseng root is available in the West in powdered form, tablets, capsules, chipped root pieces, extracts and in the form of tea. The recommended dose of a ginseng preparation depends on the reason for taking it. For a long-term tonic effect, especially for those over forty and the aged, between half and one gram should be taken twice a day. The course should last at least a month and for older people continuously. Ginseng has a cumulative effect and is a valuable aid in combating exhaustion and in coping with the effects of the ageing process. For a short-term stimulant effect to alleviate fatigue, and in case of weakness during convalescence, the dose may be increased somewhat.

Ginseng has a mild, subtle effect and is remarkably safe, even in large doses, or when taken over a long period. Modern research has confirmed that there are no known harmful side-effects.

Lee Harris

CONTRIBUTORS, p. 221
PRODUCTS, p. 225, 228

GRAPHOLOGY

Interest in the individual quality of a script has been recorded over many centuries. Chinese philosophers of the second century B.C. developed the concept that calligraphic differences were related to the character, temperament and tastes of the writer concerned. They thought that the quality of the strokes which made up a message-bearing script was of significance in its own right.

Twentieth-century research has confirmed the validity of this by examining in microscopic detail not only the subtle rhythms of tension and release, which are found to mark the execution of strokes as they move communicatively across the page, but also the degree of their liveliness or dullness.

Ideally these rhythms should be harmoniously balanced. as well as lively, so that the strokes are smoothly coherent, notwithstanding such fluctuations in letter size as may naturally occur. However, the rhythmic pattern can be rigidly regular, with negative overcontrol of movement causing the strokes themselves to show dullness; or else it may be disturbed in its coordination by such as displacement of exerted pressure, as the writing implement is directed with difficulty, in which case the strokes are likely to be broken, if they are not marked by sudden ataxic variability.

The Abbé Jean-Hyppolyte Michon of Paris coined the word graphology around 1878 from the Greek basis of its two parts. The name simply means the study of handwriting. Michon was concerned that the deviations from the copybook forms he saw should be considered in terms of specific characteristics.

Relying on the fundamental principle that any handwriting is uniquely expressive of the individual who produced it, the technique of analysis which has developed over the years provides a disciplined system for evaluating on a part-qualitative, part-measurable basis, the different components of an integrated script, which at the final count is considered as a →gestalt movement in the overall.

Nevertheless in his day the Abbé Michon was primarily concerned with the structure of letters. Thus he became associated with the rather static interpretation of graphic signs which, over the years, has resulted in much misunderstanding and abuse. The concept that one particular letter-shape could indicate that a writer possessed certain qualities, or would behave in a certain way, appealed to overenthusiastic amateurs throughout the world.

This applied more in Great Britain and the U.S.A. than elsewhere in Europe. There the German influence upon research provided a disciplined structure of inquiry into the neurological, emotional and intellectual aspects of graphic movement, which eventually gave university status to the technique. Today in many countries, including Great Britain and the U.S.A., the scientific analysis of handwriting is accepted as a diagnostic aid in cases of personality dysfunction, whether the cause is suspected to have its origin in complex psychiatric illness or is related to some more straightforward emotional maladjustment. Less often the study of a patient's handwriting is made in medical cases, either to confirm diagnosis or to provide early warning of disorder. However, significant research has been conducted in the U.S.A., and an attempt made to monitor the progressive effect on the essential stroke quality of such diseases as cancer and alcoholism.

In considering the contribution that a graphologist can make to medicine, it is important to recognize that in cases of physical illness no form of treatment can be initiated based on handwriting. All that can be done is to report observed facts to a qualified third party and provide information as to the probable cause of disturbances or deterioration. In this respect the concept that disturbances in the physical functioning of a person must upset the motor performance in the act of writing is not a difficult one to accept.

Certain disorders of the nervous system, such as Parkinson's disease, show specific graphic indications. This applies as much to the cerebral palsied at birth, who often manage to achieve an optimum degree of expressive functioning within their physical limitations, as to those suffering an accident later in life or afflicted with a tumour. Handwriting has validly been described as 'brain writing' because it is controlled by muscles that are stimulated by nerve impulses arising in cells of the ventral horn area of the spinal cord, and because the flow of such stimuli is regulated to a great extent by the motor centres in the cortex of whichever cerebral hemisphere is the dominant.

However, handwriting is a communicator of thoughts and feelings as well as a means of social contact, so that is more than just 'brain writing'. It is expressive of the mind of the writer, as of his intellectual spirit and basic soul (or psyche), so that developments in the personality through the years result in developments from the basic script forms learnt in childhood. If this were not so, handwriting would be a mechanical skill, which when learned would result in a consistency of common production as far as shape, size and slant was concerned, which just does not happen in practice.

Thus not only disorders of the mind but of the personality functioning are reflected in graphic expression. The way in which an individual deals with the information received from the world, and establishes his own place in it, is a behaviour pattern that can be traced from the way he meets the implicit challenge of projecting himself on an unmarked page. This projection is not only made in the vertical and the horizontal in terms of form, but in respect of exerted pressure in the dynamic also.

Where organic disease is concerned, there is no doubt that as an individual's functioning is affected, so the graphic trail is thereby marked. This applies to tubercular and cardiac patients and has been proved particularly through the work conducted over thirty years by Alfred Kanfer, mainly at different clinics in New York. Starting with his investigations with problems of neuro-muscular coordination amongst children, Kanfer proceeded to research into the handwriting of diagnosed cancer patients. Correlation between observed changes in the handwriting and the progress of the disease was found to occur in a high proportion of cases, irrespective of the social background or age of the patient.

However, it is necessary to make the point that because there is a psychological aspect which influences a person's functioning, the extent to which disease is present is not always directly proportionate to the degree of graphic disturbances shown. Where a patient has been able to come to terms with his terminal condition there is likely to be less evidence of stroke disintegration; while an exerted will-power can result in seemingly impossible self-determinate achievement in relation to actual physical deterioration and thereby also mask its symptoms in respect of graphic expression. Thus absence of specific indications in handwriting cannot be taken as absence of disease, although when warning symptoms are noted, they should not be ignored.

Handwriting analysis has a definite, already proven, part to play in the diagnosis of nervous and mental disorders as well as of personality stress and depressive illness. While its contribution is presently limited, clinical research into the effect of organic disease on the graphic trail is likely soon to result in advances being made in this field, particularly where the recognition of developing syndromes is concerned.

Although examination of handwriting does not have a direct therapeutic application, since essentially an individual writes as he is and cannot be changed by any alteration in graphic style, yet there is an area where some remedial work can be done, often with considerable success. This is in respect of people whose ability to express themselves on paper has either not been properly developed or has become blocked for some reason. Usually this relates to children and adolescents, although some adults may develop symptoms of agraphia, albeit false, so that they are unable to produce anything in writing.

Understanding of the many factors involved in the graphic act, of the structure of letters and of the fear of criticism often suffered by those experiencing problems of communication, is necessary if some harmony of graphic fluency is to be encouraged. Often this is best tackled by establishing a balanced pattern of tension and release in the execution of the basic directional strokes and geometric shapes which together form the alphabetical symbols of language. In doing so, confidence is developed and faults in holding the writing instrument corrected, particularly where left-handers are concerned, before actual handwriting is attempted. Usually fluency then improves considerably. It has been found that amongst children the resulting emotional release not only gives a more socially co-operative behaviour pattern but also an increased response to learning.

HAND HEALING

Hand healing is sometimes called spiritual healing but all healing could be this as the source of all healing comes from the Divine Forces.

Hand healing is so termed because the hands are placed near or on the patient's body and the healing comes through them. This is a healing art which has been known through the ages. In the Egyptian temples the Healing Priests used their hands, and in the church today we have the Laying on of Hands.

Hands were given us for a purpose and with our hands we give, whether it be solid gifts from one to another, practical gifts of binding a wound, cleaning a house, cooking food for others, painting a picture, playing music or many other ways of giving through the hands.

The greatest gift of all is what we term hand healing.

One cannot be dogmatic in telling anyone how to use the hands in healing for everyone must find what is best for them – i.e. what feels right for them.

Some healers will touch their patients by placing the hands either on the head or where the trouble is felt most. One must realize, though, when placing the hands on the supposed trouble spot, that this may be only the physical manifestation of the trouble and the cause may lie elsewhere. Some healers will feel and heal through their fingers and others through the palms of their hands.

Many healers obtain excellent results without touching their patients at all, whilst others have been equally successful by placing both hands on the head – it is for the healers to find what is right for them and one can only give suggestions and examples as a guide.

The healer should be completely relaxed so that the healing force can flow easily through him. It is easy to try and direct that force or energy but one must refrain from so doing. Remembering that energy follows thought, if one thinks of a particular part of the patient's body one can direct the energy, but this may not be the right place.

If the healer can achieve real relaxation of mind and body the flow of healing will go through the hands to the patient or, as in some cases, the reverse will happen. If there is poison, or something which requires removal from the patient, it will be dispersed. The hands must be allowed to move where they seem to want to go and this can only come with practice. It is not a question of the hands moving all over the body in all directions, but it is as if a force is directing them to certain and positive positions. Only experience can tell one where these positions are through the sensations felt in the hands.

These sensations are variable from hot, cold, prickles and pain to a creaking in one's joints. Interpretation is difficult and is not essential. What is essential is that they are accepted as signals that the places where they are felt are places that require treatment. The hands should be kept in the vicinity until the sensations cease before moving on elsewhere.

There are always times when it is not possible for the sensations to cease in one healing session, usually because the patient's condition is too bad.

It is rare to remove all symptoms and conditions and completely heal the patient at one session, although it does happen. The amount of treatment required varies from patient to patient. In very serious conditions it may be necessary every day, but normally once a week or fortnight is sufficient. In some cases once a month is enough. There are no hard-and-fast rules on this. The healer must use his intuition and common sense to decide what is required.

To be a hand healer is exciting and rewarding when one's patients respond. It is also a very responsible occupation. Many patients will rely on the advice of the healer and seek that advice, as of an authoritative source.

Therefore, it is important the healer takes his work seriously and learns to use his intuitions. All knowledge is there, if one seeks it, but it will not just come without some hard work on the healer's part.

One must learn to discipline oneself, and the more disciplined a life one leads the more one learns. Meditation and breathing exercises, preferably to start the day, are but two ways of gaining this necessary control of the physical body, and the mind or thoughts. If the day is started in a rush and hurry it often continues in this vein. If, however, the day commences in an orderly, organized, calm and disciplined fashion the frustrations, difficulties and demands made upon one will be met with confidence and tranquillity. This will be felt by the patients.

When one is working as close to a patient as a hand healer is, and using the subtle forces, the patient often picks up the emanations of the healer; so it is important to be tranquil and to ensure that nothing can get in the way of the healing force.

There are occasions when patients want to talk. This may be a great help as they may find it difficult to express their fears and worries to family or friends – it then becomes part of the healing and should be encouraged. Talking sometimes helps the healer too, by taking his mind away from the patient's physical problems.

The ideal is silence and for the healer to be an objective observer of what is happening – i.e. the sensations that are being felt and where they are felt. If one can achieve this and become an interested observer one can often learn, not only about the patient, but also to interpret what is happening. Sometimes both the hands will be completely still, other times one hand is still while the other moves, or both may move. They may move with a gentle motion towards and away from the patient, or with an up and down movement. Whatever it is, there is normally a rhythm and it is rarely a jerky movement.

There are times when one hand will be in front of the body and the other at the back, or either side of a shoulder or knee, etc. When healing eyes, one hand may be over the eye and the other at the back of the head. There are times when the arm is lifted high, as high as one can reach, and it will stay in that position for some time with the hand bent over the patient. One wonders how it is possible for an arm to be stationary for so long without tiring, but it is not part of one's physical body any more and one looks upon it as having no connection with oneself

These things are difficult to accept until one has experienced them personally. There are times too when the arm will move right away from the patient and also when the healer actually has to move away, sometimes several feet away, still with the hands giving healing. This is because around everyone are what we commonly call force fields which are made up of subtle energies. There are times when it is necessary to give healing not to the etheric, close to the patient's body, but to one of the subtler fields further away from the body.

Sometimes the patient is aware of what is happening, at others he is oblivious. When a patient asks what one is doing it is best to tell him – it is so interesting when a patient says, 'I don't know where you are but I'm feeling something in my low back,' and that is exactly where one's hands are.

Many patients feel nothing, others are ultra-sensitive and may be psychologically disturbed and say they feel faint. This happens rarely; but, in the event, it is best to stop healing, to get the patient to put his head down and give him a glass of water, and talk for a while. Sometimes, a limb will jerk even though the hands may be well away from it. Other times, when it is spinal trouble, they feel something move in their back – again, when the hands are nowhere touching the body, and they will feel better as a result. Patients often feel hot or cold over the parts being healed. Usually the healer's hands feel the reverse.

When one is healing and a sudden twinge of pain runs through the hand it is difficult not to react; but it is important not to do so, as the patient may be worried and think that they either have something awful or have been the cause of giving pain to the healer.

Some patients go to sleep while receiving treatment. This is not so much the patient as the healer who produces this reaction; and when this happens it is best to give healing with the patient lying down. Normally it is best for a patient to sit on a stool as one can get at all sides of him from top to toe. So many problems arise in the area of the spine it is essential that if a chair is used the patient should sit sideways on it.

After the healing session is completed it is beneficial for the patient to relax for a short while; patients occasionally feel sleepy, and if they are going to drive some distance it is best to rest first.

The question of payment is a difficult one and must be left to the healer. Everyone has overheads to pay and some may not have the wherewithal to do so without earning. Patients like to know where they stand, and often prefer a set fee rather than making a donation; in cases of genuine hardship all fees can be waived, remembering that in order to receive one must also give. There are cases too where the patient appears not to receive any benefit until he has first given.

When anyone feels they would like to know more about hand healing and to receive help and guidance as to how to set about it, there are some groups who will help and one or two who give courses on hand healing. One is diffident to start with and not sure of oneself, and needs guidance and basic knowledge of what one is doing; as well as someone to turn to in case of need.

Everyone could probably be a healer, but not everyone wants to be. The ability is latent until it is brought out. Sometimes this happens slowly, but a situation can arise when it is forced upon one and having taken the first step others follow.

It is not something to force oneself to do, but to go into gently. Perhaps by relieving a headache or a pain for some member of the family one realizes for the first time that something has happened through one's own hands. It is very exciting, and from small beginnings anything can develop. One's dog is also a good first patient.

Confidence is most difficult to achieve and one must never become over-confident. One must never boast or put oneself on a pedestal, because it is not oneself that has in fact done anything – one is only a vehicle and used as a channel for the one great force to help and heal others.

One is very self-conscious to begin with – conscious that one's hands are near another person; worried that nothing may happen; that the patient may not feel anything or get better.

They may be one's own hands, but they have been guided to the right places about a patient – to be kept stationary or to move, according to what is necessary. It is not one's will that has moved them, but His will; not our will that has given healing but His.

What one's own particular religion is matters not. The more simple the approach to healing the better. We are all one. The Christ Force is in each one of us. The divine spark is there for us to light or leave dormant as we will.

Elizabeth Baerlein

CONTRIBUTORS, p. 221
TRAINING, p. 232

HEALTH FARMS

Most people go to health farms to lose weight. It's a fact deplored by the devotees of healthy living who run the farms. They would prefer to stress the therapeutic value – physical, psychological and often spiritual – of peace and tranquillity, sensible exercise and careful eating. But the fact is that most of the guests regard a health-farm holiday as a penance rather than a retreat – voluntary incarceration out of the way of tempting business lunches and cream teas.

As a result there are two main types of health farm: those that recognize the material advantages of catering for appearance-conscious clients, and those that maintain an almost religious commitment to providing therapy for body and soul.

It's important, therefore, to decide which sort of farm suits your needs.

The first type provides an atmosphere rather like a genteel holiday camp. There's the same camaraderie of people 'all in the same boat together' and the forced intimacy of sauna bath and massage parlour welds many an unlikely friendship, as clients exchange notes on the progress of waistline or inner thigh bulge, and compare hunger pangs. Many of these farms are favoured by rich, single people, as a hunting ground for mates. There's always the chance of meeting a successful executive paying the price of a year's business lunches; or a rich widow shedding pounds (both sorts) before her annual fling in St Tropez. Some of the farms even lay on champagne parties (with low-calorie canapés) to help people get together.

At the other extreme, there are health hydros similar to rest homes and frequented mainly by elderly arthritic patients. It's vital, therefore, that you get full details of the health farm you wish to go to before booking. Wherever you choose to go, you will receive certain basic services. These are:

Before any treatment, and that includes starting a diet, it is necessary to have a check-up with the resident doctor. This is usually arranged automatically, on the first day of your stay. Some farms include the cost of the check-up in the holiday price. Others charge it as separate service, at the doctor's normal consultation rate. This can be quite expensive, so it's worth finding out how much it will cost before you receive your final bill.

Assuming you have no outstanding, specific health problems, the doctor will give you a general health check. He will take your blood pressure, check your pulse, heart and lungs and take a detailed medical history from you. If you have come to lose weight he will weigh you, and give you a target weight to aim for. He should also check that there is no physical malfunction – glandular trouble, for instance – that could account for obesity, and he should ensure that you are fit enough to take the strain, as it can be, of a crash diet.

Some health farms follow a →**vegetarian** régime; or provide →**macrobiotic** foods only – or any number of diets specifically tailored for the guest's needs. A diet of pure lemon juice may be recommended; or brown rice and water; or raw vegetables. Or you may choose, or be advised, to eat nothing at all, bar the odd drink of vegetable juice.

The first two days are the worst. After that you'll probably find your stomach has shrunk so much that two lettuce leaves make you feel bloated. Dramatic weight losses are possible even in a one-week health farm holiday. Certainly a person who is less than half a stone overweight should come away the right weight for their height. But if all you require is a week's starvation a health farm is an expensive way to do it. The idea of the diet is to re-educate the body, and mind, to a better way of eating, and if the moment the holiday is over you return to unhealthy, gluttonous consumption, the weight will soon return and the exercise will have been a waste of time. The attitude towards the diet is the most important thing. It should be seen as the beginning of a long-term régime, not a desperate short-term measure.

Most health farms employ at least one resident, trained masseuse. Massage sessions usually last about twenty minutes. Done properly, massage should stimulate circulation, relax muscles and soothe nerves.

You will be asked to lie on a couch, dressed in underclothes or naked with a towel over you. The limbs are massaged, then the back, neck and scalp. The experience is nearly always pleasant and relaxing, though some masseuses may think it necessary to beat the body quite hard with the sides of the hands.

Some health farms also employ a →chiropractor or →osteopath and will give special massage/manipulation for dislocated bones.

Sauna and Turkish baths are both ways of making you sweat. The idea is to lose some weight by getting rid of body moisture, and also to rid the body of impurities and dirt in the pores. Both are usually communal affairs. The sauna bath is a wooden hut with slatted benches to lie on, and a fire to heat it. The heat is essentially dry. The Turkish bath is similar, but the heat is steamier. Some farms have individual Turkish baths, machines in which you sit, the body encased in a metal cabinet into which steam is pumped. Sauna and Turkish bath sessions will be regulated by the doctor or nurses in charge and vary from five minutes to twenty-five minutes in length.

Colonic irrigation (→**high colonic irrigation**) involves flushing out the alimentary canal with water under pressure. The water is pumped into the body via a tube inserted in the rectum. It's an instant cure for →**constipation**, and some swear by it as a means of cleansing the body.

There's no point in going to a health farm if you creep out each afternoon and gorge cream buns in the local tea-shop. Some health farms absolutely forbid such secret indulgence, and may ask you to leave if they catch you at it. Others have tried instituting a fines system for anyone caught breaking the diet. But, on the whole, it is up to the individual to adhere to the farm's rules. Smoking is frowned on, at some farms actually forbidden, and early nights are encouraged.

The accommodation at health farms is usually up to good country house hotel standards. In addition, most provide facilities like tennis courts, badminton courts, swimming pools and gardens.

Rita Carter

CONTRIBUTORS, p. 221
HEALTH FARMS, p. 235

HEALTH FOODS

Going into a health food store for the first time the visitor is confronted by a bewildering display of products, many of them certainly not foods in the accepted sense. I shall guide you round the shelves of a typical health store, telling you something of the history and philosophy of the health food idea.

In Victorian times far-seeing doctors and scientists began to realize there was a relationship between food and health. This led to the development of many systems and theories as to how to live and eat. At the time there was starvation and shortage of protein amongst poor children. Practical idealists realized that fresh air, exercise and a balanced diet would do more for the well-being of these poor children than any amount of preaching. So a diet was developed based on vegetarian principles, rich in fresh fruit, vegetables, grains and beans. With such ingredients it was, and still is, possible to have a wholesome nutritious diet very inexpensively.

During the 1890s Dr Allinson demonstrated the advantages of eating wholewheat bread A few years later Eustace Miles, who was tennis champion of the world, produced some excellent high protein foods whilst his wife demonstrated delicious wholesome vegetarian (→vegetarianism) cooking at their popular restaurant at Chandos Place in London. Health stores sprang up to supply these special foods, which were in fact ordinary foods long missing from the diet. The adulteration of food had been rife for several hundred years and this new interest brought forth a parallel improvement in the standards of hygiene and purity of foods in general.

The food eaten by primitive man was natural in a way that is no longer possible. Experts tell us that there would be starvation if we did not use artificial fertilizers and insecticide sprays. There is now no part of the world where animals are free from residues of DDT. More than 3000 artificial additives are used in food compared with only 100 at the beginning of the twentieth century. It is this change perhaps more than any other which has taken place predominantly in the last fifteen years that has caused the rapid development of interest in health foods.

There are now 600 or so health stores in Britain supplying products which are as near natural as today's world permits. It is likely that the health food industry is more conscious of the needs of the consumer, rather than the conveniences of production, than in any other trade. You will find that health stores have ancillary products which are not necessarily of the highest possible nutritional quality; but these should not be taken as indicative of the main purpose and underlying philosophy.

The best health store products help you

preserve and improve your health because they contain a very high content of the naturally occurring and nutritionally effective substances, including all the most important constituent elements in nature. To achieve this there has to be careful selection of the raw materials to ensure that they are of the best nutritional quality. These are then treated, manufactured and stored in ways designed to cause little or no harm to these vital factors.

Health foods do not contain raw materials obtained by means of chemical actions that have a fundamental effect on the nature of the material in question, except when their use is necessary for reasons beyond the control of the manufacturer. Artificial additives are avoided even if legally permissible, although it must be emphasized that our polluted environment is full of residues over which we now have no control.

Just as some natural foods are harmful, no doubt some artificial additives are harmless. However, humanity has spent millions of years learning to avoid the harmful foods in the same way that it has learned to discern healing plants and beneficial foods. The health store is, therefore, a place where you can minimize your risk and maximize your nutritional status.

The corner stone of the health food store is the splendid array of different sorts of flours and exciting products both ready to make and prepare, produced from stone-ground wholewheat flour. Stone mills were in use more than 25000 years ago. Man produced flour for his bread in a split second and the heavy stones crushed and ground the wheat grain. He thrived, built civilizations and grew strong on this healthy, complete food. In the 1870s all this changed because of the invention of rollermilling. In this process the grain is rolled for a comparatively long time on cylinders with indentations of various sizes. Heat is created, the various parts of the grain separated and taken off, some as white flour, some as the fibrous bran, some as wheat germ. The white flour is used to make bread – the rest often goes for cattle food. It is from this time that many of the diseases of western civilization began to afflict us. Man needed fibre to keep him regular and the other components discarded from the flour included vital sources of trace minerals such as chromium, the B-vitamins and Vitamin E.

Although Dr Allinson and other Victorian pioneers warned against the nutritional losses from white flour, it was not until the last few years that three distinguished medical scientists, the surgeon Mr Neil Painter, Dr Denis Burkitt and Surgeon Captain Cleave, showed scientifically that nutritionists who said white bread was as good as stone-ground wholewheat were hopelessly wrong. Dangerous diseases such as diverticulitis, appendicitis and perhaps even growths of the colon were found to be associated with too little roughage in the diet. Roughage is found in the bran part of wheat in a form that is ideal.

The health store not only has the best selection of wholewheat flour together with many products made from this material, but also supplies breakfast foods, snacks and other natural foods with an especially high bran content. One problem of not shopping at a health store is that the majority of bakers selling so-called wholemeal bread provide a product containing only a proportion of the whole grain. In a Manchester survey only seven out of thirty-two wholemeal loaves contained the genuine 100 per cent flour. Your safeguard is always to obtain your bread from a health store.

It is not just wholewheat that is important. Especially nutritious and delicious is unpolished rice. The eastern disease called beri beri is a deficiency condition caused by polishing the rice and so removing Vitamin B1 (thiamin). Unpolished rice contains 10 per cent more protein, 85 per cent more essential fats and 70 per cent more minerals than the polished variety. The same general concept is true of many other cereals and pulses that are part of the health store's contribution to good, healthy eating.

There is a definite relationship between how saturated or hard the fat is and the effect on cholesterol in the bloodstream. Health stores pioneered the provision of light, delicate and nutritious unsaturated oils such as sunflower, safflower, soya and corn oils. Generally speaking animal fats are saturated, as in lard; but plant oils are usually different chemically and contain three polyunsaturated fatty acids in significant quantities. These are called linoleic, linolenic and arachidonic. They are essential for growth and strong cells. Because a food containing linoleic acid provides the body with materials to manufacture the other two, but not the reverse way round, a healthy diet needs to contain linoleic acid.

Cholesterol is a fat found in animal tissues. One egg contains about 275 mg, 4 oz. of meat about 100 mg, and a pint of milk, 50 mg. Those at risk from heart attacks are well advised to eat low cholesterol foods as this may minimize the risk of cholesterol being deposited on the walls of the blood vessels.

The theory has been advanced that if you eat a balanced diet you need no food supplements. With a perfectly balanced diet that is true, but how difficult it is today to eat the sort of food which our bodies really need. So many of us eat too much sugar and salt, have far too much fat, and eat many refined and flavour-processed foods. We are entertained with white bread and cakes and rarely enjoy the delicious fresh foods that the speed of life gives us all too little time to buy and prepare. The health store provides raw sugar which helps you to cut down your sugar intake; delicious sea salt which, with its full flavour, helps limit salt intake; vegetable oils and margarines of rich and unsaturated fats; and plenty of 100 per cent wholemeal bread.

The fat-soluble vitamins which are A, D and E can be stored in the body, so their intake can vary without any harmful effects. Vitamin A is needed for vision, growth and the mucous membranes, and is often called the anti-pollution vitamin. A great excess is not good for you; somewhere between 5000 and 40000 international units a day would be a useful supplementary dose.

Girls who work under fluorescent lights and suffer as a result from spotty skins, dandruff, acne, sinus diseases, eye weaknesses – all often benefit from Vitamin A treatment, which does not conflict with any other remedies. It is also worth trying 25000 international units a day for three days before and during a very sunny holiday, as this is a marvellous protection against sunburn.

Vitamin D is actually produced by the action of sunlight on the skin. Immigrant children in Liverpool and Glasgow are now showing frequent signs of deficiency. Vitamin D is essential to the body's use of phosphorus and calcium, vital for growing bones.

Vitamin E is mysterious and very interesting. Scientists are mixed in their views regarding it, but outstanding medical practitioners such as Dr Shute of Ontario have had excellent chemical results when using Vitamin E for aiding heart patients. He gives a minimum of 300 mg per day. Vitamin E seems to be a remarkable oxygen carrier. It is commonplace to observe the rejuvenating effect of 500 mg a day in those taking the vitamin for other purposes. Surgeons in Canada and South Africa use Vitamin E liquid (usually obtained by piercing a Vitamin E capsule) to aid postoperative wound healing. They report a remarkable absence of scarring and many health store customers use the same treatment for minor cuts, blemishes, and to protect themselves from inclement weather.

The water soluble vitamins disappear easily in cooking or in strong light. They are often thrown down the sink with the water used for preparing vegetables. The health philosophy is to prepare vegetables either raw or with slight cooking or steaming, and when there is water left over from the preparation to use it to make soup or sauce.

The B-vitamins help you to have bright eyes and a beautiful skin and ensure the steady release of energy into the organs. Deficiencies show in nerviness, lost vitality, poor skin and eyes lacking lustre. One of the best and simplest sources of B-vitamins is brewer's yeast. Another important B-vitamin is Vitamin B6, often found to be good for eczema. It frequently reduces the side-effects suffered by women who take the birth-control pill.

Vitamin C, which chemically speaking is ascorbic acid, is often found in its natural form in the health store so that all the bioflavonoids are there. Bioflavonoids have an effect on reducing the fragility of the blood capillaries and are an object of great medical interest and research. Vitamin C is essential for the healthy growth and repair of tissues and, as Dr Linus Pauling described, is very effective for preventing and controlling colds in doses of between three and five grammes a day.

Smokers need to remember that each cigarette takes about 30 mg of Vitamin C from their system, so it is important to avoid deficiency. May it be that some of the diseases that commonly afflict smokers are due to this drain on the Vitamin C resources and not just the actual effects of the cigarette itself? Stress, fatigue, infections, and injuries all require extra supplies of Vitamin C. In the natural forms available from the health store you are assured of the associated nutritional components.

There are also many minerals available at health stores.

It is a good general practice to take a natural multi-vitamin and mineral supplement each day to take care of the over-all nutritional requirements of the body. Then, should you feel that any additional supplementation is required, vary this as necessary.

Other interesting health store supplements include pollen and propolis. The bee (→**medicated bee venom therapy**) gives us so much more than honey (and health stores probably contain more varieties of honey than any other shops). Medical research has shown that these other bee-gathered substances have remarkable properties. Flower pollen is thought to help control the ageing processes in many people and also to produce an excellent effect on muscle tone. Many football teams use pollen regularly. Improved muscle tone in women is noticed in a firming of the breasts. With concentrated and reinforced pollen products many men who felt 'past it' have discovered a new lease of life. Women suffering painful periods or a difficult 'change' derive from pollen safe and effective relief.

Propolis is the resinous cement used to seal beehives. Country folk have known for hundreds of years its important anti-bacterial and, it turns out, anti-viral properties. A recent controlled clinical trial in Sarajevo by Professor Osmanagić showed that during an influenza epidemic those who had taken a course of propolis were in 95·5 per cent of cases immune from the disease whereas others caught the infection at a rate of 38·8 per cent. A mixture of propolis and Vitamin C is quite the best remedy for the common cold.

Arthritis too finds its relief in the health store. Cider apple vinegar, which taken at the rate of two teaspoonfuls in a tumbler of water during each meal is also wonderful for slimming, helps very many rheumatism and arthritis sufferers. There are other very interesting products for these conditions. One of the newest is The Devil's Claw, an African herb which has had many successful clinical trials in relieving arthritis. It is mistaken to suggest that arthritis can be cured because the bone changes which take place are usually irreversible, but great relief can be obtained with an improvement in the diet, good supplements and safe natural remedies. There have also been a lot of good reports from arthritics on the use of calcium pantothenate, which in doses of 600 mg per day is often very useful.

The remedial side of the health store accounts for almost a fifth of the space. Nowadays all remedies which claim to help you are given licences by the Department of Health and Social Security and are tested for safety, quality and efficacy. It is found that natural remedies do not always bring the rapid and spectacular cures that modern drugs lead one to expect. Their effect is on the whole person. Gentle and safe, they help to return our organism towards normality. Serious conditions should not be the subject for self-diagnosis and self-treatment. If symptoms persist longer than you would expect, see a qualified practitioner without delay.

Another effective remedial concept is based on homoeopathic (→homoeopathy) principles in that the minerals used are reduced in a complex process until they are at a concentration of only one part in a million. Biochemic tissue salts were discovered by a German, Dr Schuessler, who found that the twelve essential tissue salts could often assist the body to overcome many common illnesses. They are completely safe and do not conflict with other treatments.

Old remedies for gastric ulcers and other disturbances include slippery elm food, which enables many with weak digestion to eat normally again.

The health store is perhaps the only place where a wide range of alternative and safe remedies can be found, many of them extending back in history to the earliest recorded times. Yet this has not prevented the introduction of many interesting recent discoveries when nature's medicines have been shown to be safely effective.

Have you ever read the label listing ingredients on a box of commercial ice-cream? It looks rather like a laboratory catalogue! Many health stores, on the other hand, have ice-creams made entirely from natural materials, as are the cheeses, yoghourts and margarines.

The World Health Organization recommended many years ago that babies should not have artificial colours and flavours in their foods as these could appeal only to the parents, yet a visit to the chemist will show that most rose-hip and blackcurrant syrups are artificially coloured. The health store provides alternatives that do not contain these unnecessary hazards to the delicate kidneys of the infant. Jams too are another potent source of artificial ingredients when commercially produced, but the health store jam is made with raw sugar, without artificial colouring or flavouring. The taste is vastly improved as a result of using only traditional materials.

→Cosmetics should beautify the spirit in the same way that they make the exterior more attractive. There has been a great outcry against the exploitation of animals like whales, to produce raw materials for women to plaster over their faces. In health stores you can find a wide range of cosmetics prepared only from vegetable materials which are effective and attractive. They are cheaper than the usual commercial cosmetics and include such unusual specialities as a soothing after-shave lotion for men. Women's skin-care products contain extracts of such interesting plants as cucumbers, avocado pears, and rosemary. Many of the allergic problems associated with cosmetics are avoided when vegetable-based ingredients are tried.

So the health store is comprehensive in the wide range of stock it carries. Many stores include products specially made for diabetics, slimmers and those on salt-reduced diets. A health store contains much more than just health foods. The staff try to serve the community in an area where specialized nutritional and medical requirements are given little heed by big business, which is concerned only with the mass market and influencing the consumer to acquire new synthetic tastes. The staff need to be people who are concerned for the needs of the customer, always ready to give advice based on much experience. Staff frequently have training courses and examinations in health skills which are organized under the auspices of the National Association of Health Stores in conjunction with the Distributive Industries Training Board. They keep up to date with the latest discoveries in a dynamic, ever changing field.

Although the staff are eager to welcome the new convert to health food, many people keep putting off the moment when they will walk through the door. They want to go inside, but it is another world and they do not wish to make fools of themselves. A simple way to overcome that problem is to go in and buy a book from the book and magazine stalls that are to be found in most health stores. These publications cater for those interested in natural cooking, organic gardening, special diets and natural beauty, and will help the reader to find out about the increasing range stocked by health food shops. The cookery books will tell you what ingredients to buy and how best to use them.

Over a third of new health shop customers buy stone-ground wholewheat bread and flour. Next most popular is the entire range of wholefood breakfast cereals, particularly such traditional items as Prewett's muesli, while the choice of more than forty different varieties of pure honey attracts many others. Other favourites on the new health food shopper's list are Healthcraft's vitamin and mineral products, together with the wide range of herbal remedies which offer a safe alternative to drug-based products.

Try shopping for a day's menu from your health store – you will find plenty to tempt you when you go inside, but here is a good specimen menu for a healthy day's nutrition.

Breakfast

Wholegrain cereal such as muesli (use raw sugar if required).
Fresh fruit.
100 per cent wholewheat bread either with a free-range poached egg or honey or yeast-spread.
Herbal tea or Ceylon low-caffeine tea.

Lunch

Salad of vegetables with wholewheat bread, cottage or other natural cheese. Health store yoghourt free from artificial colours and flavours. Fruit juice.

Dinner

Textured vegetable protein made up with a tomato sauce or to extend minced meat served with wholemeal spaghetti topped with grated cheese flavoured with herbs such as oregano and basil.
Raw salad. Chocolate dessert made with Irish moss-based mould mixture.
Fresh fruit or cheese and biscuits.
Fruit juice.

So satisfying are health food meals that families frequently find a cost saving as well as a health improvement. My wish is that this description of the health store's place in alternative medicine has shown you that this is where you will find a wide range of vitally beneficial products, and where you will be tended by a dedicated staff who are looking forward to welcoming you.

Maurice Hanssen

HEBRAIC NAME CHANGING

Jewish people do not believe in magic but there is a kind of mystical symbolism about their name-changing ritual. The basic principle is asking God to grant a new lease of life to a dying person. The matter is approached as if the sick one was now a newly-born baby about to be given a name for the first time and thus a fresh start.

The old name is put aside and a new name is given in the hope that what was decreed in heaven for the old name (person) will no longer apply and that a new chapter can now be written, a future allowed to take place for one whose present life seems to be ending. The newly chosen name generally includes a reference to life or hope for life and the blessing of divine intervention, such as Chaim (Hebrew word for life), Raphael (God heals), Yechiel (God will make live) or Daniel (God has judged). The new naming ceremony is a simple service carried out in a synagogue with family and friends of the dying person following the text of a special prayer read by a rabbi. It is not a very common practice in Judaism but it has been going on for hundreds of years and is fully accepted in orthodox Judaism as a necessary act in the religion, offering hope of a new life to mortally ill people of all ages.

I went through that experience. When I was eighteen months old I lay seriously ill in a London hospital. The doctors told my mother I was dying from double-pneumonia. Only a miracle could save me. My mother and a few close relations hurried to a small synagogue in the East End where we lived, in a narrow turning off Petticoat Lane. There my old first name of Joseph was put aside and I was given a new name, the one I now use. Soon after I recovered completely.

Adam Joseph

CONTRIBUTORS, p. 221

HERBALISM

Herbalism uses medicines obtained solely from plants in treating disorders of the body. These remedies were given by the creator for this purpose. Scripture is clear as to their origin, Genesis, chapter 4 verses 11 and 12; their acceptance, Psalm 104, verse 14; and their use, Exodus, chapter 30 verses 23 and 34, and Romans, chapter 14 verse 2, leading us to the time when God's mind will be sovereign on Earth when these remedies will be used to the exclusion of all others, Revelation, chapter 22 verse 2.

Here it would be expedient to note the parallel with the healing provided for the soul of man, for all true healing must deal with the whole man and not an isolated part of him. Scripture again is explicit. In Old Testament times a sacrifice had to be made before disease (sin) of the soul could be removed, Leviticus, chapter 5.

In Isaiah, chapter 1 verses 4 and 6 this soul condition is likened to physical disease and in Romans, chapter 3 the divine remedy is given – the sacrifice of God's Son and its acceptance by those who would be cleansed. It will be noticed that one vital fact is found in both these spheres of healing – the fact of death before life or healing can be obtained.

This great principle is the basis of the herbal practice and separates it entirely from the chemical system so widespread today. In the living plant is found not only that part which is able to cure disease but also trace elements, minerals and other compounds which are totally lacking in the chemical drug produced in the laboratory. Certain herbals are used as food today as they have been in the past. When the chemist or doctor uses herbal extracts in prescriptions they are either mixed with a chemical product, or the active principle is extracted from the plant and used in isolation from the other parts regarded as having no value. In either case the herbalist claims that such treatment is not as effective as when the complete plant is used. This is borne out when the results of chemical medicine are compared with that of herbal practice.

It is interesting to note that *Potter's Cyclopedia of Botanical Drugs*, the standard pharmacopoeia of the herbalist for many years, lists some thirty-seven herbs named and used in Bible history.

If the origin of this great scheme of healing and its early use is found in the Bible its continuance and growth may be traced in secular writings. As far back as 2200 B.C. there was in existence the Sumerian herbal, and at the same period a papyrus of Egypt lists 2000 herbal doctors practising in that land. Among the Greeks, Asculapius is recorded as the first to make medicine an exclusive study and practice. His sons are mentioned in Homer's *Iliad* for their healing skill. These were followed by Hippocrates, born 460 B.C. Other herbalists were Theophrastos who wrote about 314 B.C. and is the earliest known European botanical writer. His works were printed in 1483 and translated into several languages. Pliny (A.D. 23–79) and Dioscorides (A.D. 78) both produced works on natural history and herbal medicines much valued by practitioners even today. They lived in Italy and Asia Minor respectively. The next great herbalist was Galen who lived from A.D. 131 to 200 and was the imperial physician in Rome at the invitation of the emperor. He wrote many distinguished medical books which were valued right down to the Middle Ages.

All these men used medicines derived from the plant kingdom and were in that sense the forerunners of the genuine herbalist today. Paracelsus, the Swiss physician who practised in the sixteenth century, used some herbs but also introduced such things as excreta of various kinds into medicine. He did much to popularize the Doctrine of Signatures which teaches that the appearance of a plant indicates its usage, i.e. plants with yellow flowers or roots being good for jaundice, quaking poplar for palsy and so on. This teaching was developed by Culpepper in England who also applied →**astrological** teachings to his practice. Paracelsus also introduced mercury and other mineral drugs into medical practice, burned the works of Galen, declared he had discovered the elixir of life and died at forty-eight. From this time the use of mineral, chemical drugs came into more general use until it finally reached the prominence seen

today. In England herbs were used as medicines from earliest times. Among more recent herbalists were John Gerard (1545–1611) who published *The Herball or General Historie of Plants* with 1630 large pages, and John Parkinson (1567–1629) who was the king's herbalist and a director of the Royal Gardens at Hampton Court. Nicholas Culpepper studied at Cambridge and practised at Spitalfield, dying in 1654 leaving *The Complete Herbal*, which he compiled, to posterity.

In spite of the increasing use of chemical drugs in England herbalism was the main system of healing until the nineteenth and twentieth centuries. From this time it gradually declined in popularity as the more 'wonderful' treatments were introduced, although even over this period there were always herbalists in practice and people who preferred this treatment. Over the past twenty years we have seen the backlash of chemical drug treatment with its awful side-effects from thalidomide, cortisone, gold and certain antibiotics to mention just a few. This, together with a growing awareness of the true value of the earlier system, is resulting in more people returning to the herbal treatments which are so effective without any side-effects.

In England herbal medicine was used by the ordinary housewife and countryman as part of their daily lives. In early times the priests and the druids practised the healing art, the latter venerating mistletoe which is used today in certain cancer and other treatments. There were men who accumulated knowledge and skill, eventually setting up in practice as herbalists. Their knowledge was passed down from father to son and thus the craft maintained. During the reign of Henry VIII an Act of Parliament was passed to protect the herbalist from the persecution of the chemical doctors and surgeons. This Act continued until the 1968 Medicines Act which gave the medical herbalist an official recognition unknown for centuries.

An official training school was started in 1864 known as the National Association of Medical Herbalists. This, together with the Faculty of Herbal Medicine founded in the

1940s, comprise the two main training centres for herbalists today. Over the years the standards have been raised and at the present time there are around 12000 practising herbalists trained with one or other of these two schools. There are probably other unqualified practitioners who have taken no formal training. Even a qualification or diploma only indicates that the person has attained a certain standard by training and examination. It is no indication of the ability in actual healing practice. I have come into contact with qualified men whose care I would not be at all confident about, not because the training was at fault but simply because the individual himself was not capable, by reason of his outlook or inability to empathize, of being a good practitioner. This raises a vitally important question for those who would be treated with herbal remedies: 'How can I find a competent herbal practitioner from whom I shall gain the full benefit from these remedies?'

The facilities offered are no real guide. A carpeted waiting-room with receptionist and a surgery with every modern instrument creates a good impression but, as an author in orthodox medical circles has written, 'The only qualification required for Harley Street is the ability to pay the rent required.' On the contrary, one of the most gifted herbalists in recent years, the late F. C. Carr of Shipham, would hold surgery in church halls throughout the Midlands and the west of England to which he travelled, enabling hundreds to take treatment they could not otherwise have obtained. In such conditions the very minimum of instruments were used. Frank Roberts, another well-known herbalist, never had an examination-couch in his surgery, certainly not in the early years. Both these men were able to point to patients treated and cured of conditions ranging from cancer, through gastric ulcers to simple bronchitis.

Let it not be thought that the writer is deriding either formal training or comfortable, well-equipped surgeries. With or without these it is the practitioner himself through whom healing is given – the value of the remedies is without doubt. The patient who comes for treatment sometimes for a long-standing condition is only concerned with obtaining relief from that condition.

What should a prospective patient look for when choosing a herbalist? Firstly, cleanliness. If hygiene is not observed in the area where the public have access it is hardly likely to be in the dispensary. This test should also be applied to the practitioner. Secondly, the herbalist must be consistent. Little credence can be given to advice that a patient must not smoke if the one giving it smells of tobacco. The same applies to a patient told to have his children vaccinated, a practice contrary to herbal principles. Inconsistency is a sign of instability wherever it is found. Whilst a warm personality is assuring, one should not be put off by abruptness or impatience at earlier treatment. Likewise advice must sometimes be given which cuts right across the patient's way of life. Habits of a life-time may have to be altered; and personal matters may need to be discussed.

The herbalist has at his disposal a complete range of proved remedies and it is gratifying to see orthodox medicine now accepting certain principles and treatments which have been used by the herbalist for centuries. A professor at Bath has been given a grant for research into herbal medicines to seek a cancer cure. The time and money could have been better used had he approached an established herbal practitioner for details of *his* treatments.

A vital requirement in any healer is absolute honesty. No benefit is gained by hiding from a patient the true nature of his or her disorder. When a case is fully discussed with the patient concerned, together with the treatment and the reason for this, the full cooperation of the patient is obtained. The patient himself becomes involved in his treatment which becomes more effective as a result.

When a satisfactory course of treatment has been found it is essential that the patient continues with the same practitioner as far as possible. No lasting benefit can be gained from chopping and changing as a new course of treatment has to be started and a fresh relationship built up. Individuals as well as disorders respond in different ways to treatment. Some show a very quick response whilst others require treatment over a period of many months for full relief. The patient should not lose hope. Some disorders appear to be worse before improving and symptoms sometimes alter during the course of the treatment. At such times the value of confidence in, and on the part of, the practitioner can be appreciated.

The method of diagnosis and consultation used varies between practitioners. One will use a wide range of instruments whilst another very few, the most usual being the stethoscope and a gauge for the blood pressure. Certain tests are also sometimes performed, the most common one being the urine test.

Whilst these methods may vary, certain factors are common in all cases. The patient is always given time to express him or herself, although a competent herbalist can learn a tremendous amount about a patient even before the patient starts to talk. Sometimes facts are apparent of which the patient does not speak until several visits later. Questions will be asked and even if the connection is not obvious to the patient the need for frankness in answering is very real.

What can herbalism cure? Two things it cannot do. No medicine can prolong a life beyond its allotted span. Secondly, herbal medicine cannot take the place of surgery. Whilst the herbalist contends that much surgery is unnecessary or even harmful, there are cases where operative measures must be taken.

Leaving emergencies aside, the herbalist has remedies to enable almost every disorder of the body to be treated. Results are in some cases quite dramatic. Tumours diagnosed as incurable cancers have disappeared. Operations for gall-stones and duodenal ulcers have been avoided and at least one leg has been saved from amputation to the writer's knowledge. Limbs crippled by arthritis, leg ulcers, nervous troubles, bronchitis, urinary difficulties and skin rashes are just a few disorders which have responded very successfully to herbal medication. In England it is illegal for *any* medical practitioner to claim ability to *cure* cancer. At the same time this disorder can be *treated* legally and results have been encouraging.

Any person troubled regarding health matters would be well advised to consult a medical herbalist for a full investigation of his or her problems with a view to obtaining safe, effective treatment free from the side-effects associated with chemical drug usage.

E. F. Didcott

HERBS WITH MEDICINAL VALUE

Aconite *Aconitum napellus* (Monkshead). POISONOUS perennial. Tall-stemmed; glossy leaves, dark green on top, light green underneath. Flowers like monk's hood, dark blue or purple, in June. Spindle-shaped roots.

Ointments from root relieves neuralgic and rheumatic pains. Tincture reduces fevers.

Agrimony, hemp *Eupatorium cannabinum* (Boneset). Wild perennial. Round reddish hairy stems 2–5 ft (60–150 cm). Leaves lance-shaped, hairy, covered with resinous dots. Dull purple flower heads late summer to autumn.

Tonic tea from leaves for rheumatism, colds. Cleanses wounds.

Alexanders *Smyrnum clusatrum* (Black lovage). Biennial 3–4 ft (90–120 cm). Large ternate leaves, thick membraneous stalks. Umbels of yellowish-green flowers. Ripe fruits turn black.

Whole herb diuretic, carminative.

Allspice *Pimenta officinalis* (Pimento). Tall evergreen tree of myrtle family. Berries with kidney-shaped seeds dried for flavouring spice.

Also contains volatile oil added to medicines for upset stomach, headache, toothache.

Angelica *Angelica archangelica*. Tall biennial, large leaves, strong hollow stems. Flower heads greenish-white umbels.

Tisane reduces fevers. Roots and stems useful for cooking with sour fruit to remove tartness.

Anise *Pimpinella anisum* (Aniseed). Dainty annual 18 in. (45 cm) high; feathery light green serrated leaflets, umbels creamy-white flowers. Minute fruits with seed.

Seed tea with honey relieves flatulence, asthma, bronchial catarrh. Chewing seeds helps sleep.

Arnica *Arnica montana*. POISONOUS perennial. Stem – 1 ft (30 cm) – rises from flat rosette of leaves. Flowers of yellow florets produce brown fruits.

Tincture for external use on sprains and bruises. A teaspoon in bath water and twenty-minute soak helps relax stiff muscles.

Asafoetida *Ferula asafoetida*. Tall evil-smelling perennial found wild in western Asia. Thick roots, stout stems with long leaves and umbels of greeny-yellow flowers.

Powdered root pills used for croup or colic in children.

Basil *Ocimum basilicum*. Annual about 3 ft (90 cm) high. Square stems. Flowers creamy white in whorls of leaf axils. Largish, pale green leaves with grey-green undersides dotted with oil cells. Available in frost-free months.

Aromatic leaves used in food, stimulate appetite and digestive system.

Bay *Lauris nobilis*. Bushy, sweet tree. Shiny dark green leathery leaves, pale yellowish-green beneath. Small greeny-yellow flowers followed by dark purple berries.

Leaves an important spicing agent, stimulate appetite. A pain reliever.

Bearberry *Arctostaphylos uva-ursi*. Medium-sized wild perennial shrub. Woody stems, fibrous root. Trailing clusters small white flowers with red lip May–June, followed by glossy dark green leaves, light undersides. Bright red currant-sized berries.

Leaves make infusions for urinary disorders.

Belladonna *Atropa belladonna* (Deadly nightshade). POISONOUS trailing plant with purple stem. Bell-shaped flowers June–July, followed by shiny black berries.

Alkaloid drug 'atropine' from root used in medicine as narcotic and for dilating pupil of eye.

Bergamot, red *Monarda didyma* (Bee balm). Orange-scented perennial, 18–35 in. (45–90 cm) high. Ovate lanceolated serrated leaves. Red flowers in whorls on square stem June–September.

Relaxing flower tisane, called Oswego tea, to induce sleep.

Betony, wood *Betonica officinalis*. Strong-scented wild perennial. Small crimson flowers June–August in axils of top pair of leaves, forming spike. Stemmed, toothed leaves coarse and hairy.

Healing astringent tea for catarrhal conditions, digestion, rheumatism. In ointment for cuts, sores, ulcers.

Bilberry *Vaccinium myrtillus* (Blueberry). Small deciduous shrub, ovate pointed leaves, rosy when young turning green then red. Pink flowers in May. Blue-black grey-bloomed fruits ripen July–August.

Tisane from leaves taken regularly helpful for diabetics. In syrup for urinary complaints and dysentery.

Blessed thistle *Carduus benedictus*. Medium-sized annual, large single drooping flower heads with purple florets. Dark green prickly leaves have white veins.

Infusion in mild doses, tonic and diaphoretic. Also for female complaints.

Bryony, white *Bryonia dioica*. POISONOUS wild perennial. Tuberous rootstock, climbing stems, greenish flowers in May. Red or orange berries.

Root used in homoeopathic preparation for severe coughs. Tincture effective for cure and prevention of chilblains.

Buckbean *Menyanthes trifoliata* (Marsh trefoil). Perennial water plant. Procumbent stem sheathed in long tripartite leaves. Thick spikes white flowers with red stamens May–July.

Tonic infusion for rheumatism, liver debility, skin diseases. Reduces glandular swellings.

Calamint *Calamintha officinalis* (Mountain balm). A wild mint. Hairy perennial with purple flowers, toothed broadly ovate leaves.

Makes expectorant, diaphoretic tea. Poultice from leaves for rheumatic pains and bruises.

Calamus *Acorus calamus* (Sweet flag). Reedlike waterside plant. Long sword-shaped leaves. Tall stems from creeping rootstock end in yellowish-green spikes. Only flowers in water.

Rhizomes used for stimulant and tonic. Oil essence for inhalations.

Capsicum *Capsicum annum* (Chilli pepper). Annual 1–3 ft (30–90 cm) high with white flowers. Fruits from $\frac{1}{2}$ to 11 in. ($1\frac{1}{2}$–27 cm) long, varying in colour and pungency. Paprika, cayenne, red pepper ground from pungent varieties.

For treating dropsy, diarrhoea, toothache, relaxed throat, gout. Makes strong liniment.

Caraway *Carum carvi*. Biennial $1\frac{1}{2}$–2 ft (45–60 cm) high, feathery foliage, smooth furrowed stems, umbels white flowers June–July. Seeds crescent-shaped, dark brown with paler ridges.

Seed oil contains 'carvene', a stimulant and carminative; useful for dyspepsia, nervous complaints. Tisane soothes intestinal upsets.

Cardamom *Elletaria cardamomum*. Ginger family. Tropical perennial. Tall leafy stem, small racemes yellow flowers with violet lip April–May. Greeny-grey fruit capsule with three or four brown seeds.

Infusion of seeds settles stomach, dispels flatulence.

Centaury *Centaurium umbellatum*. Low-growing annual. Pairs of stalkless oval leaves diminishing in size up square stem. Flat crown of pink star-shaped flowers which open in morning light.

Makes aromatic tonic infusion, a stomachic and blood cleanser. Acts on liver and kidneys.

Chamomile *Matricaria chamomilla* (True or wild chamomile). Small low-growing annual. Yellow and white daisy-like flowers May–September. Hollow green receptacle at base of flower contains distinctive blue healing oil.

Dried flower tisane for abdominal pains, cystitis, rheumatism, dilated veins; mouth rinse for sore gums, toothache; inhalations for head colds, catarrh; compresses for skin disorders, boils, eczema; conjunctivitis, haemorrhoids, earache and cramp.

Chervil *Anthriscus cerifolium*. Sweet-scented annual. Pale green lacy leaves, white flower umbels in June.

In food has stimulating effect on whole metabolism. Fresh herb poultice for painful joints.

Chickweed *Stellaria media*. Low, trailing annual. Egg-shaped hairy leaves, small white flowers.

Fresh bruised leaves make poultice for healing ulcers, or soothing ointment for itchy skin, chilblains. Infusion taken for kidney disorders.

Chicory *Cichorium intybus*. 3 ft (90 cm) high perennial with tap root. Hairy stems, deeply toothed lance-shaped leaves; clusters pure blue flowers in upper leaf axils.

Juice from rind or fresh root makes decoction helpful for jaundice, gout, rheumatic conditions.

Cinnamon *Cinnamomum zeylanicum*. Dried inner bark of tall bushy evergreen tree grown in orient. Long deeply veined leaves; small yellow flowers; berries dark purple.

Powder or oil a strong stimulant, astringent and carminative, good for glandular systems, upset stomach, diarrhoea, colds and sore throats.

Clary *Salvia sclarea* (Clear-eye). Aromatic biennial 15–24 in. (37–60 cm) high. Whorls of variegated flowers light purple and yellowish-white, lipped with pale blue or white. Pairs of stalkless sage-like leaves.

Decoction or infusion for eye complaints. Taken internally for digestive and kidney disorders.

Cloves *Eugenia aromatica.* Tall, tropical evergreen tree with brilliant red flowers. Aromatic flower buds called 'cloves'.

Clove oil is germicide, antiseptic and painkiller; good for toothache. In powder form or infusion for nausea, digestive upsets.

Coltsfoot *Tussilago farfara.* Creeping perennial. Yellow flowers March–May. Leathery leaves with downy undersides. Flowers and leaves never seen together.

Tisane helps tiresome coughs, bronchitis, asthma. Fresh leaves in poultice for healing dilated veins, unsightly thread veins.

Comfrey *Symphytum officinale.* Stout prickly perennial 2–3 ft (60–90 cm) high. Long hairy ovate leaves; angular hollow stem. Drooping clusters bell-shaped blue, purple, pink or cream flowers. Fibrous black root exudes milky fluid.

Contains active substance 'alantoin'. Makes tisanes, decoctions, ointments, poultices for wounds, broken bones, bronchial complaints, internal bleeding, ulcers.

Coriander *Coriandrum sativum.* Annual 1–3 ft (30–90 cm) high. Umbels pinky-white flowers July. Bright green feathery leaves. Ripe seeds small, round, ridged, sweetly aromatic.

Carminative seed tea for digestion.

Costmary *Chrysanthemum balsamita.* Perennial 2–3 ft (60–90 cm) high. Stem rises from creeping rootstock. Long slender leaves; flowers white petals, yellow centres, August, open only in full sunlight.

Powdered leaves good for dysentery, weight loss. Makes tonic tea.

Couchgrass *Agropyrum repens.* Tall, spreading grass-like weed with flat rough leaves and creeping roots.

Root used medicinally as blood cleanser, for bladder and kidney diseases and rheumatism.

Dandelion *Taraxacum officinale.* Spiky, toothed leaves; bright golden-yellow flower heads turning to fluffy down.

Leaves and root contain active substances. Makes fortifying tonic for blood disorders, skin troubles. .

Dill *Peucedanum* (or *Anethum*) *graveolens.* Annual up to 2½ ft (75 cm). Feathery leaves on stem with pale stripes, speckled blue. Yellow flower umbels June–end August.

Seeds infused in water good for indigestion, sleeplessness, stimulating milk in nursing mothers.

Elder *Sambucus nigra.* Hedgerow tree or bush 9–30 ft (3–10 m). Clusters creamy flowers followed by greenish berries ripening to black.

Vitamin-B-rich berries helpful for oedema, neuralgia. Makes good tonic tea suitable for diabetics. Flower/berry infusion a diuretic, induces perspiration. Or held in mouth relieves toothache.

Elder, ground *See* Ground elder.

Elecampane *Inula helenium.* Handsome wild perennial, downy in appearance; big fleshy root. Erect stem 4–5 ft (120–150 cm) high rises from radical rosette of enormous leaves. Bears yellow sunflower-like blooms, June–August.

Root used in tonics, antacid medicines.

Eyebright *Euphrasia officinale.* Wild hardy annual. Wiry erect branched stems; jagged leaves; tiny white or lilac flowers all summer.

Fresh juice, or infusion of herb, makes lotion for infected eyes.

Fennel *Foeniculum vulgare.* Perennial. Bright green feathery leaves; umbels flat yellow flowers July–August.

Good digestive spice. Infusion for asthmatic coughs; and soothing eye lotion. Makes infant gripe water.

Fenugreek *Trigonella foenum graecum.* Leguminous annual 2 ft (60 cm) high. Three-leaflet leaves; scented creamy flowers June–August. Sickle-shaped seed pods.

Seed tea old remedy for digestive ailments, fever. Soaked seeds make paste applied to abscesses, boils, corns. Today, valued as nourishing food in Third World. Also in birth-control experiments for its content of 'diosgenin'.

Flax *Linum usitatissimum* (Linseed). Brilliant

blue-flowered, spindly annual. Harvested August.

Oil used in medicines for constipation, sore throats, tonsillitis. Externally in poultices for reducing swellings.

Foxglove *Digitalis purpures.* POISONOUS biennial. Tall spikes of bell-shaped purple, crimson or white flowers. Hairy leaves.

Digitalis drug manufactured from flowers, used mainly in treatment of heart disease.

Garlic *Allium sativum.* Long flat grass-like leaves. Globular whitish flowers on tall stalk. Produces bulb consisting of several bulblets or 'cloves'.

Infused in milk or water for reducing blood pressure, relieving headaches, indigestion, intestinal infections, gall bladder and liver complaints, chronic bronchitis, faintness.

Gentian *Gentiana lutea.* Wild mountain variety with bright yellow flowers, large oval leaves. Root often up to 3 ft (90 cm) long.

Root containing bitter principle used for dispersing blood clots, reducing fevers. Fortifying stimulant against general weakness, nervous debility.

Ginger *Zingiber officinale.* Tall reed-like plant grown in tropics for its root.

Has antiseptic properties, used in medicines for faulty digestion, colds and coughs.

Ground elder *Aegopodium podagraria.* Troublesome garden weed but has medicinal value. Hollow furrowed stem, large ovate sharp-toothed leaves; white umbrella-like flower-heads.

Tisane, combined with hot fomentation made from root applied to painful joints, an effective remedy.

Ground ivy *Nepeta glechoma.* Trailing evergreen ground plant with heart-shaped leaves shaded crimson or purple. Blue or purple flowers April onwards.

Tisane for coughs, kidney complaints. For women, to encourage menstruation, expels retained afterbirth. Mixed with other herbs in poultice for abscesses, boils, ulcers. Fresh juice sniffed relieves congestion and headaches.

Hawthorn *Crataegus oxyacantha* (May, Whitethorn). Tall shrubby deciduous tree. Masses of white or pink flowers in spring. Crimson berries called 'haws'.

Juice extracted from haws used as heart tonic.

Henbane *Hyoscyamus niger.* Acrid POISONOUS plant, annual and biennial. Sticky hairy stem; leaves grey-green, divided; flowers yellow with purple veins May–June.

Contains 'hyoscyamine', alkaloid drug with anti-spasmodic properties used for nervous complaints, whooping cough. An opium substitute in children's medicines.

Hops *Humulus lupulus.* Climbing perennial with small yellowish-green flowers (male) and cone-like catkins (female).

Tisane is diuretic, anodyne, sleep-inducing.

Horseradish *Cochlearia armoracia.* Tall dock-like leaves; big, white fleshy roots.

Pungent root has antibiotic, diuretic stimulant properties, good for poor appetite, liver function, circulation. External remedy for stings, bites, burns, chilblains.

Horsetail *Equisetum arvense.* Non-flowering fern-like plant. Spikey green shoots; hollow, jointed erect stems end in cone-shaped catkins.

Tea good for bronchial diseases. Silicic acid content enriches blood, helpful in anaemia, blood loss, kidney and bladder diseases. Externally, staunches bleeding.

Hyssop *Hyssopus officinalis.* Fragrant evergreen shrub up to 2 ft (60 cm). Square stem, spikes of bright blue flowers.

Tisane for throat and chest complaints, irregular blood pressure, nervous disorders. Lotion applied externally relieves muscular rheumatism, cuts and bruises; ear, eye, and throat infections; insect bites.

Iceland moss *Cetraria icelandica.* Low creeping lichen, brown or grey colour, ash-like texture. Only survives in pure air in barren or mountainous places.

Contains 'cetarin'. Makes bitter tea for pulmonary complaints. Good for intestinal inflammations, dysentery.

Ivy, ground *See* Ground ivy.

Juniper *Juniperus communis.* Evergreen shrub or small tree. Reddish stems, needle leaves. Small yellow flowers May–June. Black berries take three years to ripen.

Berries chewed, or drunk as infusion, have germicidal diuretic properties helpful for infections of stomach, urinary tract, prevention of kidney stones.

Lady's bedstraw *Galium verum.* Height 1–3 ft (30–90 cm). Whorls of six to eight thread-like leaves on wiry square stems. Pannicles small, bright, yellow flowers July–August.

Infusion good for gravel stones in urinary tract. Also as laxative. Decoction makes soothing footbath.

Lady's mantle *Achemilla vulgaris.* Small spreading plant 1 ft (30 cm) high. Whole plant green, covered in soft hairs. Large kidney-shaped leaves; clusters tiny, petalless flowers June–July.

Astringent, styptic properties for healing and drying up wounds. Tisane is 'woman's friend' – restores disturbed menstrual cycle, helpful in pregnancy. Also heart tonic and blood fortifier.

Lavender *Lavendula vera.* Bushy perennial with narrow grey-green leaves, spikes of bluish-purple flowers.

Leaves and flowers of this variety make tea to calm heart palpitations, nerves, giddiness, migraine; induce sleep. Cold compress applied to temples relieves headaches. Oil heals skin ulcers, sores.

Lemon balm *Melissa offinalis.* Perennial height 1–2 ft (30–60 cm). Branching square stems, pairs of heart-shaped, lemon-scented leaves. Flowers white or yellow June–October.

Melissa tea relaxes, helps insomnia. Good for reducing fevers; settling stomach after vomiting.

Lesser celandine *Ranunculus ficaria* (Pilewort). Spreading ground plant with glossy green heart-shaped leaves. Bright yellow star-like flowers.

Decoction or ointment for bathing painful piles or varicose veins, at same time taking doses of mild infusion.

Lime *Tilia vulgaris* (Linden). Tall smooth-barked tree. Heart-shaped leaves, hanging clusters of fragrant yellow flowers.

Makes steam inhalation or tisane for bronchial and nasal catarrh, heavy colds, cramps, anaemia; also lotion for mouth ulcers, burns. Powdered lime charcoal in milk or water eliminates poisons in digestive tract; followed by laxative an effective remedy for food poisoning, migraine. Absorbs toxins in and helps festering wounds.

Liquorice *Glycyrrhiza glabra.* Tall perennial grown for its root. Leaves divided into several pairs of leaflets. Racemes purple flowers.

Used in cough medicines for expectorant and demulcant properties. Also a gentle laxative. Juice relieves pain of stomach ulcers.

Lovage *Ligusticum scoticum.* Tall umbelliferous perennial. Large celery-like leaves; thick hollow stems; umbels of yellow flowers.

Infusion stimulates digestive organs. Cleansing effect on system, its antiseptic and deodorant properties good for bathing wounds.

Marigold *Calendula officinalis.* Small garden annual with many-petalled flowers bright orange, red, yellow. Pale green oval leaves.

Petals soaked in oil or in ointment helps heal old wounds or scars. Tisane good for stomach ulcers, disorders of digestive tract.

Marjoram *Origanum marjorana* (Sweet marjoram). Low-growing bushy annual. Woody stem, small grey-green leaves; knotted flowerheads pale mauve or white June–September.

Antiseptic tisane for colds, sore throats; improves circulation. Oil extract for sprains, bruises. Makes snuff to clear nasal passages.

Marsh mallow *Althea officinalis.* Perennial wild plant, thick fleshy root, erect stems 3–4 ft (90–120 cm). Velvety hairy leaves, clusters pink flowers in leaf axils August–September.

Tea from dried root good for chest complaints; cystitis and other bladder diseases; colitis, diarrhoea and vomiting. Makes poultice to relieve burns, boils, carbuncles, reduce inflammations.

Meadow sweet *Spiraea ulmaria.* Wild perennial 2–4 ft (60–120 cm). Square reddish stems, large serrated almond-scented leaves, white and downy underneath. Cymes fragrant creamy-white flowers June–August.

Diuretic tea for fevers, digestive troubles, especially diarrhoea in children.

Melilot *Melilotus officinalis.* Tall, branching annual. Smooth trifoliate oval leaves alternately on erect stems. Racemes sweet-scented yellow or white flowers with short honey-filled heels.

Leaves in poultice applied to inflammations, cuts and bruises. As expectorant tea to relieve bronchial catarrh, or a carminative for digestion.

Mints *Mentha* varieties. Perennials. Some smooth-leaved, others woolly texture, all have own distinctive scent, e.g. peppermint, spearmint, eau de cologne, pennyroyal and others.

Well-known digestive tea, anti-spasmodic, stomach settler. Spearmint infusion for skin application. Fresh leaves rubbed on aching joints will relieve pain. Infusion of pennyroyal (*Mentha pulegium*) relieves bronchial congestion, obstructed menstruation.

Mistletoe *Viscum album.* Parasitic plant, feeds on various host trees. Hanging bunches thick leathery leaves, fleshy white berries.

Infusion of chopped leaves and young twigs in cold water a remedy for nervous complaints. Also regulates blood pressure, menstrual cycle, stimulates sluggish digestion.

Motherwort *Leonurus cardiaca.* Perennial 2–3 ft (60–90 cm) high. Erect square stem; five-lobed palmate leaves with hairy undersides. Whorls of pink flowers in upper leaf axils.

Properties: anti-spasmodic, emmenagogue, nervine, tonic. Infusion effective for female disorders and weakness, quietens whole nervous system. Mild tonic in heart disease, convalescence.

Mugwort *Artemesia vulgaris.* Aromatic perennial up to 3 ft (90 cm). Dark greeny spiky leaves with white downy undersides on strong stalks tinged purple. Yellow or purple flower-heads in terminal pannicles July–September.

Mugwort tea for rheumatism, fevers, nervous disorders. Added to water makes good footbath.

Mustard *Brassica nigra* or *alba.* Bright-yellow-flowered annual. Black variety produce narrow pods with single row tiny seeds; white variety smaller, hairy pods with larger seeds.

Used for poultices to relieve lung congestion. A general irritant and stimulant helping to draw blood to surface.

Myrrh *Commiphora myrrha.* Shrub or small tree native to Arabia and N.E. Africa. Resinous bark, knotted branches with smaller right-angled branchlets, ending in sharp spire trifoliate, oval leaves.

Volatile oil and resinous gum a healing antiseptic, emmenagogue, astringent, stimulant, tonic and expectorant for wide variety of ailments. Makes mouthwash, tincture, emulsion, liniment.

Nasturtium *Trapaeolum majus* and *minus.* Creeping climbing annual, bright green umbrella-shaped leaves; brilliant red, orange or yellow flowers.

Seasoning substitute for salt and pepper. Whole plant anti-scorbutic, is antiseptic and tonic for blood, digestive organs, nervous depression, constipation. Crushed seeds in hot poultice for skin eruptions, abscesses.

Nettle, stinging *Urtica dioica.* Familiar prolific weed. Leaves and stems covered with stinging hairs. Small greenish flower catkins June–September.

Tisane improves function of gall bladder, liver, intestinal tract. Makes gargle for sore throats. Young, salty leaves useful in salt-free diets.

Nightshade, deadly *See* Belladonna.

Nutmeg *Myristica fragrans* (Mace). Tropical tree. Large apricot-like fruits. Ripe kernel, covered in bright red net of mace, contains one nutmeg seed.

A carminative spice, good for indigestion and flatulence. To arrest diarrhoea, half teaspoon grated nutmeg in dessertspoon rum.

Onion *Allium cepa.* Grows from single small bulb or 'set' producing one leafless stalk topped with cluster of small greenish flowers in second year.

Antiseptic, diuretic, expectorant, detoxicant, antispasmodic, anthalmintic. Stimulates appetite, circulation, heart, nerves, glands; cleanses the blood, improves memory and concentration. Externally, raw juice relieves painful joints, improves brittle nails, draws out insect stings.

Pansy *Viola tricolor* (Heartsease). Wild variety with white, purple and yellow flowers. Spoon-shaped crenate leaves.

Dried powdered leaves applied to wounds; infusion for lotions and ointment. Makes tisane for blood disorders, nervous heart, exhaustion or jaundice.

Parsley *Petroselinum crispum* and *sativum* (Curled and Hamburg). Biennials, the curled with crinkly, deeply divided leaves. Hamburg has plain leaves. Both develop thin white roots.

Leaf, seed and root rich in vitamins, active substances. Makes digestive tea. Relieves kidney and bladder complaints, rheumatism, eliminates body fluids.

Plantain *Plantago major* or *psyllium.* Common wild weed. Many pinky-purple flower spikes 4–10 in. (10–25 cm) grown from radial rosette of deeply ribbed ovate leaves.

Pulped leaves external application for haemorrhoids. Tisane diuretic. Psyllium seeds a gentle laxative.

Purslane *Portulacca oleraca.* Low, spreading annual. Fleshy ovate leaves, yellow flowers on erect stems July.

Leaves make tonic tisane for blood disorders.

Rosehip *Rosa canina* (Wild dog rose). Tall prickly bush, large pink or white summer flowers succeeded by red hips containing hairy fruits.

Hips contain much Vitamin C. Makes syrup for heart tonic, dysentery, female disorders. Rosehip tea an effective diuretic.

Rosemary *Rosmarinus officinalis.* Fragrant shrub up to 5 ft (150 cm). Coniferous needles, small pale blue flowers.

Makes infusion for heart and circulation. Or tonic skin conditioner.

Rue *Ruta graveolens.* Shrubby evergreen, smooth branched stem. Bipinnate blue-green leaves with oil glands. Umbels tiny yellow flowers all summer.

Fresh or dried herb infusion or oil. Relieves flatulence, menstrual problems, croup and colic in children.

Sage *Salvia officinalis.* Perennial shrub up to 2 ft (60 cm). Hairy grey-green oblong leaves with pebbly texture. Violet-blue flowers June–July.

Sage tea as nerve or blood tonic and for sore throats.

St John's Wort *Hypericum perforatum.* Wild shade-loving perennial 1–3 ft (30–90 cm) high. Erect stems. Leaves dotted with oil glands. Yellow, five-petalled flowers July–September.

Mixed with oil for painful joints, strained muscles, sprains, bruises; wounds, ulcers, skin rashes. Taken internally on sugar cube for colic, worms in children. Tisane good for nerves, gastritis, insomnia, fainting fits, menstrual pain.

Samphire *Crithmum maritimum* (Sea fennel). Perennial 1 ft (30 cm) high. Thick fleshy stem, woody at base. Glabrous segmented leaves. Umbels tiny greeny-yellow flowers.

Infusion of whole herb a diuretic, good for kidneys. Helps lose weight.

Savory, summer *Satureia hortensis.* Annual. Slender hairy stems 1 ft (30 cm) high. Sparse narrow leaves. Pale lilac flowers in fives in leaf axils July–September.

Spicy flavour useful in salt-free diets. Crushed leaves relieve pain and swelling of bee stings.

Scullcaps *Scutellarias.* Many varieties – perennials. American *Lateriflora* known as Mad-dog or Madweed, distinguished by one-sided racemes; blue flowers bell-shaped with hollow lip and pouch.

Strong nervine, anti-spasmodic used under supervision in cases of hysteria, convulsions, nervous headaches, neuralgia caused by incessant hiccups or coughing.

Sesame *Sesamum indicum.* Tall erect annual. Deeply veined ovate leaves alternate up stem. White trumpet flowers. Egg-shaped seeds various colours greyish-white to black.

Sesame oil a mild laxative. Mucilage of leaves helps diarrhoea, kidney and bladder disorders.

Silverweed *Potentilla anserina.* Wild perennial. Small yellow buttercup-like flowers all summer. Leaves of deeply-toothed leaflets covered with silvery-white down.

Astringent tonic herb tea for cramps, diarrhoea, fevers, sciatica. Externally for bleeding piles, or as gargle.

Slippery elm *Ulmus fulva.* Native tree of N. America. Rough barked with long hairy leaves, leaf buds covered in dense yellow 'wool'. Stalkless flowers.

Makes nutritious food for infants and invalids. Hot drink compound for coughs, fevers, heart, constipation, worms and wide range of conditions. A wound antiseptic.

Solidago *Solidago virgaurea* (Golden rod). Tall perennial. Narrow pointed leaves, spikes tiny yellow flowers July–October.

Anti-inflammatory infusion for wounds, staunches bleeding. Said to dispel kidney and bladder stones.

Sorrel *Rumex scutatus* (French sorrel). Globulous perennial up to 2 ft (60 cm). Ribbed stalks, broad shield-shaped leaves, whorled spikes reddish-green flowers.

Diuretic tea for kidney, liver and blood disorders, fevers. Externally for mouth ulcers, boils, festering wounds.

Southernwood *Artemisia abrotanum.* Tough woody-stemmed perennial. Grey-green feathery leaves covered downy hairs. Yellow flowers in good summers.

Tonic astringent, stimulant. Good for ner-vous diseases. Acts on female reproductive organs.

Sunflower *Helianthus annuus.* Hairy-stemmed annual 3–12 ft (1–3·6 m) high. Huge yellow flowers up to 1 ft (30 cm) diameter. Large heart-shaped leaves. Edible seeds.

Seed oil diuretic. Also for treating coughs and colds.

Sweet cicely *Myrrhis odorata.* Tall perennial. Hollow furrowed stem, large pale feathery leaves turn purple in autumn. Clusters white flowers May–June.

Natural sweet taste useful for diabetics. Tisane for coughs, indigestion.

Tansy *Tanecetum vulgare.* Perennial 2–3 ft (60–90 cm). Erect stem, fern-like leaves, clusters flat yellow flower 'buttons' July–September. Pungent lemon and camphor scent.

Bitter tonic tea for high blood pressure, weak heart, nausea, poor appetite, menstrual disorders. A lotion for swellings, toothache, ear and eye infections.

Thyme *Thymus vulgaris.* Small evergreen bush, woody roots. Pairs of narrow elliptical grey-green leaves. Pale mauve flowers.

Distilled oil is antiseptic, anti-spasmodic, tonic, carminative.

Turmeric *Curcuma longa.* Tropical perennial, large thin leaves from base of plant. Yellowish-white flowers. Short thick underground rhizomes, grey outside, yellow internally.

Oil from roots called 'curcuma' used in Asia for colds, flatulence, liver complaints.

Valerian *Valeriana officinalis* (All-heal). Perennial 3–4 ft (90–120 cm) high. Divided leaves, the lowest with long stalks. Clusters numerous pink flowers June–August.

Roots used for sedative sleep-inducing tea. Will calm headaches, upset stomach, distressed conditions, convulsions. Lotion applied to skin eruptions, swollen joints and veins.

Verbascum *Verbascum thapsus* (Flannel plant). Tall erect biennial 4–8 ft (1·2–2·4 m) high. Leaves flannelly, broad, lanceolate covered with thick white 'wool'. Bright yellow flowers June–August.

Tisane helps respiratory troubles.

Verbena *Verbena officinalis* (Vervain). Medium-sized perennial. Stiff square stems, grey leaves, spikes scentless mauve flowers July–September.

Vervain tea a sedative, digestive tonic. Stimulates bile production. Lotion for eyes, mouth ulcers.

Violet *Viola odorata*. Wild or cultivated perennial. Heart-shaped leaves. Deep purple scented flowers.

Tea with syrup helpful in whooping cough and other persistent coughs. Soothes nerves. Good sleeping draught. Externally for eye lotion or mouth wash.

Wormwood *Artemisia absinthum*. Bushy perennial up to 2½ ft (75 cm). Tripinnatifid silver-grey leaves. Flowers greenish-yellow July–October.

Bitter properties good for stimulating appetite and digestion. Activates secretion of liver and gall bladder, cleanses intestines, improves circulation, regulates menstruation.

Yarrow *Achillea millefolium* (Milfoil). Tall creeping perennial. Bottle green feathery leaves. Heads spicy-scented pink flowers June–October.

Tisane an all round remedy, especially rheumatism. Rich in active bitter substances, minerals, vitamins.

Dr G. E. Loewenfeld
and the late Claire Loewenfeld

BIBLIOGRAPHY, p. 246
PRODUCTS, p. 224–30

HIGH COLONIC IRRIGATION

High colonic irrigation originated in Silesia about 1800. Treatment demands great knowledge, skill and the same experience as anything done by the medical profession. High colonic is done through the rectum with a 2½ ft (75 cm) catheter, which is much more pleasant than most medicines given by mouth. One can see all the waste coming through – important in case something is not in order. It is effective in completely detoxicating the intestine, getting rid of all the poisons which have accumulated over many years. After treatment the patient notices immediately the relief from wind and pressure.

Some establishments claim to do colonic irrigation, but their methods have nothing to do with high colonic irrigation – they only resemble some kind of enema. For high colonic irrigation special equipment is necessary. Skill is needed to administer a wash-out. The treatment takes 1–1½ hours, sometimes longer, depending on the patient's condition.

Treatment cannot be self-administered. It started in the U.K. in 1927 and for many years was only known in the nature-cure profession. Now many radiologists find it a great help for patients before barium enema examination. As a result the test is easier to carry out and the results more clearly seen. Many orthodox doctors recognize today the value of this treatment and quite a number have it done for themselves. High colonic irrigation is very healthy, even for those who have never had any complaint, purely for health reasons to cleanse out the system. It can be helpful for old or young, male and female, but it is not needed for children under fifteen except in special cases; it then needs to be done in a special way.

The case history should be recorded for every patient before the treatment is given. In some cases one has to refuse to carry out the treatment, after hearing the case history; patients may be advised first to have an X-ray before deciding what should be done. Diabetic patients require particularly careful handling as do those with prostatic complaints. When a doctor sends the patient one has to report to him afterwards.

There are many men and women suffering from →**constipation** associated with diverticulosis where high colonic irrigation can be of great help, if the patient follows strictly the instructions after treatment with discipline. Obesity may also be helped, as well as youngsters with acne and some other skin complaints to a lesser extent. Many patients who have constant left-sided abdominal pain may be suffering from spasm of the colon (spastic or irritable colon), frequently with constipation; such patients often leave the clinic happily relieved after the first irrigation, although in some cases further treatment may be needed once or twice a year.

Many years ago I thought women were the main sufferers from constipation, but through my years of experiences I found that many more men than women are constipated – from tension and pressures in their work. After a full day's work and worry they go home, eat without chewing their food properly, then sit watching television – without activity or exercise, and with a full stomach, they then go to bed. No wonder they suffer from indigestion and later all sorts of other complaints. Therefore high colonic patients are advised to follow, for a short or longer period, a diet which is not at all complicated. Patients have to help themselves if they want to get better.

Unfortunately many who should take care of themselves do not bother because they feel they can have another high colonic irrigation if they suffer further discomfort. If only modern society would learn that we do not live to eat, we eat to live. All food should be chewed well. When I tell patients they have to chew their food better they often say, 'Oh, I am a very slow eater.' But my reply is, 'I did not ask whether you are a quick or slow eater, I said chew the food properly.' High colonic irrigation often results in the production of pieces of orange, tomato, meat, pie, beans, cashew nuts – unchanged, not chewed at all. If people would only be more disciplined they could live a healthier, happier life.

Mrs P. Haering

CONTRIBUTORS, p. 221

HIGH VOLTAGE PHOTOGRAPHY

The weird flickering energies of lightning are now being applied in aura-research; the blue St Elmo's fire at a ship's masthead, the tingling power of the storm-charged air with its static fires and flames, the hair-raising emanation from the Van de Graaff generator in the school laboratory! All relate to →bio-energetics and high voltage photography. One may wonder whether Nature has done it all before and how Man's physical form has evolved to receive and use the energies of life.

Research into the phenomena of the →human aura required that the feeble aura energies be increased so that perception and hence analyses were more readily attainable. Knowing that one type of energy radiated by the body was ultra-violet, and that the process of resonance should exist, it was sought to flood the body with ultra-violet light so that the cells could absorb energy and re-emit it the more strongly. An old-fashioned arc lamp was used and produced a very intense beam of 'raw' energy. This beam was shone upon the hands of the subject, the effect being observed through special screens. To the delight and amazement of the observer, a 'flood of flame' was seen flashing off the fingertips, flowing down the skin and even being emitted directly from the skin. The flashes of light were *not* the same as electrical sparks but wriggled and moved as if they were alive: there was no doubt that this was a form of bioplasmic energy. Not only had the cells of the hand been energized but, unfortunately, they had been totally overloaded. Therefore, the phenomenon observed was not of the normal pale blue-grey human aura as seen by the complementary colour method (Kilner, Bagnall, Williamson) but a vastly distorted effect.

It was then decided to try creating ultra-violet for irradiation by using high-voltage corona discharges, like those sometimes experienced during storms. The equipment was designed, experiments planned, part of the circuitry was built and then funds, time and energy ran out. There has never been support for forward researches of this type in England and several groups have tried to ridicule and stop them on religious grounds. Truth *is* truth and, as with many advanced researches, investigators in other parts of the world simultaneously pursue the same channels of thought and collate data from others.

As long ago as 1898, Yakov Narkeich-Todko, and again, in 1939, S. Prat and J. Schlemmer, of Czechoslovakia, engaged in 'electrophotography'. The researches of Tesla also refer to this, with illustrations of high voltage discharges. In 1939 Semyon Kirlian noticed electrical discharges from electrodes to the skin of patients undergoing electrical treatment in a Russian hospital. Kirlian wondered if he would get pictures by imposing photo-film in the path of the discharges. He and his wife Valentina produced many types of corona-discharge instruments and many fascinating photographs. Other scientists eventually joined in the work in the 1960s. The high voltage researches of the Society of Metaphysicians had foundered and been reduced to theoretical development and research administration only due to lack of support.

Kirlian described some of his observations in glowing terms, using such phrases as, 'galaxies of coloured lines, shining, twinkling; ghostly lights, bright multi-coloured flares, dim clouds, blazing violet, fiery flashes' and so on. His description did not coincide with the normal appearance of the bluish electric discharge but had, in addition, that strange 'bioplasmic' effect that was earlier observed in the arc lamp ultra-violet energizing experiment. As with the arc lamp results, the problem lies in sorting out which of the weird lights, flames, flashes and clouds belong to purely electrical phenomena and which are biological in origin.

Many experiments have now been made with high voltage photography and there is little doubt that whilst purely physiological correlations are not obvious, there certainly are many mental influences apparent in the corona discharge photograph. Emanations from healers, mediums, and those under the influence of drugs or intense emotion, all show characteristic differences on the film. For example, intense emotional projection appears to result in red discs on the colour picture. As with the 'natural' aura seen by the use of the complementary colour methods of Kilner, Bagnall and Williamson, prognosis, diagnosis of illness and determination of various types of certain mystical and mental states are possible.

→Neometaphysics requires that energy patterns shall be capable of translation 'downwards' (lessening dimensionality) to energize the living physical body. In esoteric terms – from a spiritual, mental, astral, etheric and to a physical state. Omitting the spiritual, mental and astral states which are somewhat removed from the paraphysical (psycho-physical) realities, we can postulate a translation of energy from the psyche of a person which not only contains his psychological structure but also those patterns which determine his physical manifestation. There is evidence to support the reality of a much more stable and permanent 'energy-body' in the strange high voltage photographs showing the 'cut-leaf' effect.

A leaf has a piece cut off it and is then photographed by the corona discharge method. Allowing for quite critical experimental conditions, a picture of the energy pattern of the physical leaf is seen and, incredibly, there is also a dimmer, but still clear, picture in the area of the missing piece. Obviously the physical piece, being missing, is not the source of the energy. This experimental evidence shows that the energy pattern exists after the removal of the physical counterpart, and, therefore, that the energy pattern can and does exist alone. One might suggest that life after death of the physical body is demonstrable if the bioenergy pattern of the psyche, manifesting in some structural manner and having form thereby, can be shown to exist independently of its physical vehicle. The belief that such a superior energy system exists and is responsible for physical life, derives from neometaphysical conclusions; but many scientists, who have yet to evaluate neometaphysics, cannot accept that the cut-leaf phenomenon supports such theories. Others, however, believe in the existence of an energetic body (etheric) and are sure that high voltage photography – much more refined – will prove the matter. The implications are staggering.

Quite simple equipment can be used for experiments, but it is important when dealing with very high voltages to be *absolutely* certain that the power output of the circuits is very small and that the operator is protected both by suitable circuitry and techniques.

All types of equipment have a charged plate which can be of metal or even a saline solution between two membranes. On the plate will be an insulator. The photo-film in a light-excluding envelope is imposed, emulsion side up, between the fingertips or palm and the insulator. A short pulse of high voltage, high frequency energy is then released and the 'photograph' has been taken. Normal black and white or colour film can be used; but it is cheaper to experiment with black and white in the first instance and to use expensive colour film later when fewer errors will be made.

It is obvious that the greater control one has over the voltage, the frequency, the timing for the length of the pulse, thickness of the insulator (dielectric), atmospheric resistance (humidity, etc.), film thickness, pressure between fingertips and insulating plate and many other confusing and variable factors, the better will be the experimental data. Quite simple high voltage 'cameras' are available, and Dakin's excellent *High Voltage Photography* is recommended for circuitry and procedures. The Thelma Moss lecture slides are an experience in themselves, giving high voltage pictures from a simple coin, through to those from fingertips of people under drugs and so forth. There is no doubt that a gigantic breakthrough into a new hitherto unapproachable field of mental and, by extension, physical therapy must occur.

John J. Williamson
D.SC.(H.C.), F.S.M., M.Brit.I.R.E., F.C.G.L.I.

HOMOEOPATHY

If a person is suffering from an illness which is characterized by a certain set of symptoms, he or she will be treated homoeopathically by the administration of a substance which in health would provoke a similar set of symptoms. This concept is implicit in the word homoeopathy which is made up of two Greek words meaning 'similar' and 'suffering'. It is also often expressed in a Latin phrase coined by its founder, '*Similia similibus curentur*' – 'Let likes be treated by likes'.

Homoeopathy was first formulated as a coherent medical doctrine by a German physician, Samuel Christian Hahnemann, who was born in Meissen in 1755. Samuel Hahnemann was a man of many talents. In his youth he was an outstanding scholar who worked his way through college as a medical student by translating scientific works and giving language lessons.

He qualified as a doctor in 1779 and practised medicine for a number of years, earning a considerable reputation among his contemporaries for his medical skill. Despite his success he became increasingly discouraged by the miserable condition of medical science and gradually withdrew from active practice, busying himself in translating and writing on medical and scientific subjects.

Whilst translating Cullen's *Materia Medica*, a standard medical textbook of the time, he felt dissatisfied with the author's account of the mode of action of a Peruvian bark (*chinchona*, from which quinine is derived) in the treatment of intermittent fever. He experimented by taking the drug himself to observe its effects and was intrigued to discover that its effect closely simulated the symptoms for which it was recommended. As a result he suggested that the drug's efficacy in fever was due to the fact that it could cause fever. This aroused much opposition and persecution. Hahnemann went on to experiment with many other substances and with a group of colleagues developed his theory of 'similars' in treatment.

Putting his observations to the test he found the medicines proved effective in the conditions treated, but conventional doses of them when employed in this fashion often produced an initial worsening of the symptoms. He attempted to minimize this aggravation by reducing the size of the dose and observed that the progressive dilution of the drug could be carried to very great lengths without impairing its beneficial action. The curative action seemed to be enhanced by dilution especially if carried out in a particular manner. At the same time any harmful effects of the medicament were decreased.

Hahnemann extended the range of his experiments over a wider field of substances and diseases. By 1810 his researches had sufficiently confirmed his theories for him to give them concrete expression in *The Organon of the Healing Art*, a book which laid the foundations of homoeopathy. Hahnemann produced it in six different editions in his lifetime.

Hahnemann won over many doctors and laymen to his doctrines. With their help he began a systematic investigation of the action and effects of drugs in healthy individuals, and thus established the disease-conditions in which they would be curative. This process of 'proving' a drug, as it was and still is called, was painstaking and thorough, calling for considerable devotion and sacrifice on the part of the provers. Nearly 100 drugs were proved in Hahnemann's lifetime and the results published in his *Pure Materia Medica* and *Chronic Diseases* between 1811 and 1821. The thoroughness with which these first provings were carried out and the results noted is evidenced by their value today. Since Hahnemann's time many of the original selection of drugs have been 'reproved' and in all instances the subsequent provings have only served to endorse the accuracy of the early work. Many additional drugs have been proved since Hahnemann's time and the *Homoeopathic Materia Medica* today comprises a formidable array of medicines.

Hahnemann's system of proving medicines enables a substance which elicits its characteristic set of symptoms in a healthy individual to be used to treat disorders having a similar symptom complex. The provings are sifted, collated and combined with all the other information about the drug's effects; the result constitutes the *Homoeopathic Materia Medica*. This *Materia Medica* provides the homoeopathic practitioner with the fullest data upon a wide range of medicaments to assist in the selection of the medicines most suited to any individual patient.

The human body, the homoeopathic remedy and the process of ascertaining drug action, are entities demanding far more delicate methods of investigation than are yet available to science. Hahnemann was ahead of his time in 1810. Even now scientific research has still to develop methods of measurement and assay which will reveal the train of events leading to the curative action of 'similar' drugs. The only method of proof yet available is clinical rather than scientific, demonstrable in the patient rather than in the test-tube.

Although science cannot yet fully substantiate the thesis upon which homoeopathy is based, advances in other fields of medicine seem to have brought nearer the eventual explanation of the facts noted by Hahnemann. Since the days of Pasteur, Koch and Almroth Wright it has been known that the administration of microbial agents, or of the poisons they produce, can stimulate the body's defences against infection with such organisms; and now vaccination, inoculation and immunization are household words, exemplifying widespread acceptance of the process of utilizing a very small modified quantity of an agent which causes disease to prevent or combat it by stimulation of the body's natural defences. It is permissible to suggest that homoeopathic medicines function in much the same way, by mobilizing or stimulating the body's natural defences against illness. Viewed in this light, the homoeopathic method of encouraging the body's own recuperative powers to fight a disease by administering the right dose of a substance which in comparatively large doses could give rise to just the same symptoms, is not irrational.

Another analogy is the use of minute doses of a substance to which an individual is known to be allergic to help him overcome the allergy. This process is known as 'de-sensitizing' the patient, and the technique of its use certainly suggests that de-sensitization works by stimulating the body's resistance to the allergy-producing substances, or 'allergens' as they are called. Substances such as house-dust, cat's fur, pollen, etc., have been found responsible for such varied manifestations as asthma and urticaria, and thus the clinician utilizing de-sensitivity solutions is treating a set of symptoms with the agent initially responsible for them.

However, the importance of the word 'similar' when defining or discussing homoeopathy needs emphasis. Homoeopathy is based on the precept that substances causing *symptoms* can also be used in treatment. This is not the same as saying that what can cause disease can also cure it. In influenza, for example, the homoeopath seeks first a substance whose action simulates very closely the symptoms of the disease, for example an extract of the poisonous plant *gelsemium*. He does not usually administer a small amount of influenza vaccine. In other words, he gives a 'similar' but not necessarily 'identical' substance. Thus, it is insufficient to define the basis of homoeopathy as 'what can cause can cure'. To take an example, homoeopathic remedies are of great value in nervous conditions. Here one cannot give something which causes the illness, since its origins are so vague and ill-defined, and may not even be physical. But one can administer a medicine which has caused similar symptoms in the nervous and emotional make-up of a healthy person, and expect to alleviate them in the patient.

The aim of homoeopathic treatment is to find and administer that drug whose symptoms are recorded in the provings as corresponding most closely with those observed in the patient. This process of selection is often called finding the 'simillimum', the most similar drug. Drug-picture and disease-picture should coincide if the physician is to be sure that he is selecting the correct remedy. This is interesting because it underlines how important are symptoms to a homoeopathic doctor. It is the symptoms observed and not the name or classification of the disease which bears most weight in the choice of remedy. The homoeopathically minded physician does not for example diagnose a 'cold' and then give a remedy for 'colds'. It is well known that the so-called 'common cold' can take many forms and manifest itself in a variety of ways. It may affect the eyes, the head and the nose; the discharge may be copious or scanty, irritating or bland; the patient may feel better in fresh air or intolerant of it; thirst may be increased or virtually absent; the temperature may be raised or sub-normal; the patient may be apathetic or restless. These and many other variants are all significant to the homeopathic prescription and need to be considered when deciding on the most suitable medicine.

It is obviously helpful to classify the most effective medicines for specific conditions if practicable, *gelsemium* for influenza, *drosera* in whooping cough, or *rhus tox* for rheumatism; but several other such as *bryonia*, *eupatorium perf*, or *baptisia* may equally well be the choice in the various disease-pictures which are grouped under the broad classification of influenza. Similarly the correct remedy for a patient with whooping cough may have been selected from some dozen possibles. Homoeopathy is essentially an individual treatment and no malady can be managed efficiently with its aid unless the prescriber takes full account in the history-taking of the actual symptoms exhibited by that particular patient at that particular time.

Another reason to avoid the very natural tendency to identify a particular drug with a given condition is that the same remedy may be needed in widely differing complaints. *Pulsatilla* may be equally effective in clearing up a gastric upset as in a cold or as in certain menstrual disorders, always provided the symptoms of the condition correspond to those noted amongst provers of *pulsatilla*. This will explain why the same remedy is stated as being useful in a wide range of complaints, always with the necessary proviso that the symptoms correspond.

In assessing the significance of symptoms,

the homoeopathic physician first grades them into 'generals', i.e. those involving the whole body or personality such as 'I feel tired', and into 'locals' (or particulars), for instance 'my stomach pains me'. The general symptoms carry far greater weight than do the locals. Particular attention is paid to whatever mental symptoms are present since these constitute very accurate and sensitive pointers to the selection of the correct drug. Undue irritability, depression, odd fears, shyness, tearfulness, an hysterical tendency, over-sensitiveness to sights, sounds and smells – all are signs which will be valuable to him.

A further factor to be taken into account is the patient's reaction to circumstances and environment. Are the symptoms better for heat or for cold, are they worse in any special type of weather, are they more severe or do they occur only at any particular time of day or night? Are they better or worse for movement or are they better or worse when lying down? These are but some of the variables; the answers will assist in selecting the choice of remedy. Such varying reactions to external conditions are known to homoeopathy as 'modalities', a term the system has borrowed from logic.

To give a rough assessment of how the modalities present can influence the choice of remedy, suppose the choice of remedy in rheumatism is between *causticum* and *rhus tox*. If the rheumatism is better in rainy weather such a modality would indicate *rhus tox*; if worse in rainy weather, the choice would incline to *causticum*.

Another important feature of symptom-taking is noting what one great homoeopath called the 'strange, rare and peculiar' features. The more prominent, uncommon and remarkable a symptom, the greater its value in determining the choice of remedy. A cough is a common condition and the number of homoeopathic remedies which might be indicated are legion. But if the patient or a relative remarks on the fact that whilst coughing the sufferer holds his side because the pain is relieved by pressure, then the pointer is towards *bryonia*.

It is worth nothing here that, in the observation of what is 'strange, rare and peculiar', the patient's family can be of considerable assistance to the doctor who may not know the patient's mannerisms so well and thus not spot so easily any divergence from normal. Many a homoeopathic remedy has been successfully prescribed as a result of a member of a patient's family remarking on some small trait in the patient which has only appeared during the course of the illness.

One further point regarding symptom-taking and symptom-watching is that not *every* symptom attributed to the medicine will necessarily be found in the patient. Every individual, both healthy prover and sick patient, will show a slightly different facet of the symptom-picture, and a 'drug-picture' is a composite of the reactions of a great number of individuals to the effects of the medicament. The description of a condition given in the textbooks will fit the patient like a well-tailored cloak, but not necessarily like a glove. It is the skill of the physician which decides whether the correspondence between drug-picture and symptom-picture is sufficiently close to warrant the prescription of any particular remedy. Dr Clarke in his *Dictionary of Materia Medica* puts it thus: 'The absence of any particular characteristic of a drug is no contraindication to its use provided other indications are sufficiently pronounced.' The judgement and experience of the doctor are the final arbiters in the choice.

Although we have stressed the importance of symptom-taking in homoeopathic medicine, the homoeopathic physician is trained in and utilizes all the aids to medical practice which a medical professional qualification confers. Thus his approach to treatment will include the physical examination, such as examination of pulse-rate, blood pressure, temperature, urine, blood, and other investigations as the case demands, all of which are part of medical routine.

A few words specifically on the homoeopathic approach to chronic conditions might help in gaining a more comprehensive picture of this system of medicine. The chronic condition usually has a deeper ramification and effects than the acute. It is thus more difficult to treat successfully, especially since the homoeopathic approach is directed towards cure rather than palliation. The homoeopathic method involves a *fundamental* attack upon the illness and its origins and history-taking will demand detailed questioning, not only upon current symptoms resulting from the complaint, but also upon every other aspect of the patient's constitution and temperament wherein one may find apparently unrelated phenomena which go to make up the complete symptom-picture.

A recurrent caution in homoeopathic literature is that one must always prescribe upon 'the totality of the symptoms'. The patient's reactions to food, to different types of weather, to temperature, to stress (remember the importance of mental symptoms), the existence of any deviations from normal habits (remember the importance of the 'strange, rare and peculiar' symptoms), will all have a bearing on the choice of drug, no matter what the nature of the complaint. A dislike of music may be important whether the complaint is asthma or dyspepsia; a desire for solitude significant whether treating for painful menstruation or rheumatism.

So much for current signs and symptoms. The doctor will want to know in addition his patient's full medical history and previous treatment. He will also inquire regarding the health of the parents in case there is an hereditary factor which must be taken into account. He will probably ask too about what were the effects of any vaccination or inoculation the patient has received. The reason for all these painstaking investigations is to establish as complete a record as possible concerning the case under consideration. From this initial case-history stems the initial prescription, and subsequent treatment may be considered in relation to progress and the data on record will be used in all subsequent reviews.

In case all this investigation and matching of symptoms, both past and present, should sound too complicated and imponderable for the process to have much chance of success,

it should be mentioned that the selection of the remedy is often made less difficult for the skilled prescriber by the fact that many individuals provide in their temperaments and constitutions an early clue to the required remedy. It may be said that to the experienced homoeopath an individual 'personifies' a drug. To take an example, if a woman patient who is fair in complexion, mild by nature, easily moved to tears, fond of sympathy, intolerant of hot stuffy rooms and averse to rich greasy foods, she will probably derive benefit from a few judicious doses of *pulsatilla*, whatever the condition for which she has come for treatment. The reason for this is interesting. Ever since the earliest provings it has been observed that certain types of people are more sensitive than others to the action of any given drug. Their system appears to respond more readily to the type of stimulus which that particular remedy provides. To take an analogy, a glass tumbler can often be made to vibrate if a tuning-fork of the right frequency is sounded near it because that particular tumbler is sensitive to a note having that wavelength. If you imagine the patient as the tumbler and the remedy as the vibrating tuning-fork, you will appreciate how sensitivity to the stimulant action of a drug can occur and why if the type of patient we describe were given the right sort of stimulus in the way of a drug, this could 'trigger off' a series of reactions on the part of the mechanisms of the body which needs mobilizing and stimulating. The correct constitutional medicine seems to mobilize all sorts of recuperative processes. If the hypothetical patient mentioned were given *pulsatilla* it is probable not only would the condition of which she was complaining improve but her general health would benefit markedly.

Since homoeopathic remedies used in this fundamental fashion act upon all aspects of a person's temperament and constitution, they are often referred to as 'constitutional remedies'.

When Hahnemann was making his first tentative steps in this new field of treatment he discovered that the conventional dose of the medicine he was employing was often responsible for an initial aggravation of the condition under treatment. He found by trial and error that by reducing the quantity of drug administered he could minimize those aggravations while still retaining therapeutic efficacy. Years of patient work and carefully recorded experiments brought him to the conclusion that one of the methods of attenuation or dilution he had adopted seemed to preserve the beneficial effects of the remedy whilst eliminating harmful exacerbations of the complaint. He was also fascinated to observe that this method of dilution seemed to endow the remedy with additional efficiency and power. Since the drug became more potent as a result of dilution, he described these very small doses which he obtained from diluting the original substance as 'potencies', a name which they have retained.

Probably no aspect of homoeopathic treatment is more puzzling than the use of medicine in such minute quantities, and without actual experience of their efficacy it is difficult to explain how they can have any effect at all. However, the minute dose is not the fundamental principle of homoeopathy. The basis of homoeopathy is the use of the 'similar' drug and the employment of microdoses is a secondary development. From experience homoeopaths have found that the 'low' potencies, i.e. those in which dilution has not been carried out to very great lengths, are relatively short-lasting and superficial in their effect. The 'medium' potencies are somewhat longer-acting and appear to exert their influences on a wider and deeper range of symptoms. The high potencies are more fundamental still in their action and appear to continue the effect for a considerable period even after administation has ceased. These high potencies are those which we have mentioned as being of particular value in the treatment of deep-seated chronic conditions, and their use should be left to the physician who knows how to exploit them to the best advantage. In the home it is advisable to use one of the lower potencies and for domestic use of a homoeopathic remedy the 6c potency as a simple

generalization is recommended unless otherwise specified. A home medicine-chest containing remedies in this potency will meet most contingencies and avoid the risk of using remedies unnecessarily 'potent' for the purpose.

As to dosage, it may be taken as a general rule that it is the *frequency* of administration which is of primary importance when giving homoeopathic remedies. The material content of each dose is so small that the *size* of the dose is not so relevant. In the conditions likely to be met with in the home a remedy in the 6c potency may be given every three or four hours until an improvement is noted. If no improvement occurs within a reasonable time, say twenty-four hours, it may be assumed that the choice of remedy is incorrect.

It is usual to continue administration of the remedy *only until some improvement in the condition is noted.* As soon as an amelioration occurs dosage should be reduced or even discontinued and not resumed unless or until it is seen that progress to recovery has halted. The reason for this is the phenomenon proved by clinical experience that potentized remedies continue to act for a considerable period after administration through stimulation of the body's own recuperative powers. To continue medication once the process of recovery has set in is unnecessary.

It is contrary to the whole concept of homoeopathy to give remedies on the basis of disease names. Homoeopathic prescribing is thus less well defined and consequently more difficult to apply. It is also much more a matter of individual responsibility on the part of the prescriber. The prescription can only be successful if the practitioner, instead of relying on a clear-cut diagnosis and the appropriate medicine for it, weighs every vague and apparently unrelated phenomenon and is prepared to back his own judgement based upon his deductions from them.

A clear understanding of homoeopathic principles supported by a thorough knowledge of the medicines is required which must be applied afresh whenever he is confronted with a new set of symptoms. The results of diagnosis play a less important part in his technique than the observations and deductions made from the symptom-picture. The newcomer will say, 'How on earth can I treat a patient if I don't know what is wrong with him?', and as every homoeopathic physician knows it is most difficult to persuade colleagues that although he can and does use all the aids to medicine which are available to the doctor today, the treatment need not await the findings of diagnostic aids. In an acute infection there is not the need to await laboratory reports; of more importance is whether the patient is restless or drowsy, thirstless or thirsty, worse for heat or worse for cold, and so on. This can mean real saving in time when treatment is urgent and the bacteriologist, the pathologist, etc., have yet to give their findings.

Homoeopathy is admittedly a difficult system of medicine and this can be a drawback. A physician's task is difficult enough without all the laborious history-taking and complicated symptom-matching that we have attempted to describe, and this process may be valueless unless thorough. Unless the history-taking is thorough the symptom-picture will not be complete and selection of the appropriate remedy uncertain. Thus it is also necessary to appreciate the economic factor, for the homoeopath, needing longer to consider each case and seeing fewer patients each day, must feel extremely confident of his homoeopathic ability before he attempts to use the therapy in full-scale practice.

The major benefits resulting from homoeopathic treatment are:

It induces recovery because it stimulates the body itself to fight the disease-condition.

Homoeopathy treats all the symptoms which go to make up the whole of the condition. In a cold the remedy may be selected after consideration of the character of the symptoms of the fever, the headache, the discharge from eyes and nose, any alterations in thirst and appetite, any attendant congestion, the presence or absence of perspiration and its nature and location and so on. Since all these symptoms are treated, all may be expected to benefit if the correct remedy is given.

Because of its fundamental approach to illness, it aims at complete cure and not palliation.

Again because of its radical approach, homoeopathy can treat conditions for which there are no really curative drugs in the standard repertory. The homoeopath can treat and cure many indefinable and intangible conditions, especially in the nervous and mental spheres for which there may not be any effective standard means to cure other than recourse to 'complete rest', sedatives or in the last resort psychological treatment.

Homoeopathic treatment is safe and effective for even the youngest children, no matter which of its drugs is employed.

In treating the person and not an arbitrarily named disease, homoeopathy will benefit not only the actual disease-condition but also the general health of the patient. Homoeopathic treatment is preventative as well as curative and when used to its best advantage the system raises the general standard of health and thus prevents the development of many illnesses which usually occur only when natural resistance is at a low ebb.

Homoeopathic preparations

Homoeopathic preparations are obtained by using various methods of successive dilution and trituration from the following raw materials:

1 Mineral materials such as metals, salts, acids, as well as synthetic medicines.
2 Products of vegetable or animal origin.

From basic materials one prepares:

a) Succus and mother tinctures from fresh plants, or exceptionally, dried plants.
b) Mother tinctures of materials of animal origin.
c) Solutions or triturations of chemical products.

The dilutions and triturations customarily employed are obtained under prescribed conditions respectively in liquid medium (with succussion) or solid medium. They are called either decimal or centesimal depending on the successive operations being made in steps of 1/10th or 1/100th. The number of operations carried out in such manner determines the degree of dilution or trituration obtained in this way.

All pharmaceutical forms can be used for homoeopathic preparations. Certain forms are prepared by the specific method of impregnation of neutral forms (granules, globules, tablets, powder).

The preparations are described with the Latin name of the drug, followed by the indication of the dilution. The following abbreviations are used:

For basic tinctures   Ø or TM.
For decimals   D, Dec., or X.
For centesimals   C or CH.

preceded or followed by the figure of the dilution, e.g.

Pulsatilla 6
Aconite 30
Bryonia Ø, etc.

J. B. L. Ainsworth M.P.S.

HUMAN AURA

In recent years it has become more apparent that the human body – indeed all living things – emanate a number of forms of energy. The accurate perception and analysis of these energy-forms now comprise a most important and fascinating study of great value in all medical, parapsychological and paraphysical fields. Since 1908, when the first published researcher, Dr W. J. Kilner, commenced his special studies at St Mary's Hospital, London, where he was a radiologist, there has been a slow but certain development in the mode of detection and interpretation of life radiation. Kilner's important pioneering work, carried out in the face of ridicule from his colleagues, was followed by that of Oscar Bagnall whose work, *The Origin and Properties of the Human Aura*, was published in 1937. He was a most careful researcher and did much to verify Kilner's works and to extend the knowledge.

My own study of the aura commenced in 1947 when I realized that firm physical evidence for the validity of paraphysical effects was important if formal prejudices against transcendental research were to be overcome. My approach, as with Bagnall, differed from that of both the two early researchers. As a qualified electronic engineer and a natural psychic I was less inhibited by formal and restrictive study than many of my fellow scientists. I could, albeit with reservations, relate physical and non-physical effects to one another and postulate the need for some hitherto unknown form of energy normally beyond instrumental detection.

During the war, at the R.A.F. College at Cranwell a high-probability infinitely based general system was developed. This system, now termed neometaphysics, gave theoretical evidence, based upon empiricism both in the physical and the non-physical fields, to support new theories of the aura. Using this very important new theoretical basis, researches could proceed with a firm schedule. It was postulated that energy, the exact nature of which was presently unknown, was existent in all living organisms and that in doing work, re-manifests in various forms and eventually changes into heat.

Several years ago work was carried out on scanning the human body with infra-red detectors and led to Pyroscan. This instrument shows waves of heat emanating from the body, indicating cool areas and is now in use as an important diagnostic tool. In 1947, when verifying the works of Kilner and Bagnall, it could not be known in which part of the spectrum the perceptible aura emanated.

Using the complementary colour method or sensitizing the human eye it was determined that the aura was either near ultra-violet or near infra-red, or both. We know that it is both! Of greatest importance is the 'active' energy – that of the ultra-violet. As a consequence of these early researches a lecture was given in the Caxton Hall, London, by Dr Royston Low on my behalf. A research report entitled *Seeing the Aura* incorporated the text of the lecture and was published by the Society of Metaphysicians in August 1954.

Using special filters comprised of alcoholic solutions of various dyes, one could soon perceive the blue-grey mist around the finger-tips, between opposed fingers of the hands and around the body. The strange dark space, the inner aura and many of its characteristics soon became apparent. A careful study of photo-electric detectors and of photographic film, as then available, revealed that nothing existed of sufficient sensitivity in the frequency region concerned to equal that of the human eye. Research was therefore directed to methods of enhancing aura perception, first, by improvement of detectors, and secondly by increasing the intensity of the energy given off by the cells. Dr Muftic of the Department of Research of the Society of Metaphysicians managed to develop a photo-electric mosaic which, when scanned, gave a picture upon a cathode-ray tube screen. His research colleague was killed and their laboratory destroyed by a superstititious mob in Cairo; he fled to West Germany and was warned 'to leave such studies alone' by the pharmaceutical firm for which he worked. He left the firm and went to East Germany. So, apart from his extensive research records left to the Society of Metaphysicians, his works were lost. His first studies were published in 1960, entitled *Researches on the Aura Phenomena.*

My own studies continued with a long search for better dyes with which to sensitize the eyesight, and indeed the complementary colour effect was considerably enhanced. I then proceeded to develop methods of increasing aural energy first by irradiation of the body with 'raw' ultra-violet and secondly by creating ultra-violet with corona discharge effects; both methods were successful but in different modes. The energizing method using raw ultra-violet produces floods of strangely active sparks – later defined as bio-plasmic energy forms, and the normal bodily aura increased its intensity several times. With corona discharge as the source of ultra-violet, results were continually distorted by the discharge itself and interpretation made more difficult. Time and funds ran out and the best that could be done was to provide the many inquirers with data which had been gained and suggest paths of future research. Corona discharge research later appeared as kirlian photography, but is more correctly entitled →**high voltage photography.**

Considerable advances have been made since these early studies and there can be no doubt that improved instrumentation due to more advanced technology has made it possible to develop better scanners of the normal, non-energized (undisturbed) aura.

From ancient writings one hears of the aureole of the saintly person, also of the clairvoyance aurae with their blaze of colour but non-physical nature. Treating the aura as an *energic* emanation one may also include emanations from deep-sea fish, fire-flies, glow-worms and of course all forms of fluorescence, phosphorescence, luminosity and known modes of radiation generation. A very wide study can then be made upon which to construct accurate concepts of the mechanisms involved. The human aura appears as a relatively bright blue-grey mist about one centimetre deep around the skin. Between this mist and the skin is a strange dark space. Further out from the skin is a rough enclosing ovoid of energy; Kilner claims to have found an even more distant aura which he called the 'extra outer aura'. Whilst Kilner reports that he could see the outer and the extra outer aura and many strange effects obviously connected with mental activity, Bagnall did not see these. Reports from many clairvoyants readily confirm Kilner's more formal results. Ironically Kilner did not consider psychic solutions (as required from us by the neo-

121

metaphysical bases which gave us our research priorities) and did not realize that he had probably become clairvoyant. In his pursuit of 'seeing the aura' he was no longer perceiving in any physical manner. This does not imply that the clairvoyantly perceived aura is unreal and without its effect upon and in the life-processes; it merely tends to confirm that life is not restricted in its nature to those areas of inquiry we would *normally* define as physical.

Research by the complementary colour method of sensitizing the human eye to the near ultra-violet emanation of the living aura has given us a clear prognostic and diagnostic tool. The characteristic aurae for many different states of health have been carefully observed by Kilner and Bagnall; and considerable investigation of the striations (like self-repellent bundles of rays) of the inner aura gives much more diagnostic data. It is also apparent that various mental states have a great effect upon the quality and intensity of emanation of energy and therefore that correlations between the aural condition and psychological characteristics exist.

Early physical breakdown appears to be preceded by a lessening and darkening of the aural light over the area yet to suffer such breakdown. Prognosis of up to six weeks seems to be possible.

Breaks in the steady illumination over the skin-surface indicate a break in physical structures from which the energy emanates. For example, an arthritic joint clearly shows a sudden cessation of the even distribution of aural energy with a sudden emanation of quite brilliant rays of light with dark space between the rays, emanating at right angles from the affected joint. Dr Muftic reported that even the smallest heart section showed pulsation of light in time with the normal heart beat.

It is self-evident that further research, especially to improve our means of observing the natural or non-energized aura would be of great service to medicine, in the comprehension of the life processes, as a psychological tool and in all related spheres of bio-energetics such as →acupuncture, zone therapy (→re-flexology), ionization points on the body, →bioenergy circuitry of the body and many other rapidly expanding vistas.

John J. Williamson
D.SC. (H.C.), F.S.M., M.Brit.I.R.E., F.C.G.L.I.

HYPNOTHERAPY

Treatment of problems with emotional causes by psychotherapy may include hypnosis. Psychotherapy has been called 'talking cure'. It is usually the patient who talks rather than the therapist. Hypnosis is a self-induced state of relaxation and concentration in which the deeper parts of the mind become more accessible.

The word hypnosis was coined by James Braid in 1842 when he believed the phenomenon to be a form of sleep. Five years later, having realized that it has nothing to do with sleep, and that the patient is actually more alert while in hypnosis though more relaxed, Braid substituted the word 'mono-ideism', meaning a state of concentration. But the new word did not catch on.

In those days hypnosis was used to put repetitive statements, known as suggestions, such as 'you are confident' or 'your eczema will go', to the patient. This use persists today by entertainers and medical hypnotists. Suggestion often relieves symptoms but, like drugs, it fails to deal with the problems underlying the symptoms.

Two deaths have been reported from the mis-use of hypnosis, both at the hands of physicians. In the first case, a hospital medical practitioner consulted by a man for paralysis of his right arm put him into hypnosis and told him the paralysis would go. It did. The patient went home and cut his throat. In the second case, reported in *World Medicine*, a general practitioner told a woman in hypnosis that she would no longer be anxious about crossing the road. She confidently stepped out of his surgery straight in front of a bus. Since medical practitioners, including psychiatrists, rarely have worthwhile training in the understanding of emotional problems, medical hypnotism is very backward, though usually safer and more effective than the use of drugs to suppress emotional problems.

Yet as long ago as 1881, Josef Breuer, followed by Sigmund Freud, found that patients who respond to hypnosis will often vividly recall relevant events which they previously remembered only vaguely or not at all. Furthermore, they usually release the associated feelings. This is crucially important, because nearly all emotional problems involve bottled-up feelings which need to be released at the same time as the patient remembers their cause. This process is known as catharsis. Breuer and Freud wrote,

Not until the patients have been questioned under hypnosis do these memories emerge with the undiminished vividness of a recent event. But for six whole months one of our patients, Anna O, reproduced under hypnosis with hallucinatory vividness everything that excited her on the same day of the previous year during an attack of acute hysteria. A diary kept by her mother, without her knowledge, proved the completeness of the reproduction. . . . The patient aptly described this procedure as a talking cure, while she referred to it jokingly as chimney-sweeping.

Freud abandoned hypnosis after a patient threw her arms round him, and Breuer gave it up for similar reasons. They did not at that time understand that it is normal for a patient to have strong feelings toward the therapist, largely transferred from the parents. Later, Freud discovered that understanding these feelings was valuable in therapy and improved the relationships of the patient with people generally.

An essential part of the training of any hypnotherapist – and the British Hypnotherapy Association confines membership to therapists who have had this training – is for the therapist first of all to experience extensive hypnotherapy himself, in which he discovers his own transference feelings and investigates his own hang-ups. Only thus can he really understand and help patients.

The integration of psycho-analytic discoveries with hypnosis, which began in North America from about 1942, was in some respects a great step forward. But traditional psycho-analysis involves interpreting dreams, symptoms and statements of the patient, imposing theories and giving advice. This authoritarian approach is still used by some analysts today, and even topped up with drugs.

In 1958, the British Hypnotherapy Association was founded. It confines membership to hypnotherapists who are fully trained psychotherapists. They do not use interpretation, advice or medication, nor confine themselves to the discoveries of any one analytic pioneer. They have developed increasingly effective methods of training and treatment.

These hypnotherapists do not treat symptoms. They inquire into causes. This is important because the symptom is often only the patient's pretext for coming along. Beyond it lies a larger problem; the real one.

So hypnotherapists give the patient a thorough consultation, inquiring into his childhood, his relationships and his basic life pattern, not only his symptoms. They treat him as a whole person, not as a problem to which a person is inconveniently attached. They listen, they ask searching questions and, when appropriate, they enable the patient to put himself into hypnosis so that he can recall more readily.

This approach frequently revolutionizes the patient's life. There is no risk of mis-diagnosis as nothing is diagnosed, and bad advice or incorrect interpretations are unlikely as the therapist does not normally give either advice or interpretations. He lets the patient speak freely, with or without hypnosis, asks appropriate questions and enables him to emerge from under his accumulated fears, indoctrinations, guilts and distortions, lose his need for symptoms and be himself.

How long this takes varies from one person to another. The number of sessions required varies from zero upward. In a few cases the mere thought of treatment, or the fact of having made an appointment, or attending a consultation, prompts a patient to think over his life and resolve his problems himself. At the other extreme there are some people whose problems are never completely resolved however long they have therapy.

Hypnotherapy is frequently the quickest and most effective method available. For example, an American psychologist, who had psycho-analysis in Chicago for several years without, he said, much effect; following hypnotherapy in London, he gained insight into his problems and recovered from them in two weeks of daily sessions. His symptoms had included loss of working capacity, falling out with his wife, kicking off the bedclothes at night and eating too much.

The more relaxed and co-operative patients go easily into hypnosis. Those who could do with it most sometimes respond least. But hypnosis is only an aid in therapy, albeit an important one. If someone is unable to relax and co-operate sufficiently the answer is to find out why. The reasons are usually the reasons for the patient's problems generally, and both can be unravelled simultaneously.

The hypnotherapist does not advise the patient to try hypnosis until it is likely to be more useful and effective than keeping to other methods. When the problem can be talked out more quickly without hypnosis, or the patient is obviously not ready for it, then there would be no point in attempting it. This is common sense, but a disappointment to anyone who imagines hypnosis to be a magical process, and to those who wanted to say to the hypnotherapist, 'You have failed.' Hatred, transferred from father or mother, is the most usual cause of failure to go into hypnosis. Other common barriers are guilt or fear about having homosexual or murderous wishes, anxiety about the risk of discovering these, and fear of losing control of them.

But most people go into hypnosis to a useful extent. The mere fact of using hypnosis is relaxing. Contrary to what some people suppose, hypnosis is not addictive. When someone in hypnosis has what seems to be vivid recollections of past events, these are not always literally true recollections. They are sometimes fantasies, such as we have in dreams. Apparent recollections in hypnosis of previous lives, although sometimes very imaginative, lifelike, and containing authentic details, usually turn out to be daydreams. This is not to underestimate them, as they can be valuable in self-understanding as well as creative and enjoyable.

People who suppose that in hypnosis only truth is told, occasionally say, 'Will you put my wife into hypnosis so that I can find out whether she has been unfaithful to me?' This futile request is symptomatic of serious emotional problems in the person making it.

Self-hypnosis, that is to say hypnosis without the assistance of a therapist, has some uses, though not nearly as many as some writers of books and articles on the subject would have us believe. It is valuable for temporary analgesia; avoidance of pain. If you can use it effectively it is better than an anaesthetic when you visit the dentist, and better than a tranquilliser when you are tense. But a horror of dentistry, or persistent tension, invariably have emotional causes which need to be investigated for lasting improvement. Sometimes a fear of dental treatment turns out to be a result of bad dental experiences in the past, in which case it may be resolved as soon as these experiences are recalled, with feeling, in hypnosis. When the fear is displaced from some other problem, such as a sexual one, it can take longer to sort out.

A wide range of problems can have emotional causes. They include accident proneness, agoraphobia, alcoholism, allergies, amnesia, anxiety, anorexia, asthma, bed-wetting, blushing, car-sickness, claustrophobia, compulsions, lack of confidence, dithering, duodenal ulcer, examination nerves, failure-syndrome, fears, frigidity, frustration, guilt, 'habits', hayfever, hoarding, hysterical paralysis, impotence, indecision, indigestion, inferiority feelings, inhibitions, insomnia, kleptomania, learning difficulties, marital problems, meanness, bad memory, menstrual disorders, migraine, poor mixing, nail-biting, nervousness, nervous skin disorders, nervous visual defects, neurasthenia, neurosis, neurotic choice of partner, nightmares, orgasmic inability, over-eating, panic, phobias, premature ejaculation, procrastination, psoriasis, psychosexual problems, quivering hands, rejection feelings, sea-sickness, self-consciousness, shyness, smoking, stage-fright, stammer, tension, timidity, torticollis, nervous tremor, twitching, warts, worry, vaginismus.

Sexual problems are probably the most usual ones about which people consult hypnotherapists, and these patients are usually among the ones who get the most gratifying results. Lack of sex education is often part of the problem, so hypnotherapists then recommend the best of the currently available sex education books.

Over-eating, smoking and alcoholism are often thought of as habits. There are people who can stop eating too much, smoking, or drinking excessively, when they choose, and their indulgences are habits. But those who are unable to stop without help are addicts, and their addictions are symptomatic of emotional problems. Hypnotherapists therefore treat these patients in the same way as any others. They do not attempt to suppress the addiction by suggestion-hypnosis, though most amateurs do so.

How do we know the long-term effects of hypnotherapy, and whether there are any side-effects? The therapists in the British Hypnotherapy Association set a condition when seeing any new patient that the patient will let them know the long-term results. In some cases follow-ups have been done over more than ten years. This has contributed to the development of increasingly effective methods. There is ample evidence of lasting benefits from hypnotherapy. There is no record of self-discovery proving to be more than the patient could take. Finding out about oneself can sometimes be an unpleasant shock, but it can be an exciting adventure. As for side-effects, these are known because it is the whole person who receives the therapy, not his symptoms, and the effects on the whole person

are noted. There are often many beneficial side-effects. Since symptoms are not suppressed, they are not replaced with new symptoms. As drugs are not used there can be no addiction, overdose, poisoning or thalidomide-type disaster in hypnotherapy.

Perhaps the last word should be from a former patient of a hypnotherapist. She talked freely in and out of hypnosis, recalled dreams, told her associations with them, and reviewed her attitude to her husband and her work. Some time after completing the treatment she wrote,

The therapy has been very successful, the true test being the job I have held down now for sixteen months and also the fact that I am getting my work published again. Neither of these things seemed really possible to me when I first came to you. This has been accomplished as well as a deeper understanding. As the improvement has been maintained for so long I can say with confidence that the treatment was successful. Not only do I feel more relaxed most of the time, but it seemed to release some time afterwards a positive flood of constructive imaginative activity so that I am writing again. This pleased me more than anything. Some kind of 'block' has been removed – puzzling to know quite how you did it but one has to be glad one was lucky enough to find the right person! As you said, the treatment goes on working. And mysteriously it makes life that much more richer and more significant – perhaps because one regains possession of an important part of oneself.

R. K. Brian

ASSOCIATIONS, p. 213
BIBLIOGRAPHY, p. 247
TRAINING, p. 232

JOGGING

Arthur Lydiard, the New Zealand ex-marathon runner and one of the main promoters of jogging as a therapeutic aid, says that jogging lowers blood-fat and helps to eliminate the risk of coronary thrombosis. Jogging is an easy, relaxed and unpaced form of running.

Popular in Britain, Australia, New Zealand and the United States (a recent estimate gave the number of U.S. joggers as ten million), jogging met with approval at a seven-nation conference on physical culture in the Soviet Union where there was general agreement that carefully measured running is of great benefit to the heart and circulatory system. Professor Belaya of Moscow reported that he had successfully used jogging to treat patients after heart attacks. Other doctors at the conference recommended it for asthma and arthritis. A doctor in Tel Aviv, Professor Victor Gottheimer, has succeeded in reducing the mortality rate of post-cardiac patients to fewer than 5 per cent in the crucial five years following their attacks, by training them to a point where they jog six miles a day. This is a mortality rate five times less than for patients who do not exercise. Gottheimer bases his method on the theory that carefully selected exercise, under medical supervision, can reconstruct a damaged heart. One of his patients who had been given six months to live after a heart attack was then treated by Professor Gottheimer and eventually graduated to long-distance running, achieving a number of sports records, including covering ten kilometres in fifty-one minutes five seconds at the International Olympic Folk Sports Race at the 1972 Munich Olympics.

Among those who have turned to jogging as a life-saving therapy is Mrs Eula Weaver of Los Angeles, who suffered a stroke in her late seventies. Her doctors gave her the choice either of spending the rest of her life as an invalid or to start walking again. Vowing she would try anything to get back to normal, in time she was able to jog two miles a day. Later she entered the U.S. Senior Olympics and won the championship in a 1500-metre run for women over eighty. Today at eighty-eight she has cut down her daily work-out to one mile a day. But perhaps the most remarkable jogger of all is Larry Lewis, a former waiter, who celebrated his 106th birthday in 1976 with his daily stint of 6·7 miles around the Golden Gate Park in San Francisco.

John Newton

BIBLIOGRAPHY, p. 248
CONTRIBUTORS, p. 221

MACROBIOTICS

Macrobiotics describes an attitude to life and health that is based on an understanding of the importance of diet. It is not only a form of natural medicine; it looks beyond obtaining freedom from disease towards the more positive idea of gaining and maintaining enjoyment of our natural condition of good health and happiness.

The underlying principle which governs the selection of food in the macrobiotic diet is called the unique principle of yin and yang, the theory of the unity of antagonistic but complementary opposites. It provides a means whereby a person can judge the qualities of foods without resorting to complex tables of vitamin and mineral content. In broad terms, yin corresponds to acid, and yang to alkaline in food. Yin represents the feminine, passive principle and yin foods include fruits, drinks, summer-grown foods, foods of sweet, sour or hot flavour, large expansive texture, and purple, blue, or green in colour. Yang represents the masculine active principle. Yang foods include those of animal origin, cereals, and some vegetables. Foods that are compact and hard, red, yellow, or orange in colour, salty or bitter in flavour, and which mature in the autumn and winter are more yang.

Most illness can be attributed to an excess of yin or yang. Through macrobiotic diagnosis of symptoms it is possible to make adjustments in the diet to rectify these excesses. Because cereal grains represent the balance of yin and yang in foods that most perfectly satisfies human requirements, they are used as the principal food in the macrobiotic way of eating. They comprise usually at least 50 per cent of the diet, depending on the environment, level of activity, and general state of health. For sick people a diet including a higher proportion of cereal grains combined with some natural internal and external treatments is employed to help the body to heal itself. There are practitioners of macrobiotic healing methods, but the emphasis is very strongly upon self-diagnosis and cure. Diagnostic techniques include diagnosis on the basis of facial and physical characteristics, colour, acupuncture pulses, and digestive function as well as by considering the specific symptoms.

Thorough chewing of food is important. The first stage in the digestion of carbohydrates takes place in the mouth, so to obtain full benefit one should, in Gandhi's words, 'Drink your foods and chew your drinks.' Drinks in general are held to a low level as an excess of liquids reduces the efficiency of the kidneys and leads to fatigue, the first stage of illness. Excess liquids also create a see-saw desire for salty foods which in turn create a desire for more liquids as well as yin foods. Control of salt intake is fundamental as the level of salt consumed governs the appetite for food and drink.

Processed foods are not used. Food is taken in its most natural form, with no processing beyond cooking. Foods of local origin are preferred as there is an affinity between people of a region and the foods that grow in that region. Local foods are also more likely to be fresh, harvested in a mature state, and free of preservatives. Animal food is not an essential or important part of macrobiotics, but some macrobiotics do use occasional fish or other animal and dairy foods. Macrobiotics seeks true freedom which means neither slavery to cravings for certain foods nor slavery to a list of negative dietary restrictions. The truly healthy person should be able to eat freely of whatever he likes because his appetite will lead him to eat what is needed to maintain his existing condition. However, foods such as sugar, sugared foods, refined carbohydrates, and members of the nightshade family such as potatoes, tomatoes, and aubergines are taken with considerable caution if at all.

Quantity of food eaten can undermine the benefits of quality. Excessive consumption of food is wasteful and places unreasonable demands on the digestive organs. It also encourages intestinal parasites, which are common in affluent societies. It is best to stop eating before the appetite is completely satisfied.

Macrobiotic foods are centred on the whole grains: brown rice, whole wheat, rye, barley, oats, millet, buckwheat, and maize. These provide a wide range of flavours and uses that enable one to enjoy a varied cuisine based on whole cereals. Vegetables and pulses supplement the grains. Soya bean products used in macrobiotics are miso and tamari, a purée and a liquid soya sauce both made by the natural lactic fermentation of soya beans over a period of at least eighteen months. They are a rich source of amino acids and enhance the flavours of many foods. Other specialities include salted pickled plums called *umeboshi* which are used in cooking as well as medicinally for almost all digestive problems; mu tea, a compound tea containing fifteen roots and herbs including →ginseng; *goma-sio* sesame seed salt; green tea; and grain coffees. Wild foods are used when available and seaweeds of several types. Trace elements are obtained from these wild foods that are often absent in cultivated plants.

The ten-day rice diet is sometimes used in macrobiotics. This is a diet in which the only food taken for a ten-day period is whole brown rice. It is a useful tonic diet, purifying the blood and sorting out digestive disorders that can often be at the root of illnesses elsewhere in the body. Although it should not be practised regularly, its results can be surprising to many people in helping them to an awareness of how much diet can affect consciousness and levels of energy. The body's cleansing processes are given full rein in this diet. It can be accompanied by the discharge of accumulated residues from years of conventional eating that may take the form of spots, excessive mucus, and discharge through the kidneys. Generally however, such dramatic effects should not be sought – a reasonably healthy person will not react so strongly.

Children raised on a macrobiotic diet develop a natural and instinctive appetite for the right mixture of quality and quantity in their food. They rarely experience sickness or the cravings for sweets and other foods that are normally associated with childhood.

Macrobiotics was brought to Europe and the United States by Georges Ohsawa, a Japanese who cured his own tuberculosis using a method relying on traditional oriental medicine based on yin–yang principles combined with an appreciation of modern nutritional understanding. The system was applied in various forms in Japan. A hospital in Nagasaki where the macrobiotic diet was used as part of the treatment attributes the low level of radiation sickness subsequent to the nuclear bomb explosion to the fact that patients were on a brown-rice-based diet. (Recent experiments with rats on a whole cereal diet reveal a similar high resistance to radiation effects.) In the fifties and sixties Ohsawa travelled widely in Africa and Asia, testing his ideas against the diseases prevalent in those regions, often rediscovering traditional foods and medicines of those areas, and sometimes exposing himself to a tropical illness and then curing himself of it. His books, including *Zen Macrobiotics*, have been translated into several languages, including French and English. London saw its first macrobiotic restaurant, called Seed, in 1967 since when it has become widely practised in Britain as well as the U.S.A. and in Europe. Macrobiotic staples are available from natural foods stores and brown rice, once a hard-to-find commodity, is now even available from supermarkets.

Ohsawa's advice to his followers was, 'Go and make your own macrobiotics – I have only described the way that was suitable for me.' In this spirit the practice of macrobiotics varies in different regions and between different people. The ultimate criterion is that a person who is free of illness, sleeps well, does not worry, and lives with vitality and joy is successfully practising macrobiotics. The goal of macrobiotics is to overcome the oral problems and bad eating habits that are acquired early in life, and then to be free of the need to concern oneself overly with the intake of food. Once one's dietary system becomes second nature it is possible to devote full energies to the enjoyment of life's physical, mental, and spiritual opportunities.

Craig Sams

BIBLIOGRAPHY, p. 249

MAZDAZNAN – MASTER THOUGHT

A system of education and a way of life based on fundamental truth, which is at the back of all great religio/philosophic systems. Today, on the physical and intellectual levels, it is capable of scientific proof. On the spiritual level one can become aware of it according to the degree of spiritual understanding of the individual.

It aims at the balance between the physical, spiritual and intellectual aspects of life. Perfect health is attained and maintained by living in accordance with the laws of God (Creative Intelligence) as expressed in nature. Self-help is the rule in healing, which is mainly →**naturopathic** and manipulative. There are practitioners in Europe and elsewhere who use Mazdaznan methods.

Three great prophets have particular importance in the history of Master Thought, which is closely bound up with that of the Iranian or Aryan people and of western civilization:

Ainyahita 9600 B.C. was not a myth but a real woman. Her covenant has been adopted by the present day Mazdaznan Association: 'I am here upon the earth to reclaim the earth, to turn the deserts into a paradise most suitable unto God and his associates to dwell therein.'

Zarathustra (in Greek, *Zoroaster*) 6900 B.C., the Iranian sage, lived and worked mainly in Bactria. Observation in youth, and experiments which led to the development of wheat from a grass, artichokes from thistles, and the apple tree from the rose bush, inspired him to preach the religion of the One God.

Ahura Mazda (Infinite Intelligence) created the Universe with His Best Thought and rules it with the Law of Order, Truth and Justice. In man (the species, male and female) is a spark from that source, which enables him to distinguish right from wrong. He has freedom of choice, and if he chooses good and lives in accord with the law, man and his society can evolve towards perfection. The rule for life is 'Good Thought, Good Word, Good Deed'. That part of the *Zend Avesta* which was saved from destruction, when carefully studied, reveals the same basic aspects of right-living that were later stated by Christ.

The Master Jesus (5 B.C., as it is now believed) demonstrated what man can attain when he is 'at one' with God, when he becomes in matter what he is in spirit. This noble Master taught the Law of Love in the Sermon on the Mount, and in the Lord's Prayer (of *Ainyahita*'s Covenant). He urged his followers to 'be perfect, even as your Abba in Heaven (God within you) is perfect'. It is known that Christ visited communities in Iran, India and Egypt during the years before his ministry. These were of Zarathustrian origin, and had much knowledge of the art of →breathing and of natural therapies.

The Zarathustrian/Christian teaching was formulated for the West in a way suitable for the twentieth century by Dr Otoman Zar-Adusht Ha'nish (1844–1936). He had spent many years of his youth in a remote community in Iran where he learned to overcome a heart condition through breath control. He acquired a profound knowledge of the Ancient Wisdom, and developed his faculties to a very high degree. On his return to Europe he qualified in medicine and theology and was thus in a position to begin his work. Lecturing and working as a healer, first in Europe and later in the U.S.A., Dr Ha'nish was active in the New Thought movement, in promoting →vegetarianism, better methods of growing food plants and other aspects of Mazdaznan message. He spoke strongly in favour of women's equal rights, and parity of representation in parliament, emphasizing the importance of the mother's influence on her children – guiding them towards responsible independence – for 'the hand that rocks the cradle rules the world'. He advocated the eight-hour day with an increase in wages. In 1915 he formed a Society for the Promotion of a Federation of Nations; in the same year he was awarded a Peace Medal at the Panama Exhibition. This led to correspondence with President Wilson who later proposed the League of Nations.

It was in 1902 that Dr Ha'nish founded the Mazdaznan Association through which he taught every aspect of a better healthier way of life based on the highest principles. The first objective was to give ways and means for the individual to develop towards physical, spiritual and intellectual balance, able to rely on his own guidance from within – from the 'Divine Spark', the Avestan 'Spenta Mainyus' or the 'Christos'.

There are five inter-related subjects for practical application:

Breathing is the most important. It has two functions, for while it maintains life on the physical plane, there is a spiritual element known to the Zend people as Ga-Llama, the centralizing life principle, to Christians as the Holy Spirit, and to the Vedic Aryans as prana. Thus inspiration has a dual meaning. Prayer, singing and intoning are a feature of most religious observances and should be taken on a long exhalation. For daily use there is a choice of exercises through which one can develop the twelve senses – including those referred to as extra-sensory perception. Deeper rhythmical breathing, making full use of the lungs can effect great improvement in health and intelligence; the establishment of a longer breath rhythm – ideally seven seconds inhalation, seven seconds exhalation with one second's pause in between – will slow down and steady the heart beat. It is an important factor making for a longer and healthier life.

Personal diagnosis is an aid to understanding one's self. The shape of the head, build of body, way of thinking, organic strengths and weaknesses depend upon one's type – physical, spiritual or intellectual, with many modifications. This is a deep study which cannot be dealt with in a few words.

The *science of dietetics* is lacto-vegetarian in character. Modern methods for the production of milk and eggs make it certain that animal products will be used less and less – it is a matter of individual choice. In pastoral times it was possible to use milk in moderation without involving the slaughter of animals. Food values and combinations are dealt with. Raw foods form a large part of the régime, and in cooking, conservative methods are used to preserve the full vitamin and mineral values.

E

The medicinal use of →herbs, fasting and cleansing treatments are included – together with simple remedies. The balance of the food – between fruits, vegetables, grains and pulses – is important and varies according to the individual's type.

Glandular science: At the beginning of the century Dr Ha'nish was giving information about the endocrine glands which has been confirmed by endocrinologists only in recent years. For the harmonious working of all parts of the body it is essential that every gland should contribute its particular hormones to the bloodstream and certain volatile substances to the brain. It has only lately been realized that the thymus activity in the later years is a valuable factor, for it is part of the immune system. Dr Ha'nish taught that the thymus is the 'gland of youth' and should remain active throughout life, giving one faith, confidence and assurance and keeping one youthful in outlook.

The pineal gland was regarded as a residual organ at the time when Dr Ha'nish described it as the seat of the mind, and the organ through which the higher senses are active. It is the transmitter and receiver of messages conveyed on higher vibrations – like a radio/television transmitter and receiver. Scientists are currently studying this gland.

Exercises using singing or humming on prolonged exhalations while rotating different parts of the body and making various movements, using minimal muscular effort, all stir and activate the glands, enabling them to perform their functions more harmoniously. Daily practice proves their value.

Eugenics is the study of regeneration of the individual, and of procreation. It is of vital importance to the evolution of the human race. The wise choice of a life partner and preparation for parenthood has little place in the usual education of young people; thus they make disastrous mistakes. This must be remedied. Sexual attraction is but one ingredient in a good marriage partnership: there must be common ideals if the home is to be a happy one. Every child should be conceived with conscious thought – not by accident.

→**Prenatal (therapy)** education through the mother's thought, care for the child at birth – not cutting the cord too soon (now realized to be important) – breast feeding, and mother's guidance throughout the early years can ensure that the little one will grow into a valuable member of society. The family is the unit of which society is made; its destruction can destroy our social structure and civilization.

The value of the system outlined has been proved by daily use by associates over many years. There is no aspect of life, individual or collective, which it does not embrace. It makes progress in every field more possible.

Violet Hammerton B.SC., L.T.C.L.

ASSOCIATIONS, p. 213
CONTRIBUTORS, p. 221

MEDICATED BEE VENOM THERAPY

For six generations the medical forebears of my Austrian family evolved and developed a method of treatment by medicated bee venom which I, in turn, assimilated and greatly improved. Long before leaving medical school I was successfully treating patients, including doctors, with my bee venom therapy. Among them were the King of Italy, Professor Beneš of Czechoslovakia (afterwards President), and Professor Pirani, world top inventor of electronics.

During fifty-two years of continuous work I have successfully treated countless patients, all given up by doctors, of ankylosis, osteo- and rheumatoid arthritis, asthma, dermatitis, diabetes, eczema, psoriasis, spondylosis, thyroid deficiency and urticaria. I have had equal success with deafness, myopic retinal degeneration, blindness resulting from childhood ailments such as scarlet fever and measles, and also sufferers from retinitis pigmentosa, which is a form of blindness pronounced untreatable by doctors all over the world. [Since writing this article its author has restored the sight of Rigo Tovar, leader of Mexico's top pop-group, who suffers from retinitis pigmentosa, a chronic hereditary complaint common in Latin America – Ed.]

It is a fallacy that bee-keepers do not suffer from arthritis. After many years of professional bee-keeping they often come to me on crutches, in wheelchairs or invalid tricycles – many from overseas.

I do not use garden bees, whose stings are dangerous. The stings from my bees are not as painful and are absolutely safe. My bees are of special strains, hygienically bred, carefully selected and medically dieted to suit the type of each person's ailment. After I have fed them on the necessary medicaments I pinch the bees behind the head so they are not quite dead but not suffering. I then apply them to the patient. The bees die immediately they have implanted their sting. This type of bee does not produce honey nor large colonies like garden bees. It takes many generations of cultivation to accustom them to feed on various medicaments. They are unable to swallow many medicaments in the form I would like to give them so I have to ferment most of these feeds into fluid and much of the fluid has to be turned into fungi to coax the bees to feed on it.

I must not deplete the colony too much as if the bees get frightened they kill the queen by trying to protect her and I would have no breeding stock. I could not use more than a thousand bees from each colony for treatment as otherwise the colony would be depleted and eventually become extinct. This makes the treatment expensive.

All patients accepted by me are first subjected to blood and urine tests; also, except in eye cases, to X-ray examination. Most of them have to be treated daily which means they have to stay near my home. I work single handed and have many patients, so time is of the essence.

Treatment can last as little as three weeks, but as all my patients come to me only when they have been given up by doctors their treatment can take up to three years. Before I can benefit them I have to rid their systems of all useless and harmful medicaments administered by different doctors.

I have treated both sexes, aged from nine months to ninety-four years. No two cases are alike. The more drugs the patient has had, the more difficult it is for me to treat, and consequently the patient has some adverse reactions. These adverse reactions are not severe, and patients are only too glad that they are recovering. If there is no reaction I do not want the patient because results would not be appreciable.

It will doubtless be asked why my methods are not universally employed. The answer is that nothing is more difficult than to introduce into Great Britain any form of new and unconventional treatment because of the impenetrable opposition of the medical profession. It is worse in other countries.

I am the only person in the world who uses medicated bee venom and I regret that I am now too busy to take patients suffering from most of the ailments I have mentioned – particularly arthritis, which can be a long and time-consuming treatment. I now treat only patients with asthma; deafness, resulting from scarlet fever, measles and other childhood ailments; also sufferers from retinitis pigmentosa.

The success of my treatment for blindness is easy to establish. One has only to witness my previously blind patients driving their cars and walking about using their eyes instead of a white stick. These successes are lasting, as evidenced by people I treated thirty to forty years ago who still see wonderfully. Many of them were pronounced blind by doctors and leading eye specialists.

Doctors talk about cures that are 'just around the corner' – well, I have cut the corners. Here is one tried, tested and proven.

Julia Owen

CONTRIBUTORS, p. 221

MIGRAINE AND TENSION HEADACHE

Migraine is a name given to a collection of symptoms which when put together form a pattern that is recognizable as a specific disorder. There is some disagreement as to which symptoms are eligible for inclusion, but a definition usually accepted for the more severe or 'classical' form is where the characteristic pulsating headache is accompanied by nausea and vomiting, by interference in visual and other sensory input, and where there is difficulty in expression by either speech or movement, or both. So-called 'non-classical' migraine is really a catchment term that sweeps into the same convenient word-net the 90 per cent of cases that show variance in one respect or another from the classical definition. Some people, for example, experience an 'aura' before the attack proper – this includes events that vary a great deal from person to person, but generally speaking there is a feeling of excitement tinged with anxiety, an increase in body weight and swelling due to retention of body fluids, undue sensitivity to noise and light, tension and irritability. Others are not aware of an aura, but find that the attack proper comes on suddenly and unpredictably. So although it would be impossible to list all the symptoms that might be included in an individual migraine pattern, a working definition of migraine is any combination of associated symptoms that includes a tension headache of such severity that it interferes with or interrupts the normal process of living.

There can be no doubt that the physical effects of migraine are due to specific malfunctions of the body mechanism, which can be treated by drug therapy. Similar to those in the engine of a car, body faults can be diagnosed and modified so that there is a return to correct functioning. The tools used, instead of spanners and wrenches, are those drugs that specifically act upon the symptoms presented. But to a greater or lesser extent, they also have side-effects which in turn produce symptoms that are either similar or additional to those which were originally present. For example, the drug ergotamine which acts upon the head-pain mechanism and which is widely used in the control of acute attacks, can produce a vicious spiral of chronic headache and sickness that very much resembles the disorder it is intended to cure. Many of the psychotropic drugs prescribed for the relief of the tension have side-effects that include drowsiness, disorientation and mental confusion. But even if the pharmacological tools at our disposal were perfect, a purely mechanistic approach would still lead to total dependence upon their continued use. By treating and re-treating the same recurring symptoms, you put yourself in the same position as if you were to keep returning your car to the mechanic because the *same* parts *repeatedly* went wrong. Would you happily accept that situation, the inconvenience and loss of use involved? Instead, you would consider the possibility that factors might be involved which, although affecting the mechanism, originate from outside it. Such as the driver, for instance. Certainly in a limited sense we can be regarded as mechanisms, of a complexity that is infinitely higher than anything that can be made by man. But if we construct a model of ourselves as *nothing but* a complex of mechanical systems, then we assume not only that we have no influence upon malfunctions in those systems, but also that we are dependent upon outside help that is less than totally effective.

Current research into the wider field of the relationship between our emotions, perceptions and feelings on the one hand and body malfunctions on the other, points inescapably to the conclusion that migraine and tension headache, in common with other so-called psychosomatic disorders, are closely linked with emotional suppression and resultant anxiety. In Holland, work initiated recently at the Institute of Unitive Psychology on organic tension has shown how the energy invested in maintaining the tension originates from blocked feelings and emotions. This forms the basis of a therapeutic approach that treats mind and body, psyche and soma, as an integrated whole. It utilizes methods and techniques derived from phenomenological and →gestalt psychology, existential psychotherapy and biodynamics (→bioenergy and biodynamics) to uncover the origins of the physical tension and pain. Whether the process turns out to be short or long depends upon the rate at which each individual is prepared to travel in what amounts to a journey of self-exploration and discovery, so that he or she can re-live, re-experience and finally come to understand and to resolve the inner conflicts that originated during infancy, childhood or puberty, and which lie at the root of the migraine. The format can either be that of a series of individual sessions or group seminars (usually limited to fifteen people) with an appropriately experienced psychologist or psychotherapist. Individual sessions obviously tend initially to cost more, and many people prefer to join the group seminars, which create an atmosphere of mutual understanding and support during a transitional period. Once undergone, the therapy to an increasing extent can be self-applied, and therefore does not lead to a dependence upon continued treatment.

That there is a growing demand in this country for this alternative approach to the age-old problems of migraine and tension headache is largely due to the way in which it facilitates changes in perception that can lead to a more satisfying, fulfilling and tension-free way of life. Though it is often used initially as a supplement to drug or diet-based therapy, in many cases it eventually obviates the need for these treatments.

Charles Bentley M.A.

CONTRIBUTORS, p. 222

MULTIPLE SCLEROSIS

Roger MacDougall was a leading British playwright and film-writer in the early fifties. Then in February 1953 he was diagnosed as suffering from multiple sclerosis. Within a few years he was almost completely paralysed, his voice was affected and he was virtually blind. Through a process of self-experimentation he adopted a diet which at first stabilized his symptoms and then slowly brought about an improvement in his health. It took fifteen years before he achieved his present state of

fitness. Now in his late sixties he leads a normal active life.

He based his efforts towards recovery on the assumption that multiple sclerosis is caused by a chemical imbalance which results in the body being unable to create replacement tissue for the myelin layers surrounding the nerves. He felt that the disease might be controllable by an adjustment of diet which would correct the imbalance. As a result he adopted a dietary régime which excluded gluten (a substance found in the flour of wheat, rye, barley and oats), which was low in sugars and animal fats and high in unsaturated fats. Vegetables, fruits and fresh fish were included in the diet. To ensure that the restrictions involved did not result in a deficiency of vitamins or minerals he devised a vitamin and mineral supplement to make good any such deficiencies. Mr MacDougall explains that his diet is not a cure but a control and has to be rigidly adhered to at all times.

Another dietary approach to multiple sclerosis is that of the West German physician Dr Joseph Evers, founder of the only clinic in the world to specialize in the treatment of the disease. Dr Evers has published results of his successful treatments. The diet he gives patients, which is not gluten-free, includes raw fruits, root vegetables, raw milk, raw eggs, raw rolled oats, honey and water. Sprouted seeds and raw fermented foods are also given.

John Newton

BIBLIOGRAPHY, p. 248
CONTRIBUTORS, p. 222

MUSIC THERAPY

The therapeutic value of music has been recognized from time immemorial and used throughout the world in magic, religion and medicine. Magicians used music in their rites to cast out the spirits of disease; music carried to the deity the prayers of the man sick in mind or body; the ancient philosophers believed in the action of music on the behaviour of man. In the eighteenth century medical men began to study the effects of music on bodily functions and on the mood of their patients. Today music therapy has become a discipline of its own and is related to the recent trends of physiological and psychological medicine in many countries of the old and new worlds.

Man is a resonant body able to perceive and emit sounds. Sound, or music which is made of sounds, makes a powerful effect on him. It can penetrate at different levels of consciousness and provoke many physical, mental and psychological responses. Music is man's creation and answers his basic need to organize his experiences and make them meaningful. This need still exists in the most disorderly or disintegrated being, who can benefit from the elements of safety and predictability which exist in music. The vibrations of sound create a two-way communication from within and without.

Music therapy works on the four elements contained in any sound, pitch, duration, tone colour and volume. They are present in any music. Each of them affects the patient in a specific manner, irrespective of his musical ability or education. The response to music is individual even when it has been conditioned by education and prejudice.

Single musical experiences affect the whole man, his mind, body and emotions, music therapy uses them as an integrating force, as well as a means of communication at any level of intelligence or education. A musical experience often reveals in the patient some affinity with a specific sound, with an instrument, with a tune or a rhythm which indicates the way he relates to music and can identify with it, whether he listens to or makes music himself.

There are two main techniques in music therapy, the receptive and the active methods, complementary to one another. Both aim at opening channels of communication with people whose ability to communicate has been impaired or lost through illness or handicap: the paralysed, the psychotic, geriatric, spastic, →**autistic,** and the subnormal who have lost or never had the ability to relate normally

to the world around them. Music therapy can help them to communicate and to restore or develop means of perceptual, physical or mental contacts necessary to communication, or help them to find compensatory means or substitute for what they cannot have.

In the active method, the patient is engaged in making music, singing or playing an instrument, whose technique may be at the most elementary level. The experience involves physical and mental activity, sensory motor control in time and space which should be developed as much as possible. Even on a single sound, the patient can express feelings of anger, fear, timidity, hatred or sweetness. The method is not to teach him but to leave him play as spontaneously as possible. Then he can without fear let out in a socially acceptable and non-verbal way unspeakable feelings he should become aware of.

Active techniques help the physically affected patient to use whatever movement he can make and to develop a better sensory motor control. Music generally provokes a strong activation towards movement of any kind and can be of special assistance in physical rehabilitation. It can give to the patient a sense of achievement which can be measured and assessed, built on slow but well-graded progress, within the limits imposed by the handicap. Compensatory means or substitutes can be provided by music if it becomes an individual means of self-expression and a pursuit to be followed in a satisfactory way under the direction of the therapist.

In the receptive method, the patient is a listener to music. It can effect a change of mood or behaviour in the patient, provided that the music is chosen for the purpose. It should be of the kind that the patient can relate to at the time and reflect his actual state of mind and body. Soft music is not soothing to an agitated patient, nor can gay music make him feel less depressed. Contact must be made first before any change of mood can be expected.

When the patient identifies with a strong musical impact, he may experience a catharsis, as was witnessed in ancient Greece or in the rites of the Tarantella. The experience helps the patient to get rid of unbearable tension. The beauty and harmony of great music can help the patient to communicate with deep human feelings. He can also relate to other people through sharing the common experience of listening to music.

Receptive techniques are often linked with psychiatric treatment through the unconscious process which takes place when the patient listens to music which leads to the expression of buried emotions. It works on the immense power of penetration and association of sound. Music can sink into the subconscious, hidden and forgotten until some kind of association brings it up to consciousness, still charged with the same emotion. The discharge of such feelings may bring much relief to the patient, and is in any case valuable material for the psychiatrist. Music therapy is sometimes the only means to operate a breakthrough with a non-communicating patient.

Music is a social art, and music therapy can be one of the best means of social rehabilitation with any kind of patient, children or adults. It unites them and provokes communication within an accepted situation. The experience is a shared one in which the discipline is imposed by the music itself. It helps patients to relate, to feel useful and needed by the group, to have responsibility and to possess their own identity through the part they have to play on their own instrument, or to sing with their own voice. Musical abilities vary considerably in such a group, and great musical and psychological skills are needed to make it truly therapeutic, and not just recreational.

The music therapist is not a teacher, but a musician who shares musical experiences with the patient, sometimes in a one-to-one relationship, or with the whole group. He or she is a member of the therapeutic team who treats the patient in various ways. Rarely can one of the para-medical therapies claim to have effected a cure by itself. But when music therapy cannot deal directly with the disorder itself, as would be in surgical cases, it can deal with the psychological, mental or social consequences of the illness or handicap and bring comfort to the patient. Music therapy is one of the most noble functions of music. It works on an immense range of human responses to the elusive substance of sound embodied in positive and concrete experience.

The training in music therapy is undertaken in several countries, including Great Britain where the Guildhall School of Music and Drama, in association with the British Society for Music Therapy, offers a diploma course leading to recognized qualification in the subject. Meetings at national and international level have taken place in the last twenty years. There is a large bibliography of publications on music therapy.

Juliette Alvin F.G.S.M., M.T.

ASSOCIATIONS, p. 213
BIBLIOGRAPHY, p. 248
CONTRIBUTORS, p. 222
TRAINING, p. 232

NATURAL CHILDBIRTH

The aim is to enable pregnancy and birth to proceed with the minimum of interference. For this the mother needs to be confident, aware and responsible. Help is given to prepare a mother in understanding the bodily changes and emotional experiences of pregnancy; to become aware of her responsibility to herself and the developing baby; and so to be an active participant rather than a patient, so that the birth experience is one of total fulfilment for mother and child.

With the acceptance of pregnancy the couple need to make plans early, deciding whether to have the baby at home or in hospital. At home the mother is more relaxed in familiar surroundings and with freedom to do as she wishes. In hospital she is a 'guest' and is required to conform to rules and procedures. For medical, social and practical reasons a home birth may not always be possible. Mothers may not always feel confident that this is what they want. They may not even be aware that the choice exists, especially in the case of a first pregnancy.

For a home birth the mother's choice of doctor and midwife is very important. They must be people with whom she feels relaxed, free to express herself, and in whom there is trust and understanding. A bond is made between mother and midwife enabling her to grow without fear through the pregnancy.

Relaxation is the first lesson. Many women worry that they will be unable to relax; that it requires a special sort of muscle control which they have to achieve during labour. This is not so. If the woman attends a good antenatal class she will learn techniques of breathing, singing and simple exercises. With this the muscle contractions during labour can be experienced without tension, and the body is in harmony with the activity of the uterus.

As the baby grows and the figure changes the mother needs to pay particular attention to the way she sits, stands and moves, taking care not to strain the joints and muscles or to move clumsily. She needs to allow changes in the patterns of her movements and posture and so prevent strain and backache. For some mothers practising prenatal →yoga, the →Alexander technique and some →Tai-chi sequences has been helpful in learning to let go. Letting go relieves pressure on the internal organs, creating balance and stillness in the mother so that she is more in touch with the baby. It releases tension in the pelvic region, preparing muscles that will open the birth canal. Care must be taken to avoid over-eating as this can hinder both pregnancy and labour. In general, the mother *must* be in good health. She must be prepared to give up some of her activities in the later months of pregnancy so that she can have sufficient rest.

One of the biggest steps women have to take is to overcome fear – fear of pain, fear of the unknown. In the early months there are often anxieties that the baby will be deformed, that the mother herself will die during labour, and that the labour will be very painful. Old wives' tales add to these anxieties. In addition the mother-to-be may worry that she will become fat and unattractive to her partner. Fear and anxiety are transferred to the baby in the womb and must be worked through with the support of the father, midwife and the doctor. Spontaneous and gentle love-making helps the couple in releasing tension, and men need reassurance that they will not harm the baby. In the later months there are positions best avoided but the doctor and midwife will advise.

The father and any children should be encouraged to participate in antenatal examinations by feeling the baby's position and listening to its heart beating. In this way the whole family is preparing for the birth and strengthening bonds.

With the understanding that the baby is ready to leave the mother the work of labour begins. The mother's attitude during the first stage affects the way she experiences the pain of contractions. If she is afraid, tense or exhausted the muscles are no longer in harmony with the movements of the baby and she experiences great pain. On the other hand, she can remain calm, walking around freely and using any relaxation methods she has learned. In this way there is instinctive cooperation between mother and baby. Pain is recognized as natural, and birth can become a wonderful experience without the mask of drugs.

Once the head is born the mother can be instructed by the midwife to lift the baby onto her abdomen. It is important to pause at this moment to allow the baby to experience its first sensations in the world and through eye contact for the mother and baby to say hello. The baby needs time to go from one experience to another in an unhurried way. Sensitivity to what it is experiencing is essential; harsh light and noise can shock the baby and stop the gentle awakening of its senses. The cord remains uncut until it ceases to function and the baby is ready to separate from the mother. Babies are naked and vulnerable and need the most gentle handling by as few people as possible. Skin contact between mother and baby is essential at this moment. If the baby lies on the mother for at least the first half hour of its life it will feel secure, whilst the mother experiences an instinctive maternal bond which lasts a life-time.

To ease the transition into the world the baby can be placed in a warm bath of water. This helps free its body of tension and allows expression of movement. The father can be instructed in bathing the baby and holding it against his chest afterwards – skin to skin. The baby is then given back to the mother to suckle and rest.

A number of conditions have been outlined as essential to enable childbirth to be natural; a healthy body; a preparation and education of the mother for pregnancy, labour and motherhood; self-understanding on the part of the mother; good relationships within the family and with midwife and doctor; and a sensitivity to what the baby is experiencing at birth.

Margo Hogan s.r.n., s.c.m.

ASSOCIATIONS, pp. 216, 217, 219
BIBLIOGRAPHY, p. 245
CONTRIBUTORS, p. 222

NATURISM

The benefits of nude swimming and sunbathing are almost exclusively psychological. Some proponents argue physical benefits. Sun on skin produces Vitamin D. But you can get all the sun you need wearing a bikini, so why strip completely?

There is only one answer: it makes you feel good. Letting fresh air get everywhere is exhilarating. There is no quicker way of feeling ten years younger. And surprisingly it is very relaxing. That may seem odd since most non-nudists become nervous at even the thought of undressing in public. Yet once over the initial hurdle a deep, beautiful peace will surely sweep through you. As the last vestige goes so does a lifetime of conditioned tension.

You are bound to notice how many people have operation scars and other imperfections. This is where nudism makes for healthier, more balanced thinking. It is not the end of the world for a woman to have a caesarean scar, nor for some men to have one testicle lower than the other. You begin to see people as people, not as packaged symbols of people. Deformity, middle-age-spreads, breasts that no longer point forward like dainty door knobs, are all part of life. When you have seen one set of genitals you have seen them all, so you start looking at people's faces.

Naturist children develop a special kind of confidence. Around puberty some youngsters, through raised in naturism, suddenly develop shyness. Go easy on them. They grow out of it in a year or two. *Nudist Society*, an American study published by Crown Publishing Inc. of New York, asserts that the incidence of delinquency is significantly smaller in children from naturist families.

Historically the clothes obsession is new. The Greeks did not suffer from it. Neither did the Romans until the fourth century, just before their decline. The first prosecution in Britain for nude sea-bathing was not until the early nineteenth century. Naturism as an organized movement began in Europe early this century, first in Germany. In Britain there are now one or two remote beaches where the police turn a blind eye, but clubs are everywhere. In the more developed European countries huge beaches are set aside for naturism. Yugoslavia has enormous motel-complexes. France offers nudist-villages and four-star hotels. You can cruise in naked luxury from Hamburg to New York in a special German liner. In the U.S.A. you can live, retire, work, go to school, get married, and fly around your private airplane in great nudist parks.

Dr Auguste Rollier in Switzerland took sunbathing very seriously. Thousands of people went to his clinic at Leysin where controlled sunbathing was part of his rejuvenation programme.

Never forget that the sun can burn. The right amount will leave you feeling great. Too much can actually kill you. Take it easy. Relax. Above all, enjoy!

C. M. Hills

ASSOCIATIONS, p. 214

NATUROPATHY

'Vis medicatrix naturae' (HIPPOCRATES, the Father of Medicine, 400 B.C.).

If one can grasp the meaning of Hippocrates' reference to the life-force, the healing power present in all living things, one comes close to understanding the essence of naturopathy in the light of which all its principles and therapeutic methods form a clear, common-sense approach to self-healing. It is the inherent tendency of living cells to function towards the good of the whole body, which in turn works towards the maintenance of healthy cells and the rejection of waste products.

Animals in their natural environment are rarely diseased, instinctively choosing when and what to eat, feeling their surroundings as an ecological whole and responding to them accordingly, reflecting Nature's laws of cause and effect without question. Occasionally finding themselves deviated from this balanced state probably due to the interference of man, they stop and listen to Nature's guiding voice, letting the life-force renew their bodies by seeking solitude and fasting.

Nature cure may be described as a way of life in which man also opens his awareness to these energy processes and shares with the animals a harmony within himself and his environment and is thus able to live a healthy life, though the present end-effect of so-called scientific technology is one of pollution. The nature-cure lifestyle requires no external therapeutics as such, since a healthy body is self-balancing and self-healing, elimination being carried out to ensure freedom from the build-up of waste which provides the breeding ground for nearly all disease.

When man falls away from his natural path, symptoms appear and provide painful signals, warning him to reflect upon how he is the creator of his condition.

Nature cure probably originates from a time when man was a fully instinctive creature and natural healing was a part of everyday life. Recent history illustrates a new revival. Before Hippocrates' time the healing priests of the Aesculapian Order established temples of healing, often near mineral waters or hot springs which were used therapeutically along with fasting and massage. Healing water, widely used by the Romans for social and therapeutic purposes, was partly absorbed into orthodox medicine when the medical profession took control of the Roman baths at Bath, but hydrotherapy was originated in its own right in the early 1800s in Germany as a water-cure by Vincent Priessnitz and developed by Kneipp, leading to the emergence of distinct naturopathic centres such as those seen today.

Naturopathy embraces all the therapeutic methods by which the human organism may be guided back to its original state of wholeness. Essentially it aims at freeing and restoring the life-force by natural means. In this light specific diagnosis becomes less significant, for while allopathy names and attempts to suppress symptoms, naturopathy seeks to recognize and remove the causes of these symptoms, seeing them in the form of blockages to the energy-flow originating within the body. These blockages may occur at various levels of the functioning body and reflections in the individual emotions will be revealed to the perceptive eye.

There is no such thing as specific disease as an entity other than the apparent condition which manifests temporarily in the body as a result of one, or a series of these blockages. Disease really means dis-ease or ill-at-ease.

Naturopathy is primarily concerned with wholeness and balance, and the principle that only health can result from such a state of being. The parts of the body are seen not as separate but as interdependent aspects in relationships forming the whole, the quality of each part affecting the whole and vice versa. The naturopath attempts to restore the wholeness so that the life-force may flow fully. To do this he aims at purifying the system by removing obstructions and the causes of the 'diseased' condition.

The approach to health is made on all levels; one adjusts the diet, corrects any structural imbalance such as spinal osteopathic lesions which prevent the innervation and subsequent well-being of the corresponding organ, and attempts to bring to the subject's awareness light on psycho-emotional tendencies affecting the body.

The removal of toxic waste products which constitute the main cause of ill-health is encouraged by fasting, hydrotherapy, Vitamin-C-containing fruit juices, →osteopathy and massage. The next step is to restore the vitality of the tissues by means of diet, with possible supplementary vitamins and minerals previously deficient, proper elimination, abstention from harmful substances, i.e. bad food, suppressive drugs, tobacco, alcohol and other stimulants; and psycho-emotional reintegration.

The most direct route to health by elimination of unwanted waste matter is by fasting or abstention from all foods for varying periods during which only water is drunk, though in a less severe régime diluted juices of freshly squeezed fruits are used, being cleansing to the system and containing Vitamin C which assists with the catabolic or breaking down process of metabolism.

Left free from the anabolic or building-up processes concerned with ingested food, the gastro-intestinal system has a chance to rest, enabling the body to focus its energies on clearing out its waste residues accumulated over the years through stress, eating adulterated, unwholesome foods, lack of exercise and so on; these are released from the tissues into the circulation to be eliminated through the appropriate organs: the kidneys, bowels, lungs and skin. This sudden release brings about the fasting syndrome and the subject should be warned about these early stages of fever, nausea, headaches, diarrhoea, depressions and fatigue as long-suppressed symptoms are brought to the surface, manifesting in darkening urine, foul breath and sweating. These symptoms should be welcomed as the unburdening of past mistakes and these healing crises will pass if the fast is endured, leaving the individual purified and filled with new vitality.

These eliminative processes are encouraged by assisting Nature with hydrotherapy to further release through the skin by the various applications of hot and cold water, and with the warm-water enema to stimulate and assist the activity of the bowels.

Fot those aware of the principles of nature cure, therapy may be carried out at home; otherwise guidance is essential. The longer the preceding unbalanced state or the older the patient the more gradually should one enter into a fast, building up the vitality beforehand with cleansing diets previously discussed with the consulting naturopath.

On the other hand the younger individual as a rule has a far higher level of vitality to begin with and may launch straight into the fast, though in all cases great care should be taken when breaking the fast, making a gradual return and building up to a balanced diet. Children, so much closer to their natural instinct, nearly always automatically fast when sick, and having good vitality quickly return to health.

These observations lead up to the naturopathic principle concerning acute and chronic states and how the suppression of the acute symptoms of childhood with drugs and/or superfluous or harmful food, only drives the poisonous waste deeper into the system to emerge later in a different form. This continued suppression leads to chronic conditions with an associated reduction in vitality. Acute conditions include fevers, colds, diarrhoea, skin eruptions, inflammation and scarlet fever and are all signs of vitality trying to manifest through the body; whilst chronic ones are bronchitis, valvular disorder of the heart, diabetes, kidney disease and rheumatism.

Misguided surgery may often be a cause of chronic disease, e.g. tonsilectomy where the orthodox school has confused the tonsils with the causative factor of the condition and removed them, whereas the real cause of tonsilitis is systemic, an imbalance of the organism as a whole, reflecting as a focus of infection in the tonsils of which the inflammation is the body's attempt at elimination.

This example exposes a basic underlying difference between alternative medicine and allopathy. The general practitioner approaches the infected part at a chemical level, destroying much toxic substance but also damaging organisms present in every healthy body essential for the maintenance of health and balance of vital fluids. The body now has to get rid of this unusable drug as well as its already unwanted load. On the other hand the naturopath takes a view of the system as a whole with its interdependent parts in relationship, seeks the underlying causes at work and removes them.

During the course of the fast, then, symptoms long suppressed in the past may rise to the surface in reverse order to that in which previous ignorance initiated them; the inherent vitality works through each corresponding organ in turn until all obstructions to health are cleared. At this turning point the individual may start afresh, maintaining a high level of positive health providing that he lives along the lines of a nature-cure lifestyle and that he has also rid himself of the self-destructive habits, mental or dietary, which originally led to his downfall.

It is as well to be aware that the continued intake of synthetically manufactured substances, especially sugar, excessive meat, alcohol, tobacco, all white flour and white sugar products, and all suppressive drugs, lead to nearly all the conditions found in today's hospitals, where the healing processes of acute conditions are not recognized as beneficial and are suppressed, later to become chronic.

Naturopathic education is brought mostly to public awareness through diet with the present-day popularity of →**vegetarian** wholefood restaurants and →**health food** shops, whilst ways of fasting are less widely known, being sought after by the more intent seekers of health, a term that many consider as merely a state where they are not stricken with an actual disease.

No specific diet may be detailed here. Personal guidance from a naturopath is much more practical and individually suitable. But the emphasis is on wholeness, retaining as much of the life-force of food as possible between its extraction from the environment and its consumption. Therefore fresh green leafy vegetables, preferably those organically grown, are recommended; a certain proportion should be eaten in the raw state or as close to it as possible. Fruit and vegetables are eaten along with whole grains, beans and their products, with the addition of proteins as individually required, bearing in mind that most of the necessary requirements may be found in grains and vegetables, despite so much misguided publicity about the apparent necessity of so much meat and starchy foods.

One has to understand that the energy derived from eating does not increase with the amount consumed. The energy with which we express life is the result of the interaction between the life force working through the metabolic processes in the individual and the life-force inherent in the food; therefore too much food merely clogs the system, dampening the vitality, rendering the consumer weak and lethargic until a suitable period of abstention allows the digestive system to work through this burden. On the other hand, eating the correct amount of food in balanced ratio gives the human organism the greatest performance.

This amount and ratio is a matter of individual choice, for it is only one's intuitive self-examination that can determine a factor which may be of great help, but to be healthy one has to listen to one's inner voice and to be receptive to the guiding feelings constantly changing within the body. Basically we all have the knowledge of what we should and should not eat and do; it is a matter of tuning into it and distinguishing it from all the other external stimuli which crowd modern-day living. When the keen initiate of nature cure finds within himself the energy source which permeates every level of his being and links him with all living things, then he will know what and when to eat and how to live. He will have no desire to inhibit this wonderful state of well-being with any harmful substances. He will have developed a healthy desire for that food and life which is good and an automatic discrimination as to what is unusable. Such a man needs no physician, being his own self-balancing self-healing organism.

Naturopathy is therefore mainly concerned with the prevention of disease by means of education in nature cure to maintain a maximum level of health through correct living, eating and thinking; and it encourages the growth of an ever-widening awareness of the cosmic harmony.

Nigel P. Castle

NEOMETAPHYSICAL CONCEPTS OF PSYCHOLOGY

Neometaphysics, as an infinitely based general system, seeks fundamental principles underlying all human experience and presents a coherent science constructed from these general principles and their inter-relationships. Each principle is verified for generality by ensuring that it remains true within all spheres of action one may contemplate and for all time; that is, each principle is infinitely based in space and in time. The inter-relationships and interdependence of fundamental laws give rise to a simple system wherein the dynamics of all changes of state become apparent, so not only is a pure state of infinitely based law observed, but also the processes governing its manifestation. Thus we gain a logical system empirically based upon both mental and physical experience and of use as a high probability tool in any form of problem-solving, be it in the physical sciences or the so-called transcendental ones.

Some of the more important fields of application lie within the spiritual, mental, parapsychological and paraphysical sciences and clear methods of application are perceivable in political, economic, business, governmental and many other everyday structures. These do not exclude physical science and, in fact, the growth of any science is a consequence of its unification with other data sources and the magnitude of its empirical information.

By a process of 'neometaphysical translation' from the 'pure' statement of Law to the 'relative' or conditional statement, neometaphysics is applicable to any field of inquiry.[1] One of the more important studies of neometaphysicians at the present time is to seek ways and means to understand and so promote mental health; to increase the awareness within an evolving and harmonious environment. Neometaphysical translations from fundamental energy studies into psychological spheres reveal fascinating new modes of psychological exploration.

In an optimum mode of life wherein mental health was at a 'maximum possible' level, the understanding by the individual of himself and his fellows within an infinite and eternal state, temporarily limited by physical environments, would be a constant, conscious experience, his reactions to his environment being generally instinctive, rather than inhibited by the shortcomings of formal learning and enforced law. Yet these instinctive reactions would be capable of easy analysis at any time, should conscious evaluation be necessary. Such evaluation, without a unified system, would require a knowledge of many different subjects, far beyond the learning and intellectual powers of any person. In fact, such intense study of itself would constitute an inhibitive danger to the freedom of the mind. One simple general system, being a synthesis of all others, completely meets such requirements. Synthesis of the many general systems is vital and in the act of synthesis a statement of fundamental law appears which one can readily comprehend and apply without a lifetime's study. The very simplicity of neometaphysics and its utterly generalized structure make it an ideal method of gaining answers to any problems. More important, the actual perception itself of fundamental laws constitutes the best possible therapy against psychological impediment because of the ease of application of fundamental concepts in the solution of personal problems.

The postulates of mental energy formed into patterns which are of varying magnitudes and states; energy in a constant state of change and which, by multi-dimensional resonances, transfers various modes from state to state, and many other energic concepts well established in formal science, lead to a new approach into the nature of the psyche and its functioning. Insight is gained into the internal structure and function of the psyche as well as the external mental-energy environment wherein the psyche functions.

A unit of mental energy may be called a 'psychon', when it refers to the living mind; and an awareness of the characteristics of any singly perceived mental fact, requiring conceptual ability, suggests the term 'conceptuon' for a unit of organized mental energy.

Translating from energic fundamentals one may then postulate a force, an opposition, a type of change caused or work done, a flow, a rate of flow, and indeed all other fundamental processes of energy in action. The units flowing, doing work and so on, being 'psychons' or 'conceptuons' according to the depth of one's inquiry.

The implications of such translations to physicists well acquainted with energy processes and neometaphysics will be immediately apparent. The requirements for transfer of energy by resonance, wherein the 'transmitter' and 'receiver' must possess the same energic structure in order for a transfer to occur, shows how communication of complex energy patterns takes place. The amount of mental energy and its intensity govern the nature and intensity of awareness. For example, the psyche may be said to possess 100 per cent mental energy, about 98 per cent may be 'held' in problems in the mind, some 1 per cent or more also withheld by the awareness of the physical sense-data, leaving a very small measure of one's total energy for creative purposes. A very small improvement in one's mental environment will result in a large proportionate increase in 'free' mental energy and creative ability. The restraint placed upon human unity and progress by psychological obstruction is of appalling proportion. Meditative practices can, therefore, temporarily release mental energy for use; either for a higher level of mental activity or for a

widened field of perception. The enhanced ability to engage in mental activity and the improved faculty of scanning a wider area of data, in themselves, enabling many previously insoluble problems to be eliminated. Similarly, harmonious art forms, contact with tranquillity in Nature, the experience of spiritually based physical love, bring the identification of fundamental laws into the psyche, minimize mental activity, enhance one's creative ability and provide fundamental data in therapeutic form.

Mental energy is not restricted to one individual or the other but, by its nature, is shared by all. The same theories gained by neometaphysical translation remain true and at once cast great functional light upon such matters as group experience, formation of higher 'group minds', telepathy, clairvoyance, clairaudience, astral projection, →**radiesthesia**, psycho-kinetics, and indeed all parapsychological and paraphysical phenomena. The mental energy theories also cover the old 'magicks', throw light upon mystical experience, give solutions to bio-plasmic energy forms, can account for the manner in which energy patterns can be created at will and projected to a 'dimensional location' to produce some pre-determined effect. In producing bio-plasmic and psycho-kinetic effects a restructuring of mental energy into forms able to manifest (resonate) in the mode required at its new location is gained. This re-location and re-structuring requires new concepts of 'dimensional transformation processes': the mind and the will (mental potential) creating such transformations. Such an experimental technique lies in 'thought photography' – or changing the state of ionization of a photographic film by the imposition of a mental image.

We find that not only are many new therapeutic techniques made available by development of new modes of psychology through neometaphysical translation, but also that the actual study of neometaphysics itself constitutes such an optimum therapy. The perception of any fundamental law is simultaneously the perception of solutions to all problems caused by the previous non-perception of that principle. Many neometaphysical concepts are gained with a vast release of mental energy, due to the mass solution of similar basic mental problems and this increase in awareness is consistent with the mechanism of revelation and deep religious experience.

John J. Williamson
D.SC. (H.C.), F.S.M., M.Brit.I.R.E., F.C.G.L.I.

ASSOCIATIONS, p. 218
BIBLIOGRAPHY, p. 248
CONTRIBUTORS, p. 222

Note

1. New terminology has had to be developed to prefix any study re-presented from the standpoint of neometaphysics as a consequence of translation, with the word 'neo' (Greek, *neo*, new). Thus, psychology seen from the standpoint of neometaphysics becomes 'neopsychology'; physics becomes 'neophysics', and so on.

ORTHOMOLECULAR PSYCHIATRY

The term orthomolecular psychiatry (or megavitamin therapy) was introduced in 1968 by the American scientist, Professor Linus Pauling, 1945 Nobel prize-winner in chemistry. It has been defined as 'the treatment of mental disease by the provision of the optimum molecular environment for the mind, especially the optimum concentration of substances normally present in the human body'. The guiding principle followed in the method is that the mind's functioning is dependent on the nutritional and chemical state of the brain and that in a variety of conditions large doses of vitamins, particularly the B vitamins, together with other therapy where necessary, can improve the brain's functioning.

Although orthomolecular psychiatry began as a treatment for schizophrenia (treating it as a disease of chemical imbalance), the conditions now being treated cover a much wider field and include anxiety and depression. The child psychiatrist, Dr Allan Cott, reported in the American journal *Schizophrenia* that he

had treated 500 children over a period of five years suffering from childhood psychoses, hyperactivity and brain injury, with the orthomolecular approach, and found that this treatment showed greater promise than any other he had tried.

John Newton

BIBLIOGRAPHY, p. 249
CONTRIBUTORS, p. 222

OSTEOPATHY

As a result of its remarkable successes in the treatment of back pain and so-called 'slipped discs', osteopathy has become a household word. Unfortunately, because of its reputation in this one class of ailments, its scope of action has tended to narrow down conversely with its increase in popularity. Orthodox medically trained osteopaths largely promulgate this concept, i.e. a system of manipulation, adjunctive to orthodox medicine, with its main field of action in orthopaedics and rheumatology which as such provides a more successful approach to such conditions than do the accepted orthodox techniques, thus filling a blank spot in classical medical practice. It will be seen, however, that the practice of osteopathy according to this concept, whilst providing a much-needed service to the general public, is nevertheless very limited and far removed from that of the founder of osteopathy.

It is interesting to note that the much wider scope and clinical possibilities of osteopathy, especially in the field of much functional disease, is often wrongly attributed by allopathic medicine to psychogenic factors. The clinical experience of osteopaths often show to the contrary that traumata and their clinical sequelae are commonly responsible. Trauma engenders mechanical disturbances and imbalance, particularly in the pelvic, spinal and cranial fields, thus giving rise, particularly in sensitive subjects, to abnormal reflex patterns which can express themselves in terms of autonomic nervous system, neuro-hormonal and neuro-circulatory dysfunctions of various kinds. These clinical possibilities have been well discussed and described in terms of the then prevalent basic sciences in the early osteopathic textbooks, but adequate scientific explanation was sometimes lacking for the simple reason that many of them were written over half a century ago. A modern and scientifically up-to-date literature has now become available. For example, *Osteopathic Medicine* by Drs Hoag, Cole and Bradford, published by McGraw-Hill, is a contemporary work that should be read by everyone who is seriously interested in learning about the wider scope of osteopathic practice.

A number of publications particularly emphasizing osteopathy as a system of medicine with a wide field of clinical application are now available from the publishers, The Maidstone Osteopathic Clinic. Osteopathy is therefore applicable to:

The diverse structural problems arising in and affecting the musculo-skeletal system itself, e.g. low-back pain and sciatica; brachial, appendicular, muscular and ligamentous problems, headaches of mechanical origin, post-surgical conditions, etc., which classically come within the purview of orthopaedic medicine.

In addition it can be exceedingly helpful in the considerable field of functional, or rather as they are more commonly known today as 'psychosomatic', diseases. Sometimes they are, of course, but in the clinical experience of osteopaths practising according to original and wider concepts of the founder of the system, Dr A. T. Still, they are more often not. Some common conditions coming under this heading are: →**migraine** and reflex headaches of various origins, asthma, functional heart problems, gastric-ulcer, various gut disturbances, and what patients often describe as 'nerves'.

More established chronic problems which although manifesting pathology as such, nevertheless are characterized by a considerable functional element, e.g. chronic bronchitis, sinusitis and heart disease.

Some of the conditions that come within the

aegis of the medical specialities, gynaecology, ophthalmology and ear, nose and throat. Many occupational and industrial hazard complaints that affect the musculo-skeletal system and that cause the loss of many man-hours of work. Osteopathy is also effective in some acute diseases, but is seldom applied in this respect for the simple reason that (i) the public are unaware of its potentialities in this respect and (ii) most osteopathic practices are widespread and operate more on a consultative than a domicilary basis.

It should be particularly noted that osteopathy is not a substitute for medicine and/or surgery, although it is often an effective alternative in the above-mentioned conditions where allopathic medicine is either ineffective or less effective.

Patients normally attend osteopaths in private practice, or at the several clinics for persons of limited means which exist up and down the country. Since osteopaths have no statutory recognition and practise under Common Law, their services are not available within the National Health Service (see Foreword, p. 11). Copies of directories of qualified osteopaths may be obtained from The Society of Osteopaths Ltd, Osteopathic Education and Research Ltd (European Osteopathic Register), General Council and Register of Osteopaths Ltd, whose members designate themselves M.S.O., M.E.O.R., and M.R.O. respectively. Unfortunately Common Law allows anyone qualified or unqualified to call themselves an osteopath. In consequence several thousand people of indeterminate ability practise osteopathy and other forms of manipulative therapy under the guise of osteopathy. Unfortunately there is no way of knowing whether they are competent or not. The public, however, may be assured that an osteopath in one of the directories mentioned above is adequately qualified to a known and determinate standard of training. Membership of these three groups jointly represents about 500 practitioners, approximately 450 of whom are practising in the U.K.

Osteopathy is applicable to all age groups of either sex. Old people's troubles, women's complaints and problems of growth and development in children have particular emphasis respectively. Elderly people, although often incurable as far as their chronic ailment may be concerned, can frequently be maintained, reasonably pain-free and comfortably functioning during the last years of their lives. Children equally may be helped to achieve adulthood, with their spines and other structures in good developmental and mechanical condition, thus minimizing the possibility of mediocre or even ill-health in later life.

Osteopathy originated in the U.S.A. just over a century ago. The founder, Dr Andrew Taylor Still, born in 1830, was the son of a clergyman who also practised medicine. In his autobiography, Still, who studied engineering for five years, explains how he started to examine the human body as if it were a machine, paying attention to all the various anomalies of the different parts and comparing them with all the different devices used in engineering. He approached the human body in the same way as an engineer sets about finding out all the defects that impair smooth running and functioning, in order to prove his theory that the human body could suffer all sorts of mechanical disturbances which might eventually cause disease.

Still's methodological researches led to the discovery of certain abnormalities (later called 'lesions') which could be systematically palpated. He adopted this procedure of diagnosis and evolved various manual procedures for their treatment and built upon it his system which became osteopathy.

Still made a special study of functional disease and the structural disturbances, particularly of the spine, which accompanied them. Out of practice eventually arose the need for a theory on which Still could base these ideas destined to become osteopathy.

In 1870 he proclaimed the rule of the artery, this being the great basic principle of osteopathy – 'Wherever the circulation of the blood is normal, disease cannot develop because our blood is capable of manufacturing all the necessary substances to maintain natural immunity against disease.' It must be stressed that all this happened at a time when much less was known about the blood and the rôle that it played in the human organism. Obviously Still was only able to express his ideas in terms of the current knowledge of those times.

Following his eventual realization of the idea of a comprehensive therapeutical system, and in order to differentiate it from the others, Still conceived the word osteopathy, this being a combination of two Greek words, *osteos* (bone) and *pathos* (disease). It has been said that his choice was unwise since the word itself simply means 'bone disease'. Perhaps there is justification for this criticism; many people who are not fully acquainted with the subject think of an osteopath as some kind of bone doctor. Inherent in this conception is the implication that osteopathy has a very narrow scope indeed, which is not borne out by clinical fact.

In its broadest sense an 'osteopathic lesion' is any structural abnormality that may lead to functional or subsequently organic disease. Osteopathy regards the change from the quadruped to the biped stance as one of the main predisposing aetiological factors in man's ailments. Add to this the effect of macro- and micro-traumata, either acute or chronic, and mechanical imbalance quickly follows. In the biped stance, gravity has a continuously deleterious effect on man's structure. For instance:

The intervertebral discs and the apophyseal joints of the spine have become weight-bearing, tending to make the junction areas extremely unstable, especially the lumbo-sacral and sacro-iliac articulations.

It is on account of the continuous strain at the level of these articulations that low-back pain and sciatica are so common. This constitutes a typical osteopathic mechanical lesion of the low back, and is very amenable to osteopathic treatment. Furthermore, gravity tends to make the abdominal and pelvic viscera, including the diaphragm, sag inferiorly. This predisposes man to visceroptosis, hernia, portal hypertension, haemorrhoids, →**consti-**

pation, varix and other conditions due to intra-abdominal compression and stasis.

Much of the cardio-vascular system is obliged to function against gravity, and equally has constantly to adapt to man's changing postures. Similarly with the respiratory system, the bronchi must drain against gravity, i.e. by means of coughing, sneezing and the actions of the ciliated epithelium.

Should there be any excessive or mechanical distortion on a spinal articulation, the weight of gravity will tend to hold the joint in stress, usually at an extreme point of its normal range of movement, and reduced mobility ensues.

This becomes one type of 'osteopathic lesion'. This term also includes any state of stress involving any structure and its function. For example, articulations other than in the spine may be included, such as in the extremities: other examples include the fascial planes, muscles, legs, viscera, endocrine glands, etc.

In the history and development of osteopathy, perhaps the least understood and most controversial factor has been the 'osteopathic lesion'. In medical literature, the term 'lesion' simply means 'abnormality and/or injury' but, in the osteopathic sense it becomes much more complex and is far removed from the grosser forms of mechanical disturbance such as dislocation of the joint surfaces, with pressure on the nerve fibres. In such conditions, the problem is surgical and not osteopathic; in the latter condition, paralysis would supervene. Briefly, the osteopathic lesion may be described as a modification of normal joint movement, all structures surrounding, and attached to the vertebral area are involved and such terms as stress, strain, thickening, shortening, swelling, etc., give the clue to what is really a physio-pathological and mechanical condition and not a mere anatomical deviation, although of course, these can and do occur. It is from these several factors, collectively or singly, that the functional activity of the body begins to suffer.

Lesions of recent occurrence are usually called 'acute' lesions; long-standing lesions are described as 'chronic' lesions. Both types of lesion can occur in the same patient, the chronic developing from the acute, or the acute can manifest, from time to time, within the chronic state. The point to be made clear is that the lesion-state is progressive and that the acute condition is often an expression of compensatory failure in the presence of long-standing lesions. Whatever type of lesion we have to consider, the causes are several and must be traced to their source. Primary lesions frequently arise from accidents, blows, torsional stress, improper posture, nutritional errors, infection, or from metabolic retention and auto-toxaemia. Mental and emotional factors such as anxiety, fear, frustration, resentment, etc., may also lead to disturbance of the spinal balance. Whatever the primary aetiological factor may be, whether it be traumatic, postural, dietetic or psychological, the functioning of the body is impaired, and if this is continued over long periods organic tissue changes are likely to occur. From the osteopathic point of view, the osteopathic spinal lesion represents the largest single aetiological factor in this vicious circle of functional and organic disorder, and it is here that corrective and normalizing influences of manipulation can be brought to bear, to restore the natural defences and to allow the self-regulating tendency of the body to come into operation.

Therein lies the rationale of Still's original hypotheses.

The rôle of the osteopath is to normalize these structural relationships; such treatment being called an 'osteopathic adjustment'.

All that has been said in this respect may be additionally expressed in terms particularly original to Denslow and Korr concerning the 'Facilitated Segment'. By definition an intervertebral osteopathic lesion means that there is a tissue stretch on one side and a shortening on the other side. All the para-vertebral structures (including muscles, ligaments, etc.) are richly supplied with sensory nerve endings, which are sensitive to such changes of tension and are of the non-adapting type.

For example, let us suppose a vertebra side bent on the one below. The proprioceptors on the lengthened side (neuro-muscular spindle, golgi tendon receptors) will continuously bombard the spinal cord segment to which they are related. We are here assuming that the upper vertebra is fixed in side bending, this being called in osteopathy a spinal side-bending rotation lesion.

Denslow, Korr and others have shown experimentally that this afferent bombardment facilitates the neuronal pool of the related spinal cord segment. This facilitation implies that these neurones are maintained at or near threshold level. In the neuronal pool, there are three important types of neurones: motor, sensory and autonomic. Korr described how facilitation through the different fibres affects all three types. Normally the sympathetic neurones have only an intermittent effect on the viscera, as during stress and exercise. However, under these circumstances they may stimulate the viscera, not only during stress and exercise, but they are also facilitated in response to any increased nervous activity in the body.

If we take for example the gastro-intestinal tract, this sympathetic facilitation results in decreased peristalsis and glandulomotor activity as well as vaso-constriction in the gastro-intestinal tract. Osteopathy regards this as an important aetiological factor in many G.I.T. (gastro-intestinal tract) conditions. There is a marked trend in modern medicine towards regarding autonomic disturbances, especially sympatheticotonia, as important aetiological factors in many visceral conditions. (Kuntz pioneered these researches.)

Still did not believe in those early days that the use of any auxiliary method or aid to the body was necessary. Perhaps he had good reason, but on the other hand he lived in different times. More will be said about this later. It will be evident, however, that spinal treatment may not always suffice to bring the body back into a state of permanent balance if gross nutritional disturbances, either by excess or deficiency, are present, or should prolonged and intense mento-emotional disturbance exist. Under these circumstances, spinal treatment may do no more than temporarily relieve the symptoms unless the primary causes can be removed. The adoption of a suitable régime or psychological treatment may be indispensable if permanent results are to be obtained. Similarly in a purely structural sense, lesions that are being maintained by tension or by bad posture for example, if corrected, will only tend to return if nothing is done to correct the bad posture. Relaxation treatment and postural re-education on Eeman and Mathias →Alexander principles are indicated in these circumstances.

These facts have not been ignored by any means and in more recent years there are few osteopaths who do not use some form of adjunctive therapy. The concept of the Total Lesion and the Total Adjustment have long been established in osteopathy and are expressed in the idea that a person may, apart from structural lesion, be disturbed both biochemically and psychologically. Therefore, to restore the balance of a person as a whole, apart from structural adjustment, biochemical and psychological adjustment may be necessary; adjustment on all three levels being the Total Adjustment.

The reader may think that the spinal column alone is the main concern of the osteopath. Although this is in part true, the pelvis, the feet and the other joints may equally receive their share of attention. Osteopaths also pay attention to what are known as the soft tissues, i.e. muscles and ligaments, and much osteopathic technique is concerned with these in addition to treating the purely bony aspects of the articulatory system.

Osteopathy is in a constant state of evolution in terms of modifications in existing theory and technique, for example the newer concept of →'cranial' osteopathy. Over the years specialist approaches to gynaecology, ear, nose and throat, cardiology and orthopaedics have been developed and serve to enrich and widen the already vast scope of osteopathic general practice.

The theory of osteopathy is firmly based on the sciences of anatomy, physiology, pathology, general medicine and the pre-medical subjects of biology, chemistry, zoology, physics, histology and embryology. A. T. Still was, however, a devout Christian and he saw the sum total of his life's work in those terms. The human being represented God's Great Handiwork, and the complexity of the human body and its mechanical intricacies as being the final product of the Great Architect. Today, now that knowledge about eastern religions is freely available, the mutual 'holistic' philosophy which exists between these and Total Lesion osteopathy is apparent within the context of these different religions. The author believes that certainly a spiritual connotation if not a mystical exists, but many osteopaths may well not agree.

Osteopathy was first brought to Great Britain from the U.S.A. by graduates of the first osteopathic school in that country. This was round about the years 1902–3. The British School of Osteopathy was founded in 1918.

A session with a practitioner will take twenty minutes to half an hour, and in some cases may be followed by a short period of rest after the treatment before departure. Over what period a patient will need to attend is not easy to determine: it depends on (1) the condition being treated, (2) its chronicity, (3) the age of the person, and (4) the attitude and general health aspects of the patient. In other words there are a number of variables. Several months' treatment at probably weekly intervals is average. Sometimes a problem will clear with several treatments only. Treatment rarely extends to years. Some very chronic and/or elderly patients may need a continuity of treatment in a maintenance sense. Due, however, to the small number of properly qualified osteopaths in practice, and the enormous and growing demand on their services, patients are perforce treated and discharged as quickly as their condition permits, in order to allow other patients to be seen and treated without delay.

Osteopathic treatment is always preceded by a consultation/examination, the latter being primarily manual, but equally supported by the diagnostic methods of general medicine, physical, laboratory and X-ray as indicated.

Patients can often feel worse before they are better, but this is by no means a general rule.

Sometimes there is just a progressive 'getting better' or an instantaneous relief of symptoms, the latter not necessarily to be confused with total cure. Tissue reactions do often occur locally where the particular manual procedures have been applied. Sometimes the symptom-picture changes and pains are temporarily felt elsewhere prior to resolution. Patients are suitably reassured by their practitioners.

There are no successes on record nor any valid statistics as such, for the simple reason that since the profession and its schools have no statutory recognition, there is no public money available to carry out the necessary research and statistical studies. However, for over seventy years osteopaths in Great Britain have carried out a service to the public, the demand for which has progressively increased over the years – obviously because they get results and satisfy their patients. Today more and more doctors and consultants are referring patients for osteopathic treatment. Recently a well-known osteopath gave a reception for all the doctors in his area who had referred him patients. There were thirty-two present. The General Medical Council has recently relaxed its former prohibitive attitude, thus making it possible for doctors to make referrals.

The success of osteopathy is inherent in its clinical record over three-quarters of a century.

Osteopathy is neither in opposition nor at variance with conventional medicine, surgery or any other system of medicine, e.g. →**homoeopathy**, →**acupuncture**, etc. It does not, however, actively support or give credence to extreme, cranky and messianic 'fringe medicine' practices, although it does not necessarily condemn them, for the unorthodoxy of today invariably becomes the orthodoxy of tomorrow. While enjoying our newly-found respectability and wide acceptance we must never forget that in its early days our movement was also subject to intolerance and ridicule, and that its pioneers were looked upon as cranks and charlatans. Tolerance should therefore give warmth to our attitudes towards all other practitioners of medicine, orthodox and unorthodox, who are engaged in helping to relieve and cure the suffering of their fellow creatures.

It is the author's firm belief that all systems of medicine are complementary and neither is adjunctive one to the other, and that one day there will be one medicine and one medicine only. The recent acceptance as official policy by the World Health Organization of the need to mobilize all traditional systems of medicine in the Third World, in addition to the practice of western medicine in those countries in order to ensure 'total health-care delivery', is a firm pointer that the trend in official international circles is now definitely in that direction.

Thomas G. Dummer D.O., M.S.O.

PRENATAL THERAPY

Based on the original idea of the ancient Chinese foot massage, prenatal therapy evolved from the observation that the reflex of the spine in the foot was also the reflex of the gestation period.

Conception corresponds to the first vertebra of the spine, and birth to the coccyx; the whole thirty-eight weeks of gestation being divisible in the length of the spine.

According to the Chinese foot massage technique, manipulation of the foot reflexes loosens and releases tensions in the respective parts of the body. Manipulation of the spinal reflex releases stress in the spine, it also releases stress – or blockages – in the gestation period. The gestation period is the time during which we build our body, during which the characteristics of our mind are established; it is the prenatal pattern on which our postnatal life is established.

Prenatal therapy is based on an understanding of the attitudes of mind developed at the different periods of gestation that are generated from the inherited characteristics, racial characteristics, 'karmic' traits, and any other factors which may influence the moment of conception. This may also include the influence of medical drugs and environment.

These attitudes of mind are as real to the newly developed consciousness as those that we may feel during the events of an average day in our postnatal life. What is important to our understanding of this work is that they become the attitudes of mind which control our daily lives.

There are five noticeable stages during gestation in which this patterning takes place. The first is before conception when the consciousness is approaching the single cell of its new life. If the inherited traits and environmental influences are against normality there is a 'reluctance' to enter the life. This inhibition of the spontaneous action of the consciousness produces the severely inhibited and retarded child.

The second stage is that of conception. This is the first real challenge to the consciousness; it is the entry into matter, which is also the beginning of the time factor of life. The consciousness which fails to handle this stage of his development can never really handle the factors of space and time; the reality of life is limited.

The third stage is that of postconception and covers the period of time from conception to about the half-way, the nineteenth week, the quickening stage. Inhibiting influences at this stage produce either pulmonary troubles or immaturity of character and of physical development of the chest.

The fourth stage which starts at the quickening is one in which the consciousness changes his focus from himself to the objective world around him. This is the first social challenge, the first impact of the outside world. It is the solar plexus syndrome.

During this fourth stage – particularly between the sixth to the eighth months – the very real attitudes of mind of the new consciousness are formed. He is like a child going into an examination room when, for some reason or another, he has not mastered his studies; he feels procrastination, fear, and reluctance; he cannot find the energy or will to go forward.

It is at this stage that he develops the tensions which affect his intestines, his bowels, the female generative organs; it is here that low-back troubles begin. It is also at this time that we establish our ability to handle the action principles of life, the ability to move into a situation and complete it. The baby will show every sign at this stage of reluctance to emerge from the womb. It is largely him, and not his mother, who makes the act of birth difficult and painful.

The final and fifth stage is that of birth. Birth is the fulfilment of all that has gone before. The initial reluctance of the first stage, the challenge of the second stage, the development of the third stage, the attitudes of mind of the fourth stage, all contribute to the ability to complete this final fulfilment of entry into the outer world. The baby is a consciousness formed by the characteristics foregathered at conception and developed during gestation into a living being.

This prenatal pattern is the established mentality and physique of the new baby. He may be retarded, inhibited, unable to develop; he may be full of fears and reluctances. But all of these are changeable.

Because the gestation period has the same reflex area as the spine, and because manipulation of the reflex area releases stresses and blockages, we are able to loosen the structure of this period of time.

Manipulation on a reflex area activates a pattern of change in the patient and it is his own inner motive patterns and will that enable him to change. Manipulation of the body direct (or any form of external treatment) effects this change for him. The difference between the two is that if he is able to make a change in himself the change is a re-creation; it is absolute and becomes a change in generic structure. If the change is done for him it is merely superficial patterning of the outer structure and has no permanent value.

It is the nature of prenatal therapy that the patient is able to make his change within himself, that even in small and tentative ways he is able to unlock the doors of his enprisonment and emerge little by little into the outer world; that the blocks formed during and before gestation are loosened and released and that even the worst of retarded conditions are changeable to those of complete normality.

This inner ability to change applies to every case, whether it be a mongoloid child, spastic, →autistic, paralysed; whether the condition is asthma, bronchitis, glandular; whether the condition is purely physical or a mental one, the principle is the same, change is possible from within the child and, by his own ability, to re-create his primary structure.

Treatment is by manipulation or massage of the reflexes of the feet. But also the same reflexes which exist in the hands and the head are used. Reflexes in the feet have a direct effect on the action principle of life, those in the hands have an effect on the executive ability, and those in the head have an effect on the mental ability. All three of these functions are used in any action that we make; the blockage can be in one or the other.

Whether we base our observation on the clinical results of this work or on the principles involved, it is evident that most forms of physical and mental defectiveness can be changed, usually to normality. The limiting factors in the accomplishment of a complete change are in the environment, in very extreme defectiveness, and in the age of the patient, the younger the better.

See also →**Natural childbirth.**

Robert St John

ASSOCIATIONS, p. 217
BIBLIOGRAPHY, p. 245
CONTRIBUTORS, p. 222
TRAINING, p. 233

PRIMAL THERAPY

The term 'primal', which comes from the Latin *primus* (first), means 'primitive' or 'primeval' or 'primordial'. It was used by Freud in the phrases 'primal horde', a group consisting of a dominant male, the primal father, a number of females he kept to himself, and a number of males he kept in subjection; and 'primal scene', the child's idea of his parents having intercourse, around which phantasy ideas have been woven.

Primal therapy is a treatment which connects present feelings, behaviour and experiences with feelings, behaviour and experiences in childhood, infancy, at birth and in the womb (primal experiences).

There are two main theories on which deep-level intensive therapy is based. One is the Primal Formulation, put forward by Arthur Janov of Los Angeles, author of *The Primal Scream*,[1] and the other is the Intensive Thesis,[2] formulated by the present writer.

The Primal Formulation can be summarized as follows:

Experiences which are harmful or hurtful to the embryo, foetus, infant or child create a pool of Primal Pain.

An overload of primal pain disrupts the smooth unifying functions within the brain and literally produces a split personality – someone with a non-integrated dual consciousness each part of which acts as an independent entity. . . .
Unless unresolved painful memory circuits (and past feelings *are* memories) are integrated, neurosis will not be cured. . . .
Pain seals events into the unconscious, and feeling pain in titrated doses opens up the unconscious. . . .
We can view neurosis as a series of buried reactions: where there were stimuli without the possibility of proper response. . . .
It is a specific feeling which binds together various experiences; and the feeling has its lower-line elements which can be triggered by the events in the present. . . .
The treatment of neurosis does not involve having certain kinds of social interactions, whether it be having your transference or intellectual defences analysed by a psychoanalyst or in confronting someone in group therapy. . . .[3]

Janov's treatment of neurosis consists of a three-week period of isolation from work, family, wife, husband or lover, friends, tobacco alcohol, drugs, entertainments, reading, television, radio, and any other ways of suppressing or avoiding the Pool of Pain, during which

the patient has week-day sessions with the therapist and can contact him in moments of crisis.

This period is followed by nine months or more of 'primalling' in groups, each patient going into his own pain and allowing himself to feel it, to discharge it by sobbing, screaming and other expressions of reactivated pain, and to make connections with the present. The therapist goes from one group-member to another in an auxiliary rôle, not directing or interpreting, but encouraging the free expression of his/her pain.

Janov is uncompromising in his dismissal of all other forms of therapy. Speaking of sex therapy, he says:

Any approach to sexual problems, such as that of Masters and Johnson, which treats sexual difficulties apart from a person's history, must ultimately fail.[4]

He says of psychoanalysis, meditation and Behavioral Therapy:

The patient . . . may sincerely believe that he has been changed and helped by anything from meditation to psychoanalysis because he has been able to use some new ideology or mantra as a tranquillizer, diffusing and suppressing the pain . . .
In other forms of psychotherapy such as Conditioning or Behavioral Therapy one rearranges the symbolism so that the homosexual person no longer thinks 'cock' and goes on homosexual quests; he now thinks 'women'.[5]

For various reasons he also dismisses Reich (→**Reichian therapy**), the Reality Therapists, →**gestalt** therapy, →**biofeedback**, →**encounter**, rational emotive and →**psychodrama**.

The alternative to Janov's theory is the Intensive Thesis,[6] which is the basis of the treatment method of the present writer.

According to this thesis, neurosis is caused by excessive undischarged Fear.[7] Fear (with a capital F) is the continuum of conscious and unconscious fear. This Fear produces malign (or undesirable) inhibition of impulses, or in other words, *blocking of benign connections*.[8] We can understand impulses and their inhibition in two ways, psychic (direct experience) and neurological (scientific). We know from direct experience what it is to have an impulse (say, to laugh, or to strike someone) and to inhibit the impulse, and we know from neurological experiments that inhibition can be produced by high frequency stimulation (overloading) of parts of the brain.

Overloading, then, is one important way of causing inhibition. If someone faints when pain reaches a certain threshold, there is massive inhibition and loss of consciousness (shut-down). This may not be malign, as it saves the organism unnecessary suffering. If someone faints at the sight of blood, however, the shut-down is likely to be malign, because the person is totally dependent at times of emergency.

The inhibition caused by overloading at times of crisis in the womb, at birth, when breast- or bottle-feeding, when deprived of contact or affection, when hurt or injured or humiliated, can be reduced and made selective by the adult if he succeeds in connecting the deep, mid and high ranges of his neural organization. (The rhinic, limbic and supra-limbic lobes of the brain.) Then the capacity of his cerebral cortex to discriminate can be connected with the deep engrams (neural memories or circuits).

He can then begin to replace the *dam*[9] (indiscriminate blocking) with a system of *locks* (selective blocking). He can allow benign inhibition (control of sphincters, control of destructive expressions of fear, rage, lust, grief or exuberance) and reduce malign inhibition (compulsive and inconvenient opening or shutting of sphincters, inability to have erection or orgasm, or to express fear, rage, lust, grief or exuberance in non-destructive ways).

What is blocked is not simply pain. The bliss and ecstasy of good womb experience, of good moments in a difficult intimate relationship, the free and liberating discharge of fear, rage, grief and exuberance, the current or orgasm, may also be blocked and may also be re-experienced when malign inhibition is lifted and connections restored.

The therapy based on the Intensive Thesis is called Intensive Rhythm Therapy,[10] and it consists of several phases. It begins with individual sessions which prepare the person for the three-week Launching Period.[11]

The Launching Period is a period of isolation from all distractions and drugs, and of intensive individual therapy, as described in relation to Janov's therapy. The person now begins to make connections at a deep level, and continues the process both in group and in individual sessions, usually with both a male and a female therapist.

There are important differences between the therapy as described by Janov and Intensive Rhythm Therapy, which preserves all the insights of Freud, Reich, Rank, Melanie Klein, Winnicott, Kurt Lewis, Perls, Lowen, Moreno, Albert Pesso . . ., and does not dismiss alternative therapies such as →**bioenergetics** and sex therapy.

One important difference is that individual therapy is continued after the three-week Launching Period for at least one and usually two years. It is not then ended in such a way that the lifting of malign inhibitions is terminated. It is phased out gradually, and Reciport, a method of reciprocal support introduced by the present writer, enables the person to continue the self-liberating process with a partner who has had similar experiences and has been trained to give and receive support one hour each way every week for as long as the partners need it.

Another important difference is that the Intensive Rhythm Therapy recognizes the danger of Primal Therapy: the person may become stuck in a Primal Rut. This means that one lock in the dam may be opened (say, the Anger Lock), and he or she continues to release energy through that lock, expressing anger but blocking grief, fear, laughter, joy and exuberance.

If this happens to Intensive Rhythm Therapy, there are methods of making the person aware of the Primal Rut, of helping him to open up the other locks, and of reviving good body-memories which unify and vitalize the whole organism.

There is also a profound difference between Janov's theory of neurosis and the Intensive

Thesis. According to the Intensive Thesis there is a channel connecting all good experiences from conception to the present day. The cell memories which constitute this channel may be blocked, and excessive emphasis on the Pool of Pain may help to keep them blocked.

It is the aim of Intensive Rhythm Therapy to open up the bliss, happiness and exuberance channel by making neural connections in a state of deep relaxation. In this way Fear (the continuum of conscious and unconscious fear) is systematically reduced, malign inhibitions are lifted, benign inhibitions are restored and strengthened, and the person finds his own unique personal rhythms.

He ventures out and takes risks more and more, but retreats into womb-like security when he is hurt or tired. He establishes relationships of many kinds, but can withdraw into voluntary solitude. His eating, drinking, sleeping, working rhythms gradually become adapted to the needs of the total organism.

The Intensive Thesis has identified the main Fear-draining, therapeutic elements, all of which contribute to the effect of Intensive Rhythm Therapy: they are benign transference, which does not keep the person in over-long childish dependency, and which is phased out without rejection of or by the therapist and without terminating the self-liberating process; benign incentives combined with opportunities within the person's scope; the support and encouragement of a group which meets weekly over a long period; a three-week break with the inertia of drugs and routine; the facilitation of verbal, vocal and bodily expression of feelings which have been blocked; the rejection, by the therapist and group, of the false self, and the support and encouragement of the authentic self; the temporary removal of performance fears (fears of failing sexually, in examinations, in work, in social contacts); the eroding through self-questioning, with the aid of the therapist, of unrealistic expectations and self-destructive idea-systems; establishing benign connections between deep-, mid- and high-brain activity

through regression and reliving; and the ability of the therapist to change direction in order to pull the person out of malign regression (the prolonged clinging to childish irresponsibility), or out of malign expression and discharge: the primal rut.

As Fear dissolves, 'problems' slowly fade away.

G. *Seaborn Jones* B.A.(Oxon.), PH.D.(Lond.)

BIBLIOGRAPHY, p. 249
CONTRIBUTORS, p. 222
TRAINING, p. 231

Notes

1. Janov, Arthur, *The Primal Scream*, Abacus, 1973.
2. Seaborn Jones, Glyn, 'The flow, the dam and the locks', *Energy and Character* (ed. D. Boadella, Abbotsbury, Dorset), January 1975.
3. Janov, Arthur, and Holden, E. Michael, *Primal Man: The New Consciousness*, Crowell, New York, 1975.
4. ibid.
5. ibid.
6. Seaborn Jones, Glyn, 'Launching', *Energy and Character*, January 1976.
7. Seaborn Jones, Glyn, *Treatment or Torture: The Philosophy, Techniques and Future of Psychodynamics*, Tavistock, 1968.
8. Seaborn Jones, 'The flow, the dam and the locks'.
9. ibid.
10. Seaborn Jones, 'Launching', 'The flow, the dam and the locks', and 'Intensive rhythm therapy', *Energy and Character*, January 1975.
11. Seaborn Jones, 'Launching'.

PSIONIC MEDICINE

There is a tradition in medicine extending over centuries which ascribes to the vital force the most significant rôle in health and disease. It is not the part or the symptom which commands the attention of the physician but the patient as a living whole. Thus both diagnosis and treatment are directed to what Hahnemann, the founder of →homoeopathy, called the vital dynamis.

In this tradition there is no question of mere suppression of symptoms by drugs or surgical intervention: the objective is the restoration of the patient to full vitality. And this involves the discovery and removal of the toxic factors which are inhibiting vitality to cells, tissues and organs and to the patient as a vital functional and perceptive being.

Over the last half century or thereabouts, a number of doctors and others working in the medical field have become increasingly interested in the recovery of knowledge of this tradition. Among them are Abrams in California, Guyon Richards and his colleagues in London, Edward Bach and more latterly George Laurence. They have drawn on the work of Steiner, Reich (→Reichian therapy), McDonagh, Mermet and others, as well as on the classical medical philosophies and their own experience to lay the foundations of contemporary practices based on the need to restore and sustain optimum vitality.

George Laurence, physician and surgeon with wide experience in British medicine, came to the conclusion after many years in practice that he did not know why many of his patients were ill. This was particularly true of chronic illness. He realized also that his contemporaries were equally in the dark as to the basic causes of chronic disease. So he decided to devote the remainder of his professional life to the search for a method which could reveal and at the same time remove such causes. He was determined to avoid as far as possible the use of drugs and surgery which he knew so often produced dangerous and debilitating side-effects, often worse than the disease itself, and related only to effects.

After fifteen years of patient and dedicated work he evolved a system of medical diagnosis and therapy which he called psionic medicine. His method was based on the sensitivity which enables the dowser or water diviner to find water, minerals, missing objects and so on, often with the use of a map only

(→radiesthesia). He found that the vital energies which maintain the integrity of the body can be dowsed. To apply this sensitivity to the study of imbalance in this vital dynamis and to find the cause, with the medical knowledge and experience he had as a doctor, was but a short step.

Laurence and his colleagues developed the system in such a way that it could be interpreted in terms of orthodox medical and surgical findings and terminology and could thus be made available in established medicine. His method added a further dimension to existing diagnostic possibilities in clinic and laboratory, a dimension which embraced the basic pre-disposing causes of illness in the individual patient, thus making possible treatment at a more fundamental level, without the necessity of using dangerous drugs and other damaging procedures.

Furthermore he demonstrated the value of the traditional homoeopathic *materia medica*, derived from natural sources and used in minute doses. He recognized that these medicines related in an almost miraculous manner to the subtle causes of disease.

Laurence's contribution to medicine is based on the fact that everything in nature vibrates and emits radiations which may be perceived, given the required sensitivity. Thus he brought back the basic art of medicine and re-established the rightful marriage between art and science without which there can be no real medical practice.

In practical terms, diagnosis is carried out with the aid of a small blood sample on absorbent paper, together with details of the complaint and medical history of the patient. The presence of the patient is not essential to diagnosis and thus psionic medicine is available anywhere in the world provided the necessary sample and detail is available. The techniques make use of 'witnesses': samples of tissues, organs, diseases and material taken from the three kingdoms of nature, usually in homoeopathic potency. A dowser's pendulum is also used. The bloodspot is equivalent to a map which a dowser uses. But in this case it is a 'map' of the patient.

It is possible for the trained practitioner not only to detect imbalance in the vital dynamis but also its degree and distribution throughout the organ system. Further, the cause of the deviation from normal may be established and the simillimum found: that is, the combination of remedies or single homoeopathic remedy that will remove the cause and correct the vital imbalance. Treatment is not usually prolonged, requires no hospitalization and is effective at all ages.

Inherited miasms or acquired toxins residual from acute infections constitute the major causes. Certain chemical and other radiations may also produce an imbalance of the vital dynamis and eventually produce symptoms of chronic disease.

The term miasm was used by Hahnemann to denote a departure from vital dynamic balance due to an infection in a forebear. Thus, certain chronic diseases may have their root in a previous generation and may manifest symptoms at any time, not necessarily in childhood, because of the predisposition established by the miasm. Trigger or precipitating factors in the environment, including diet, climate, pollution or emotional stress, may bring on an attack of symptoms. When this occurs, or even before it occurs if vital imbalance has been diagnosed, psionic medical treatment is instituted to remove the basic cause, thereby resolving the symptoms often without further aid.

To advance Laurence's work, The Psionic Medical Society was formed in 1968 with medical, dental and lay membership. Later, The Institute of Psionic Medicine was founded, the aims of which were to train doctors and dental surgeons in the techniques, to maintain a register of qualified practitioners and to pursue research in psionic medicine.

By removing the causes of chronic and degenerative disease the need for complex and costly replacement surgery and supportive therapy is reduced. A high proportion of mental illness is initiated by inherited miasms and acquired toxins and the need for mental hospitals and allied provisions could be effectively eased by psionic medicine.

Psionic medicine dispenses with the need for animal experimentation and the production of standardized synthetic drugs. There is no standardized diagnosis or therapy. Both are entirely relevant to the individual patient.

The techniques may be used to test effects of standardized drugs and individual intolerance and also sensitivity to aluminium, fluorine compounds, mercury, lead, radiation and other toxic elements, and to determine neutralizing remedies.

Psionic medical treatment effectively paves the way for self-help. The latter can never be entirely effective if miasms and acquired toxins are still present. Their removal, by increasing the overall vitality, produces the most fruitful base for subsequent self-help.

Carl Upton L.D.S.(Birm.), M.I.Psi.Med.

ASSOCIATIONS, p. 217
BIBLIOGRAPHY, p. 249
CONTRIBUTORS, p. 222

PSYCHIC SURGERY

Essentially we are all spirits inhabiting earthly bodies. When we die we discard our bodies like clothes that have gone out of fashion and progress to another realm of existence. This belief is central to most of the great religions but little has been done to try to prove it. There are, however, men and women around the world – of all religious beliefs – who have the ability to see, hear and communicate with people whom we call dead but who have merely gone on ahead to a new life.

A former fireman, I am now consulted by people around the world in their search for better health. The reason is that a surgeon who used to practise in England and who died in 1937 now continues to treat the sick through my mediumship. I was sixteen when William Lang died. Our paths never crossed on earth, for I was born in Merseyside and spent all my early life in the dockland area, living with my grandparents. On leaving school I took various jobs – as a garage hand, butcher and dockworker – before joining the R.A.F.

where I became an instructor in gunnery, boxing and battle drill. I was still in the Air Force when I married in 1944. My first child, a daughter, lived only a month and it was her death which led me to question whether there was a life after death. I soon received evidence that convinced me there is a next world, and I was told by the various spirit communicators that they would form a spiritual healing band, operating through my mediumship. As a result of my inquiries I developed trance mediumship during which I lost consciousness, and spirit people spoke through my lips. On my return to normality I had no memory of what had taken place. It was during these sessions that William Lang first made his presence known. Although I was caught up in these experiences I demanded proof that the communicators were the people they claimed to be. The appearance of Lang provided an opportunity to check his claims. So often the 'spirit guides' who establish a link with mediums claim a former earthly existence beyond the range of human memory or even shroud their identities in mystery. But here was a man who claimed to have been a surgeon until his retirement in 1912 (nine years before I was born) and to have lived for a further twenty-five years.

My research satisfied me that I was in touch with William Lang, who became ophthalmic surgeon to the Middlesex Hospital in 1880 and who moved on to the Central London Ophthalmic Hospital (later Moorfields Eye Hospital) in 1884. He was senior vice-president of the Ophthalmological Society in 1903, and acted as president of the Ophthalmological Section of the Royal Society of Medicine. According to Lang, he wanted to continue helping people who were ill while, at the same time, providing proof of an after-life. Therefore I willingly provided an earthly body for this purpose and our remarkable healing partnership began. The critic, of course, might suggest that I had picked a name from a list of past medical men, researched his life and now act the part of Lang when in a trance. In other words, that it is no more than a clever charade. That might explain the accuracy of dates and events which Lang recalls – assuming I have a brilliant memory – but there is much more to the return of William Lang than that. Doctors who worked with him, patients who consulted him, and members of Lang's own family have all visited my home at Aylesbury, Bucks., and spoken to Lang. They have been left in no doubt that it is Lang. Not only does he have the extensive medical knowledge one would expect from such an eminent surgeon but he recognizes people with whom he enjoyed an earthly association. His grand-daughter, Susan, is among the people who have testified that Lang is who he says he is. He speaks with the same voice and has the same mannerisms. He even 'operates' with his left hand, as he did on earth, though I am normally right-handed. There have been a number of books published about the Chapman–Lang partnership which give a detailed account of the overwhelming evidence that Lang has survived death – among them *The Return of Dr Lang* and *Extraordinary Encounters*.

Lang continues to use his medical knowledge in treating the sick and he brings about improvement and cures by 'operating' on his patients – but not with a physical scalpel. The reason is that he is no longer concerned with the physical body. Instead he takes advantage of his new vantage point in another realm, to effect changes in the spirit-body which is a go-between for the actual spirit of each individual and the physical body. According to Lang the spirit-body shapes itself around the physical body, contracting beneath the skin but able to expand to the skin's surface. It is composed of electrical cells and supplies energy to the physical body. This view, incidentally, appears to be confirmed by Russian researchers who have found a way of photographing the 'aura' of living things, producing beautiful, multi-coloured complex pictures of this electrical energy (→**high voltage photography**).

A magnetic force holds the spirit-body's electrical cells together and, indeed, throughout life the physical and spirit-bodies cling together like magnets. When we die the spirit-body continues to cling to the physical body for a period but it, too, eventually is shed, for the spirit has no need for it in the next world. If, during our lives, the spirit-body is not in harmony with our earthly bodies, for whatever reason, we develop an illness. Similarly, if something is wrong with our bodies this brings about a corresponding change in the spirit-body. So, William Lang explains, by putting right the conditions of disharmony in the *spirit-body* he endeavours to correct physical ills. Though there is never any guarantee of success, and some patients do not respond to this treatment for reasons we do not understand, there are on record many cases, backed by medical reports, which show that desperately ill people who have consulted William Lang as a last resort have greatly benefited or have been totally cured.

To receive treatment the patient lies, fully clothed, on a medical couch. Lang then uses my body as though it were his own as he discusses the condition and makes a diagnosis. Lang uses spirit instruments to correct the trouble and though these are not seen by the patient there is little doubt about what is happening as my entranced hands go through the motions of operating just an inch or so above the physical body. Surgery on the spirit-body leaves a scar and just occasionally a corresponding scar, which is short-lived, appears on the human body too. It is usually sufficient for a patient to see 'Dr' Lang – as he is affectionately known by his patients – just once, but each continues to receive healing from him over an extended period. Indeed, distant healing is given to any patient who consults Lang, regardless of whether he or she is given an appointment. Though it can in some instances bring about a cure on its own, better results are produced where the spirit surgeon sees the patient and has the use of the medium's body to convey the treatment.

I have always welcomed examination from the medical world and as a result I now work closely with doctors in a number of countries. In France and Switzerland, for example, I hold regular clinics at which doctors bring their patients for treatment from Dr Lang. Medical etiquette prevents the use of their names in most cases, but one or two doctors have been so impressed by the spirit surgeon's results that they have spoken publicly about his treatment. Lang and I have treated the sick in other countries, too, including the United States of America. And, from my Aylesbury base, where I continue to see English patients, I deal with a huge postbag from people all over the world.

Many famous people – actors, sportsmen, T.V. personalities among them – have turned to Lang and myself for help. Typical of their attitude to this remarkable partnership is the tribute paid by Queen Anne of Romania who in a foreword to *Extraordinary Encounters*,, told how she and her husband first heard about it through a book, adding, 'We came to know personally George Chapman and William Lang, and were most impressed by Mr Chapman's simplicity, sincerity and love for his fellow men; dedicating his daily life so that Dr Lang could work through him, to cure and help us mentally and spiritually. Dr Lang and his work put the fourth dimension in our grasp through spiritual healing.'

George Chapman

BIBLIOGRAPHY, p. 249
CONTRIBUTORS, p. 222

PSYCHODRAMA

Ideally psychodrama is something not to be read about, discussed or even something to 'know about', but to be felt and experienced. Psychodrama is an action-orientated therapeutic method in which an individual enacts scenes or problems related to his past, present, or future life-situations. It is a method which approaches human interaction in a practical, concrete manner by looking at a person's life as it is and as it could be. A psychodrama scene is an individual's own creation, spontaneously enacted by group-members who either act out their own problems or help others to do so, by being in certain necessary rôles. This method also allows the exploration of alternative ways of expressing feelings in rehearsing new rôles in a safe, controlled, and supportive atmosphere.

The psychodramatic approach is suitable for a wide range of problems, people and purposes. It has been successfully used with 'normal' children, adolescents and adults, with families, and with people who have moderate problems in living, as well as the highly disturbed individual or chronic hospitalized patient. It is also effectively used in industry and education, and in examining social problems (sociodrama). The psychodrama session is normally from $1\frac{1}{2}$ to 3 hours, and an on-going group would probably meet once or twice a week. Members may remain in a group from approximately six months to three years. Psychodrama is also involved in the human potential movement, either in the form of on-going groups or one or two day workshops.

Historically psychodrama owes its existence to a Viennese psychiatrist, Jacob Moreno, born in 1892. He received his medical degree in 1917 and five years later founded the Theatre of Spontaneity in Vienna. In 1925 he moved to the United States and continued his work in psychodrama and published one of his better-known works, *Who Shall Survive*, in 1934. In 1936 he established the Moreno Sanitorium in Beacon, New York, which became a training centre, a hospital, and the first real theatre of psychodrama. Moreno's influence in the field of psychotherapy is well documented; many of the psychodramatic techniques are found in other forms of psychotherapy.

Moreno believed that people have difficulties because there is rarely any sphere of life, whether physical, mental, social, or cultural, which is totally free from disequilibrium or conflict in a person's life. Everyone has their 'public' rôle, but all of us have different rôles which, at various times, pressure to become active (much like a potential volcano). It is this pressure from within which may be a source of anxiety. In psychodrama these 'hidden individuals' can become present and one can safely explore ways to use them in the real world.

Moreno searched for a medium that permitted work on the verbal and non-verbal level, in both fantasy and reality, and would also facilitate a powerful and total emotional release which is called mental catharsis. This intense emotional release cannot be reproduced wholesale, nor can it be stored in our emotional or personal reservoir; the release must be applied concretely and specifically to each conflict area. With this release of emotional energy comes clarity. Each person becomes clearer about their own solutions, choices and directions.

Important changes can occur in a person as a result of their psychodramatic work. Some possible outcomes to psychodramatic events are:

1 Each individual's sense of choices in her/his life-situations is increased because of an exploration and familiarity with a wide variety of alternatives.

2 The use of spontaneous play, dance and imagination develops creative responses and reduces feelings of inhibition.

3 Through identification with others in the psychodramatic action, there is an increased capacity for empathy, and this quality of empathy is an important element in human relationships.

4 There is a greater validation of one's own sense of vitality, and of being more in touch with feelings, thoughts, imagery and authenticity.

5 There is an increase in flexibility; the individual develops a greater sense of mastery over a variety of rôle-situations, e.g. father, lover, student, friend, etc.

6 Psychodrama presents an opportunity to work towards fulfilling our basic needs and expressing impulses which are at our very centre.

Psychodrama is very effective in bringing about these changes for a variety of reasons. It does not allow an individual just to talk about his problems in a defensive, vague or circumstantial manner, instead it calls for concrete behaviour. By re-creating and re-enacting a disruptive event, the individual may become more aware of his/her own contribution to the problem. Thus a person may discover that when he/she asks for warmth, care and affection, he/she is ignored because his/her posture, voice, tone and gestures deny the very need that he/she is expressing with their words.

In psychodrama, possible solutions to problems can be rehearsed in a safe, simulated situation before experiencing them in the real world. People in the group can also learn and develop the behaviours which they find lacking in themselves and can then apply these to their own life-situations.

To facilitate the understanding of a psychodramatic action (an enactment) it might be useful to imagine a situation where a young man (John) in a group comes forward and indicates that he wishes to enact a scene related to the death of his mother for which in real life he was not present. At the time of her death he was eight years old. A mattress is placed on the floor and a group-member that John had selected as being most similar to his mother lies covered on the bed. By a variety of techniques, John is helped to be and to feel as he did when he was a child. John begins to talk with his 'mother' about his love for her, his sorrow and grief and in the description which follows it may be useful to keep this scene in mind.

John's action will take place on a 'psychodramatic stage'. The stage is free from constrictions and stresses of real life and provides an opportunity to experience feelings and new rôles in a safer place.

John is known as the protagonist, the main character – the one 'working' on their problem. The protagonist portrays scenes and incidents from his own private world which for each of us is unique. John is brought to a state of emotional readiness by describing the relationship with his mother when he was eight years old. He is 'warmed up' to a greater extent by describing the hospital-room as John imagines it to be. He is aided further in this process through contact with his 'mother'.

John's work will be facilitated by the director, who in a sense is the 'chief therapist' and 'producer' of the psychodramatic event. This person must have a high degree of skill, the sensitivity and training of a therapist, but also must be comfortable working in highly emotional and volatile situations. The director must also inspire trust and confidence as he/she has ultimate responsibility for the overall psychodrama session. He/she must also remain aware of the audience's mood in order that they too benefit from the action taking place. Finally in the period of sharing which will follow John's psychodramatic enactment, the director must also facilitate the group discussion so that the maximum benefit can occur for all the group-members.

The person being John's mother is known as an auxiliary ego. This is most often the people (but sometimes an object) who are essential for re-creating the psychodramatic scene (the rest of the cast). In some situations the auxiliary may be called upon to play a non-specific or general rôle, e.g. a policeman, a client, student, etc., rather than a specific person: 'my mother', 'my boss'. Auxiliary egos may sometimes be inanimate objects such as the desk that the protagonist uses at work, his/her car, or a fantasy figure such as Prince Charming who will come and rescue the protagonist, or the devil, God, etc. The auxiliary ego's major function is to help the protagonist to enact his/her scene, but they may also help to release the protagonist's emotions. John's 'mother' may, for example, express some of her own sadness and thus encourage her 'son' to cry in order to relieve blocked grief.

Those not directly participating in John's psychodrama are known as the audience. They may give feedback to the protagonist in the sharing period which will follow the completion of his scene. They will probably also benefit from John's work, as most of us can powerfully identify with the very emotional scenes. John's work with his mother may facilitate the clarification of other group-members' own relationships with their parental figures.

A variety of techniques are employed to

facilitate the psychodramatic process. One is known as a soliloquy which would involve John speaking aloud about his feelings as he walks down the 'hospital corridor' leading to his dying mother's room. It is used most effectively in situations where there is a high state of emotional tension because it allows the protagonist safely to vent his/her feelings and thoughts.

Another technique is known as mirroring. Here another person or persons would imitate the protagonist's behaviour. This is an effective way of giving feedback and understanding to the protagonist as to how others see and react to him/her. It may also give the protagonist a different viewpoint and shed a new light on a situation. The individual, for example, may discover that people become annoyed with him/her because of his/her whining, compliant manner.

One of the better known and essential methods is that involving the use of a double or alter-ego. The major function of the double is to help the protagonist express emotions. In a sense, the double is one's own invisible, unexpressed self. In our example, the double stands next to John and another lies next to his mother and copies their body postures. An additional function of the double is to provide support, give empathy, and to express and dramatize unexpressed feelings. At times, the double may interpret our resistances and defences. In John's psychodrama, when he suddenly stopped talking, his voice quavering and choked, his double quietly said: 'I feel terribly sad and I want to cry.' His double began to make sobbing sounds to encourage a release in John.

Another key technique is the use of rôle reversal where the protagonist literally places himself in another person's shoes, taking on their emotions, attitudes, etc. In the situation described above, John became his 'mother', taking her place on the mattress and she became John. From this perspective, it is possible to create a situation that decreases anxiety by allowing for greater empathy and understanding between the people involved.

Other techniques include working with fantasy material, the enactment of dreams, and the rehearsal of a coming event, e.g. an interview with a boss. Frequently, the ultimate reason behind many of these techniques is to bring about emotional release and/or reduction in fears and anxiety.

Psychodrama then can be seen to be a very effective method in helping people to grow, and to lead more fulfilling and richer lives. At the same time it must be kept in mind that it is a very powerful technique, and should only be practised by those who have had experience with the technique as well as training in the use and directing of psychodrama.

Joel Badaines Ph.D.

ASSOCIATIONS, p. 211
CONTRIBUTORS, p. 222

PULSED HIGH FREQUENCY

Pulsed electromagnetic energy is developed by a machine which emits short bursts of high frequency radio waves. The bursts have a duration of 65 microseconds with an interval between pulsations of 1600 microseconds. This unique pulsing effect causes any heat generated with the energy to be dissipated by the body so that there is no temperature rise in the tissues. Pulsed high frequency (P.H.F.) has been extremely effective in treating sinusitis, bursitis, rheumatoid arthritis, osteomyelitis, disorders of muscles, tendons, and bones, such as sprains, strains, and fractures. P.H.F. therapy is completely safe. After many years of application there are no reported contra-indications to its use.

The B.B.C. programme *Tomorrow's World* reported on research at Leeds Infirmary showing how P.H.F. can regenerate peripheral nerves; it demonstrated the clinical use of P.H.F. in treating a recently sprained ankle. The *British Medical Journal* published the results of a study at Leeds on soft tissue injuries which showed that patients who received P.H.F. therapy experienced definite biological improvement, especially in the reduction of pain and disability. The *New*

Scientist has reported how P.H.F. is gaining increasing use in both conventional and heterodox medical centres, especially for reducing tissue swelling following injury. The article described how the calcification which develops with swollen joints (synovitis) disappears with P.H.F. Other examples of its use included reduction of excess tissue fluid (oedema or swelling) associated with cellular damage, quicker formation of new skin in burns, dispersal of normal bruising which follows some types of surgery, and increased speed of healing in many conditions. One finding of particular importance was that symptomatic relief in patients suffering from peptic ulceration could be speeded up if P.H.F. was combined with a normal medical régime. The control group of patients, those who did not receive P.H.F. therapy, needed up to twice as long to obtain the same relief.

P.H.F. also combats infection. The results of a study at a New York hospital published in *Clinical Medicine* described how pelvic inflammatory disease in forty-five patients was treated with pulsed high frequency energy in addition to routine hospital therapy of antibiotics, sedatives, and bed rest. These patients recovered more quickly (7·4 days in hospital) than those receiving only the routine treatment (13·5 days in hospital), an average saving of six days in hospital per patient with P.H.F. therapy.

I have been treating patients with P.H.F. for over five years, and have been able to observe clinically how effective it can be when dealing with deep-seated infections. When treating complaints such as prostatitis, marked improvement has been noted after three to four treatments. P.H.F. is most effective when dealing with an acute injury, such as sprained ankles, wrists, etc. With broken bones it is possible to treat directly through plaster casts. The healing time can be reduced by as much as 50 per cent. Dramatic relief from pain has been obtained with severely painful complaints such as broken ribs.

It is not necessary for patients to undress; treatment can be given through clothing or surgical dressings. A treatment is normally for one hour, unless more than one area requires attention. The number of treatments required naturally depends on the condition being treated and whether it is acute or chronic. Here are some examples:

Sinusitis: acute, seven treatments upwards. Chronic, at least twenty treatments.
Prostatitis: twenty treatments, but there will be a marked relief of discomfort after one or two.
Sprain, such as sprained ankles. Five or six treatments, but relief from pain after the first treatment.

Kay Kiernan

L.C.S.P.(Phys.), M.F.Phys., I.R.M.T.

CONTRIBUTORS, p. 222

RADIESTHESIA

Radiesthesia is the use of the sensitivity to radiation possessed by living creatures and includes not only the ancient art of rhabdomancy or dowsing but also the more modern radionics, or 'instrumentation of radiesthesia'.

From simple dowsing – to search for water, buried objects, minerals, oil, and archaeological remains – to the more sophisticated work of seeking lost people, prognosis and diagnosis of illness, transmission of cures, and even less physical things such as investigating mental states, foretelling the future, assessing the past, detecting strange other-world energies, and seeking mineral deposits from a map of a distant place . . . we are in the world of the radiesthetist.

Most equipment, be it a hazel fork cut from the hedgerows, a simple pendulum, divining-wand[1] or the latest 'black box', will work for 90 per cent of people and certainly for 100 per cent of psychics. Bob Welling of B.B.C.'s *Nationwide* managed to find a penny in the gravel of Archer's Court. At a meeting of twenty guests only one failed to use a divining-rod within thirty minutes; the failure was afraid of psychics. The reaction gained by this failure gives the quite technical answer to the

F

dowsing phenomenon: the major part of it is psychological, but nevertheless real.

The psyche as a complex, constantly evolving mental energy-pattern directed by desire and will, can reach out into its external world of similar energies and patterns and, in making contact, gain modifications which represent information. The flow of this energy is directed, promoted or blocked by patterns in the mind; by psychological structures. These obstructed blockages can readily be modified.

Early attempts to provide instruments for radiesthesia (the simple pendulum, for example, can only convey limited information in laborious ways) sought explanations within the boundaries of formal science and inevitably failed. Many strange instruments were produced and soon many users were asking, 'Why does it work without the plug in?' or, 'I took out the insides and it made no difference.' Why, indeed?

Radiesthetic detectors, amplifiers, transmitters, rate instruments (to collect numerically based data about various states) and others were produced, often at great expense and many times leading to complaint, frustration, loss and even High Court[2] cases when it was discovered that the instruments were random in operation and often non-operable. If you believed in them explicitly they worked; if you lost faith in them they did not. There are, in scientific evaluation, simple basic processes such as ratios, percentages, degrees of value and intensity, and so on. If these aids to evaluation were consciously or unconsciously apparent in the instrument concerned, then the psyche's conditions were satisfied and the instrument could function. All conceptually insignificant parts of a black box were thrown away, and the proper suggestions imposed by printing the circuit for the psyche to enjoy. Printed dials and connectors were made and rotating knobs connected to nothing were put on the dials. The printed picture of a ratio, percentage, detection, output, radiating or any other system worked just as well. Mnemonics,[3] the study and application of the psychological element in radionics, was born.

So far as you can conceive the exact structure of your needs, be they personal or to help others, and, so far as you can find good reasons psychologically to do so, then mental-energy patterned and real can be projected. Dowsing generally refers to the use of simple instruments to achieve one's aims and the more complex and meaningful radiesthetic instrumentation (radionics) uses not only simple dowsing detectors but psychologically orientated instrumentation. The more advanced neometaphysical theories suggest that with a little more psychological advancement healing can be direct and better, that we might remain healthy or regain health as a consequence of our own mental powers.

Try the dowsing technique for yourself. Make a simple pendulum by hanging a large bead on a thin cord about one foot long. Hold it over any object and, if necessary, give it a deliberate swing. This will eliminate any psychological obstruction you may impose. Try again and note *how* it swings. There are four modes: straight left-to-right across the body; to-and-fro away from the body; clockwise circles; and anti-clockwise circles. These four modes can combine to give slanted or elliptical movements. Also, responses may come singly, or in repeating pairs, triads, tetrads and so on; they can be small, medium or mighty.

Now determine which type of response corresponds to the things you wish to identify. With pad and pencil ready, head the page with *Table of Correspondences* and then proceed with the first test. Take a coin, hold your pendulum over it and mentally ask, 'Is this a coin?' The answer must be yes. Note the swing and enter, say, 'Yes – straight to-and-fro swing.' Now ask, 'Is this a piece of cheese?' Enter, 'No – anti-clockwise swing.' Continue, 'Is this copper?' Enter, 'Yes/no – partly – angular straight swing.'

Try the mnemonic system. Write the names of illnesses and hold the pendulum over each in turn, noting the responses, such as, influenza – clockwise, straight, to-and-fro, anti-clockwise, triads. Proceed with medication, vitamins. Iron: cascara. Note the correspondences; or ask, 'Is iron needed?' holding the pendulum over 'common cold' and noting whether the response gives yes or no. →**Homoeopathic** medicines are peculiarly suited to pendulum tests. You can also test food for its value to you by simple yes–no tests on the spot.

Further personal data can be gained by holding the pendulum, say, over the hand and noting reactions from each of three parts of the digits and from the palm. You may notice some strange effects, like the same response from your heart coming from a part of a finger! This leads to the study of radiesthesia of →**acupuncture** and zone-therapy (→**reflexology**) points and much else.

Be careful when studying the results of others. It is far better to develop your own responses because they, and they alone, are in attunement with your own personal psychological patterns.

Let us applaud the long and dedicated efforts of the radiesthetists. Albert Abrams for his black box; the electrician at the Walton House Institute, London; George de la Warr, Ruth Drown, Guyon Richards, Curtis Upton, Maby, Bovis, Brünler and many others. We must not forget that now-deceased, crusty character, Reverend Cameron[4] of Elsinore, U.S.A., nor W. E. Benham,[5] physicist with a radiesthetic bent, and others too numerous to list but not forgotten. Nor the learned bodies, whose ignorance and prejudice did more to promote angry researchers more than the degradation of non-formal subjects. Above all give credit to the non-recognized, non-earning, non-profit, totally dedicated groups and individuals who fought the prejudice/truth fight so well since 1946 and onwards, whose data is now the basis of a rapidly developing spiritual science.

In spite of the neometaphysical[6] solutions to psychic aspects of radiesthetic work, there remains a special area of research to which the term 'borderline science' was given: it was later re-named, inadequately, paraphysics. This special psycho/physical region is involved with the study of the exact manner in which mind and matter co-mingle. For example,

thinking correctly – remember the psychic element – as an ionized photoplate[7] causes images to appear on the developed film; physical phenomena in the sceance-room[8] causes charged electroscope-leaves to collapse; mental projection at critically balanced bridge-circuits causes variation in output (the basis of so-called spirit-ratio),[9] psychokinetic projection[10] can cause metal-bending and many other physical effects.

If we accept the neometaphysical suggestion that mind transcends but includes matter, then all physically described energies and things are the result of mental energy transformed and held, as it were, as a physically appearing process. The next step would be to seek direct mind/matter phenomena and to try to get a clear view of the exact functioning of transformation processes which all appear so far to involve ionization functions.

From the radiesthetic side of the paraphysical fence one finds evidence to suppose that radiesthetic energy travels at 200000: times the speed of light. In hologramic mode, all parts of a radiesthetic spectrum[11] contain all other parts! This was a totally unexpected result gained from biometric studies, because the electromagnetic analogue leads one to expect that harmonics of a fundamental frequency would be separate, whereas in radiesthesia they are not so separated. Such a result, against the expectations of the scientist-observer, suggests his own impartiality and gives added reality to the infinitely dimensioned matrix[12] required in mental processes, wherein all points co-exist in space and time.

Allowing for the distortion that non-perception of psychic aspects brought about (distortions due to a too strict formalism) there are very many wonderful results and much authentic data to support radiesthetic healing, although a wider view of the many inter-related fields suggests that both the terms radiesthesia and radionics are being lost in the need for more embracing terminology occasioned by neometaphysics and its application in mental energy,[13] bio-energetic and other spheres. Such wonders as photography of human organs, many cures, prognoses and diagnoses all carried out at a distance by mental projection conditioned by mnemonic instrumentation; special correlations between zone therapy, acupuncture, chakras, the →human aura and many other phenomena, inspire the dedicated to pursue their course towards a vast and mysterious vista, a broad understanding of a new approach to medicine both mental and physical.

John J. Williamson
D.SC.(H.C.), F.S.M., M.Brit.I.R.E., F.C.G.L.I.

ASSOCIATIONS, p. 218
BIBLIOGRAPHY, p. 250
CONTRIBUTORS, p. 222
PRODUCTS, p. 227
TRAINING, p. 233

Notes

1. Elio, Pasquini, and Rome, *The Amplifying Pendulum*, 2nd edition, Society of Metaphysicians, 1972.

2. Reports on G. de la Warr case, *The Times*.

3. *Research Papers on Mnemonics*, Society of Metaphysicians, c. 1952.

4. Rev. Verne L. Cameron, *The Cameron Aurameter* and various research papers, Society of Metaphysicians, 1971.

5. W. Benham and John J. Williamson, *Handbook of the Aura Biometer*, 2nd edition, Society of Metaphysicians, 1968; W. Benham and J. J. Williamson, *Biometric Analysis of the Flying Saucer Photographs*, 2nd edition, Society of Metaphysicians, 1968.

6. J. J. Williamson, *An Outline of the Principles and Concepts of the New Metaphysics*, Society of Metaphysicians, 1967.

7. Research papers, *Wainwright Report*, Society of Metaphysicians, c. 1962.

8. W. J. Crawford D.SC., *The Reality of Psychic Phenomena*, 1918.

9. 'Spirit radio', in *Empire News, News of the World, Metaphysical Digest*, c. 1947.

10. John Taylor, *Superminds*, Macmillan London, 1975.

11. J. J. Williamson, research papers, *Radiesthetic Spectrum Analysis*, unpublished

archives, Society of Metaphysicians, 1968.

12. *Cranwell Lectures*, Parts I, II and III, Society of Metaphysicians, 1970.

13. Mental energy studies: many articles in *Metaphysical Digest*, journal of the Society of Metaphysicians, 1946–60.

RADIONICS

Will Osmond, a lawyer in his late thirties, had been plagued for nearly ten years by recurrent bouts of agonizing and incapacitating cystitis. A particularly refined form of medical torture called prostatic massage and many courses of ever more lethal antibiotics had apparently served only to enhance the severity of subsequent attacks. Osmond was nearing desperation when a friend gave him the name and address of a radionic practitioner. At that time he had never heard of radionics and, judging by his friend's description, the method struck him as nonsense.

However, he arranged to call. After a discussion he concluded that the practitioner was a person of unimpeachable sincerity and he decided to put radionics to the test. He duly received treatment for the next few months during which time he had no personal contact with the practitioner at all. That was over twenty years ago and he has not had a suspicion of cystitis since that day.

Will Osmond's case is typical of thousands. Many people who turn to radionics have failed to obtain relief elsewhere. Many are sceptical, yet many derive great benefit from it. It is now becoming more widely known and a growing number of practitioners of other forms of alternative medicine, such as →chiropractic, →osteopathy and medical →herbalism are coming to recognize the value of radionics as an adjunctive therapy.

Radionics is the method started fifty years ago by which a practitioner using a pendulum or stick pad in conjunction with a hair or blood specimen of the patient and a means of creating patterns of non-physical energy, identifies the causes of illness and provides remedial treatment, all in the absence of the patient. What then is this apparently mysterious process and how does it work? It only appears to be mysterious because man has only just begun to re-discover the natural laws and processes which make phenomena of this kind explicable. It is now emerging that, whereas science used to regard the ultimate constituents of the universe as energy and matter, the truth is that matter is itself only crystallized energy, that the ultimate irreducible components of all creation are energy and consciousness, and that the whole phenomenal world, human, animal, vegetable and mineral, is shot through with what one great scientist, Erwin Schroedinger, called 'mind stuff'. This is recognized by the new inter-disciplinary science of psychotronics, which was recently described by Doctor Zdenek Rejdak, President of the International Association for Psychotronic Research, as follows:[1]

Psychotronics is the science which in an inter-disciplinary fashion studies the distant interactions between living organisms and their environment, internal and external, and the energetic processes underlying their manifestations. Psychotronics understands "consciousness" in unity with "energy" and "matter". The studies of these interactions contribute to new understandings of the energetic capabilities of the human being, life processes and matter in general.

Radionics sees the cosmos as a unified system in which no part is entirely separate from any other part. That view has always been good mysticism and today it is good physics as well; and radionics has some affinities with both. As Arthur Koestler was recently reported as saying:[2]

It's amazing how many physicists today are interested in extra-sensory perceptions and all that kind of thing. Today, physicists are mystics! Modern physics has destroyed materialism. Matter evaporates. It runs through the fingers like sand. . . . It's an Alice-in-Wonderland universe. The unthinkable propositions of modern physics make the unthinkable concepts of para-psychology a little less unacceptable.

Once one can begin to visualize the universe as an immensely complex network of interlocking and interacting energy fields, the concepts of radionics begin, in Koestler's words, to become 'a little less unacceptable' The energy it is concerned with embraces not only the physical energies known to mainstream science – electromagnetic, nuclear and gravitational energy – but also the non-physical or subtle energies. These include, for example, the energy of life known in Hindu medico-philosophy as prana, the yin and yang of Chinese →acupuncture and many others. Indeed, while physical and non-physical energy intermingle, radionics is relatively more concerned with the latter than the former.

The reason is that the subtle energy-field in any biological system, say a human being, is antecedent in point of causation to the physical electromagnetic energy field. Radionics sees the energy of the cosmos condensing into progressively more solid forms as the processes of creation proceed further and further from the source of all that is, and so the relatively more rarified has a conditioning effect on the relatively more dense. Thus, a human being, in whom the structure of the cosmos is reflected on a microcosmic scale, comprises configurations of subtle energy as well as electromagnetic energy; and, as radionics seeks always to get back as far as possible to first causes, it is at the subtle energy level that its analyses are made and its treatments are given.

So what is a radionic analysis and how is it made? We have seen that the cosmos can be viewed as a network of interlocking energy currents of which the observer (in this case the radionic practitioner) himself forms part. At the non-physical level, everything is connected with everything else and there is no separation. Each individual, as a point of consciousness, is enmeshed in what Pir Vilayat Inayat Khan calls the 'collective conscious', a phrase which provides a more helpful construct than Jung's 'collective unconscious' as it emphasizes the active, dynamic, creative aspect of the mental component of the universe. Theoretically, therefore, information about anything which is happening anywhere is available to me at all times. Information about distant events does not, however, enter my conscious mind because all input data has normally to go through the sieve of my five physical senses which are specifically designed to protect me from bombardment with an excessive quantity of data by filtering out all but a comparatively narrow band of physical energy effects.

If, therefore, I want to obtain information to which my physical senses do not have access I have to make use of the inner, non-physical sense (sometimes inaccurately described as the sixth sense) with which man has always been endowed. That sense can be tuned, by a direction from the conscious mind, to select from the multifarious streams of non-physical energy in which it is immersed the one which carries the required information. The incoming subtle energy signal then has to be converted, or transduced, into physical (electromagnetic) energy so as to make it comprehensible to the conscious mind.

For this purpose the pendulum or stick pad is used as a detecting device. A very small current is generated in the neuro-muscular system which, independently of conscious volition, causes the pendulum to move and, by the direction of its swing or gyration, to indicate yes or no responses to consciously held questions. Professor W. A. Tiller PH.D., Chairman of the Department of Materials Science at Stanford University in the U.S.A. and a prominent figure in the field of psychotronics, has categorized the processes for registering and decoding non-physical energy signals as follows:[3]

There are three categories of devices one may use for monitoring non-physical energies: (a) a human being who has already developed other sensory systems and makes observations with them and provides a verbal readout (a medium); (b) a living system (animal, plant or human) plus an attached electromagnetic or mechanical device, so that the living system transduces the non-physical energies into readout via a purely physical path (kirlian devices) [high voltage photography]; and (c) a totally inanimate device based upon a different logic system than that which we call physical, which acts both as a transducer and a readout mechanism (no instruments in this category).

The case of radionics clearly belongs to Tiller's second category: a human being, using a mechanical device in the form of a pendulum, transduces the non-physical energies reaching him from the 'collective conscious' into readout in the form of oscillations or gyrations of the pendulum. Thus, when the practitioner who treated Will Osmond analysed that case he would no doubt have used his pendulum to obtain information about the condition of Mr Osmond's bladder, kidneys and other relevant internal organs, his psychological state and any other factors (such as his diet and alcohol intake) which might have contributed to the symptoms. This process, which depends largely on focussing the mind, is an entirely natural, rational and logical one and, as Arthur Koestler has indicated, no more extraordinary or 'mystical' than contemporary physics. Similarly, Professor Tiller has said:[4]

I wish to underline or re-emphasize that one-pointedness of mind (directed application of mind) is the key element in enhancing one's radiesthetic sense [radiesthesia], one's ability meaningfully to use special instruments like a radionic instrument, one's ability to tune directly into the universal information source or one's ability to tap primary energy streams in the cosmos. Perhaps we can also see here the influence of one's attitude as he performs a function upon his adaptability to perform that function effectively. I wish also to strongly emphasize that it all occurs in a very natural way via natural processes having firm foundations in physics. However, much of what I have discussed concerns 'tomorrow's physics'– pointed to by discoveries today.

Radionics is now, however, concerned only with analysing a case in order to determine the underlying causes of the symptoms: it would not have done Mr Osmond much good merely to be told, for example, that a distortion in some part of his subtle energy field had resulted in a disturbance of the balance of his intestinal fauna, or something of that kind. He needed, and obtained, first treatment to rectify the para-physical disharmony and, secondly, hard practical advice to lay off alcohol.

The distinctive contribution of radionics to

the healing arts is twofold. First, in the search for the ultimate causes of illness it penetrates far deeper than any other system into the psycho-spiritual constitution of man. Secondly, it is the only system to have developed a complete methodology for making analyses and applying remedial treatment at the subtle energy level.

In order to do this it simulates, as may be required, all the patterns or configurations of non-physical energy associated with all the features of the subtle anatomy (such as the so-called astral and causal bodies and the chakras), the physical anatomy, the psychology and the various disease conditions to which man is prone. The traditional way of setting up a required pattern, or subtle energy field (e.g. in Mr Osmond's case the pattern of the bladder), is to use a device consisting of a series of calibrated potentiometers (resistances) with pre-determined rates (i.e. dial settings) representing the various features. A similar result can also be obtained with certain distinctive geometrical designs. The practitioner makes an analysis in order to identify the points of weakness in the system and then seeks to strengthen them by irradiating the patient (using a hair or blood specimen as a witness) with an energy pattern specifically designed to correct the distortions in the patient's own energy-field disclosed by the analysis.

This process can be roughly illustrated, at the level of physical (magnetic) energy, by reference to the experiment every schoolboy has carried out with iron filings, a sheet of paper and a magnet. If the magnet is held under the paper the filings arrange themselves in a symmetrical pattern along the lines of force. If the magnet is taken away and the paper is moved, the pattern is distorted, but its symmetry or integrity can be restored by re-asserting the magnetic field.

Radionics can be used for the treatment of any condition, without exception, but that is not to say that it is a cure-all: on the contrary, it is not claimed as a cure for anything because results depend largely on the response of each individual patient, quite irrespective of the name by which his symptoms are known by orthodox medicine. In other words, as with all true healing methods there is a large subjective factor in the situation which makes it quite impossible to generalize about the prospects of success in relation to particular named ailments. All that can be said is that clinical experience over about half a century shows unmistakably that a large proportion of patients derive substantial benefit, very often in cases where conventional medicine has nothing to offer or, as in Will Osmond's case, had failed to alleviate the condition.

Among the other advantages of radionics are that it is equally suitable for the treatment of male and female, young and old alike; that it is free of unwanted side-effects; that it has a valuable preventive rôle because, as most illness is generated at the para-physical level of the organism, signs of trouble may be radionically recognizable at that level sometime before the appearance of physical symptoms; that, in a case where various different therapies might be appropriate, it can be used to determine which would be the most valuable; and that treatment is given *in absentia* and distance is immaterial.

How long treatment will take depends on a wide variety of variable factors. In a short sharp acute condition such as a local infection which would subside in a few days anyway, radionic treatment may be able to hasten natural recovery. In other cases of a more deep-seated or chronic nature it may take months or even years to obtain the fullest possible benefit. It should not, however, be thought of as merely an aspirin substitute; it is based on fundamental concepts relating to the essential nature of man and the cosmos and therefore offers a learning experience as well as the alleviation of symptoms. Thus, it may frequently lead to the development of a deeper philosophy of life on the part of the patient and modifications of his life-style, both of which may react favourably on his general state of health.

Radionic treatment normally combines well with the other forms of alternative medicine. It is less happy in the company of allopathic medicine as it is essentially based on a pro-biotic rather than an antibiotic philosophy; but radionic practitioners do nevertheless of necessity regularly treat patients who are undergoing orthodox treatment at the same time and the results are often entirely satisfactory.

All that is required in the first instance to obtain treatment is for the patient to write to the practitioner indicating broadly his problem and inquiring whether the practitioner could help. A list of practitioners is obtainable from the Radionic Association whose entry appears in the Directory of this book.

John Wilcox M.A.

Notes

1. Z. Rejdak and others, Announcement concerning Third International Conference on Psychotronic Research, *International Journal of Paraphysics*, Vol. II, Nos. 1 & 2 (1977).

2. A. Koestler interviewed by Norman Moss, *The Times*, 21 February 1977.

3. W. A. Tiller, Are Psychoenergetic Pictures Possible?, *New Scientist*, vol. 62 (1974), p. 895.

4. W. A. Tiller, *Radionics, Radiesthesia and Physics*, Academy of Parapsychology and Medicine (Denver, Colorado), 1972.

RECESSED HEEL FOOTWEAR

The basic concept of recessed heel footwear is now almost twenty years old, and last year in North America an estimated twenty million pairs were sold. →Yoga practitioners and nature enthusiasts as well as the medical establishment now look favourably on this type of footwear.

It was, in fact, a yoga teacher in Denmark who first developed a commercially successful recessed heel shoe. She had remarked several things which the reader can also easily recognize. When standing barefoot on soft ground, one's heel sinks slowly into the ground more deeply than the rest of the foot. As the heel sinks, the pelvis tilts slightly, the spine straightens, and one is more erect and breathing more easily. When walking on a soft surface, the heel's impact drives it deeper into the ground than the rest of the foot, and there is a rolling motion as the weight goes forward to the next stride. The imprint left by the foot clearly shows that deeper heel imprint and the roll forward. The yoga teacher who remarked on this combined four elements: the recessed heel, an arch support, a rocker sole, and a wide toe area. She was trying to duplicate, as best possible, the positions the foot would take in normal walking and standing when the ground beneath is naturally soft, a forest's ground, a meadow's grass, or a beach's packed sand. Since on hard pavements the foot cannot seek a natural position, she put her idea of the position into the sole of her shoe.

The recessed heel footwear which we know today has been refined and further developed by a number of firms. Taken into consideration have been optimal angle of inclination for the recessed heel for each size of shoe, the type and degree of arch support, the curve of the rocker sole, and the shape of the toe area, as well as the grip and support of the heel counter. All of these factors are important if 'natural' walking and standing positions are to be possible on 'unnaturally' hard surfaces, such as pavements and concrete floors.

Is it really 'natural' to have one's heel lower than the rest of the foot? Haven't people been walking with heels for centuries and without major problems? Well, not quite. Most people worked in soft farm fields and wore flat wooden shoes which did sink in at the heels in the soft ground. Others rode horseback, and their high heels were used to prevent them from slipping through the stirrups. Only in relatively modern times has man tried to spend a lifetime wearing high-heeled shoes on hard walking surfaces. The result has been a very high incidence of foot and back problems among city dwellers.

Most people take walking for granted but with little understanding. When walking the foot moves in three directions, forward, up and down, and side to side. As the foot is lifted into the air and then starts its descent towards the ground, the foot structure becomes loose and flaccid, almost like a bag of bones. Then, while on the ground the foot changes into a firm lever, rigid enough to propel you off on your next footstep. (This changing skeletal structure is one reason a foot can vary as much as half a size depending upon whether it is measured with or without body weight on it.) During the walking motion the pressure, the weight of the body, goes first on the heel, is transferred diagonally over the outside of the foot to the big toe, and then springs off for the next step. This changing path of weight and the transfer from flaccid to rigid state is a marvellously complex operation, as long as it continues to work properly. Occasionally problems arise. Sometimes the foot will attempt a take-off while it's still in the limpid state. This creates hypermobility (too much moving around). The result can be corns and callouses, and possibly more serious troubles. This is one of the reasons for the support counter of the heel. The arch support also minimizes hypermobility by keeping the inner foot structure from flopping around. However, it is possible to go too far. Some shoes have too much and too rigid supports, thus preventing the foot from being flexible when it should be able to loosen up for the down-step. This technical, medical knowledge of how the foot functions and the different way it functions in the air and on the ground are relatively new and only recently recognized by medical authorities.

It is with such new knowledge of the foot's functions that a noted American authority recently wrote:

A shoe in which the sole is higher than the heel would actually be the ideal footwear in the erect position, in that it would throw the weight of the body on the heels and make it necessary to bend the truck slightly forward in order to maintain the centre of gravity. This would relieve pressure from the back edges of the vertebral structures which lie behind in the low back. Obese individuals, as well as pregnant women, both carry an extra load in front for which some backward compensation must be made.[1]

At the Sports Medicine Clinic, Carleton University, Ottawa, Canada, leading North American orthopaedists conducted clinic tests on a large sampling of healthy, active competitive athletes who wore recessed heel shoes during those periods of the day when they were not training or competing. It is recognized medically that it is extremely important for athletes and dancers to exercise properly their heel cord tendons and muscles. The clinical tests showed that the recessed heel shoes provided the kind of stretching that the doctors felt was important for the athletes and that no problems were caused as a result of wearing the recessed heels. Less than 1 per cent of those in the test found them to be uncomfortable after the short, initial adaption period. Tests of recessed heel shoes at the California College of Pediatry have, also, generally been interpreted as favourable to recessed heel footwear. One of the doctors participating in that test programme pointed out particular advantages to pregnant women. During pregnancy some women experience pain in the lower back, have tired legs, and have sore feet with pronating or flattening of the arches. One of the major reasons is that such women are simply not prepared to carry the extra weight of their pregnancy. With recessed heel footwear, such women find a slight tilt to the pelvis and a straighter posture which, thus, better enables them to carry the added weight of pregnancy. Additionally the broad toe area and the flexible, contoured arch support help prevent the painful pronating or flattening. The toes are able to move and to support the added weight.

With many 'nature' or 'natural' shoes on the market the consumer must be wary. Only a few combine all important natural features:

1 A recessed heel in which the level of the heel is sufficiently below the level of the ball of the foot and where the angle of inclination is neither too severe nor too flat.
2 A flexible, contoured arch support which gives proper support to the longitudinal arch without being excessive.
3 A broad toe area in which the toes can

properly flex as they go through the flexible-flaccid to rigid state and back again.

4 A snug, well-fitting heel counter which prevents the heel from rocking side to side or falling off the back of the sole.

5 A well-proportioned rocker sole which assists the foot with the transfer and forward propulsion of the body's weight.

Within the range of manufacturers who do provide all of the above features there is, of course, a range of prices depending on the quality of materials and workmanship. Unfortunately, in Great Britain several major shoe manufacturers have introduced shoes with the wide toe area and general outward appearance of 'natural' shoes but without the critical recessed heel feature. They have put such uppers on conventional wedge soles, thus negating the natural aspect.

For all its positive features, the main claim for recessed heel footwear is that most normal people find that after a day of walking and/or standing, they are less tired than when wearing raised heels or flat soles.

Certain people should not wear recessed heel footwear. Those who have irritated or damaged Achilles tendons must not wear them. There are certain foot deformities and certain special structural problems which do not lend themselves to the wearing of recessed heels, and in such questionable cases a doctor must be consulted. Such exceptions apart, recessed heel footwear seems generally beneficial for the public at large.

Alan K. Jackson

BIBLIOGRAPHY, p. 246
CONTRIBUTORS, p. 222
PRODUCTS, p. 229

Note

1. Paul C. Williams M.D., *Low Back and Neck Pain*, University of Texas Press, 1975.

REFLEXOLOGY

The founder of what is popularly called zone therapy was an American ear, nose and throat specialist, Dr William H. Fitzgerald. At the turn of the century he introduced to the western world the technique that he had studied extensively and which had been practised in China and India for thousands of years. Fitzgerald pointed out that the application of fingers and thumb pressure accompanied by massaging motions on some parts of the body could have a positive effect on the physiological function of certain other parts, however far removed from the actual treatment zone. This sounds as if it might be related to →acupuncture; but no direct connection between zone therapy and acupuncture is established so far. It is accepted that there might be some relationship with Hatha →yoga.

In the 1930s an American lady, Eunice D. Ingham, considerably developed the Fitzgerald technique, but with almost complete concentration on the zones of the feet. She contributed so much to the technique that it has carried her name ever since as, in full, the Ingham Reflex Method of Compression Massage. It is an extremely sensitive and precise form of foot massage for which considerable knowledge of anatomy and physiology is required. Because of the interpretational skills required it is not the kind of treatment one could expect from a chiropodist and the reputation of the technique, at one time, was in jeopardy because of its misapplication by inexperienced people who had been badly trained, who then trained others with inadequate background knowledge of the basic medical sciences. This is not to say that skilled chiropodists cannot do much useful work in connection with the technique; but the purpose and procedures are quite different.

A number of British people went to America to receive their training direct at the hands of Miss Ingham herself; but during the 1940s and 1950s interest and activity in this country declined. Then in the sixties came a reawakening of interest, at which time the author contacted Miss Ingham after seeing how the technique could successfully and dramatically treat →constipation. The author, a qualified osteopath and medical →herbalist, has been practising and also teaching the foot-reflex technique ever since. Several hundred French and Belgian physiotherapists have been trained by the author and other teachers, and a number of qualified practitioners in other natural therapies have been trained in the United Kingdom. It is regarded as most important that any prospective student is already qualified and experienced in some accepted therapeutic modality such as physiotherapy, →osteopathy, →homoeopathy, etc.

The whole principle of the Ingham technique is that there is a direct reflex action between the nerve endings in the feet and the various organs of the body. The soles and parts of the upper foot together make up a complete 'chart' of the vital organs – a picture of the body. The therapy works on a functional level. It can be used for diagnosis, as a preventive therapy and as a direct treatment system of reflexology. It has a balancing effect, assisting the natural homeostasis of the body and its organs by remote control from the feet. The practitioner holds the patient's feet, one at a time, and uses sensitive fingers to read the surface, almost like a blind person reading Braille. The experienced practitioner actually feels a difference in the affected area through the surface of the foot. Sometimes it may feel like a shallow depression in the skin or more often like crystals under the skin. When such an area in the foot is subjected to pressure the patient may feel intense pain. Other extremely sensitive patients may even feel pain in the organ that is out of balance, but this is exceptional. Patients have described the sensation as being like having a needle, or broken glass, stuck into the foot when even quite gentle finger pressure is exerted on the functional point.

During treatment the pressure is maintained on the appropriate point while a clockwise rotating movement of the hand is applied continuously, without sliding away or losing contact. Pressure must always remain the same whichever part of the foot – i.e. the body-map – is being manipulated. Treatments usually last about twenty minutes and it is customary for a second treatment to be given, if necessary, after a few days unless there has been a complete recovery, which can easily occur, depending on the condition being treated. If pain is still present when pressure is exerted this is an indication that the therapy should be continued; but it is not usual to give more than one or two treatments in any one week. The author has found that both the Ingham technique and total reflex therapy are particularly useful in her own practice when used in conjunction with other natural therapies. Compression massage on the feet has proved very effective in gall-stone conditions and has stimulated the passing of very small gravel stones and even kidney stones. Sometimes the treatment helps to build up a healing crisis to the point where it can be stopped to allow the body resources to take over the natural function of healing, perhaps gently aided by other therapies such as diet control, homoeopathy and hydrotherapy.

The author's own foot chart indicates in detail where all the reflex points of the feet are situated, based on the original findings of Miss Ingham and Dr Fitzgerald. Although these points are extremely precise in diagnosis and treatment terms it can be shown that, for example, the heart area is approximately in the centre of the instep of the left foot; the liver zone is on the outside centre of the sole of the right foot; the ascending colon zone is on the sole of the right foot; the descending colon on the left foot; and the transverse colon zone runs across both feet. Sinus reflexes are in the upper part of the toes, the pituitary gland reflexes are in the balls of the big toes, and so on, with left-hand organs on the left foot, right-hand organs on the right foot and 'central' organ reflexes overlapping from foot to foot.

One of the most significant aspects of the Ingham method for diagnosis and treatment is that the patient feels pain when the crystal deposits in the feet are subjected to pressure, and relief when these deposits are dispersed by simple massage and manipulation of the appropriate reflex zone. Although these phenomena are felt locally on the zones of the feet, the organic or system-disorder of the patient is corrected at the same time on the physiological level, sometimes quite dramatically.

Foot reflexology brings relief for many conditions, particularly those involving congestion. It will unblock sinuses, relieve →migraine, assist the function of the pancreas, liven up a sluggish liver. It is very effective with constipation and in disorders of the kidneys and will perform many other useful therapeutic tasks that will greatly assist the practitioner in his efforts to return the patient to full health more quickly and more effectively. Many of the technique's successes have been in the dispersal of toxic elements that so often affect the organs of the body and affect the natural energy flows. Again, however, it should be emphasized that such techniques should be applied by properly qualified practitioners who are aware of the sometimes unexpected complications and reactions.

No two patients are alike in the way they react to reflex therapy. Naturally the more toxic the substances that exist in the bloodstream and elsewhere in the general systems of the patient the more dramatic are the reactions likely to be. Sometimes, for example, a patient will feel intensely cold. Another patient may experience symptoms of emotional distress. It is essential for the practitioner of this technique to remember that although apparently simple, it is in fact quite drastic in its effect and care should be taken with particularly sensitive patients. Most of all, it must be understood that what the practitioner is aiming to do is to assist the normal course of nature to affect a proper restoration of circulation by the elimination of stagnant poisons blocking the life flows of the body.

Diagnostically all the parts of the body and all the organs have a reflex point on the feet. The more extreme the reaction when pressure is applied the more serious is the disorder or malfunction. As the pain of the pressure point decreases during treatment so does the health of the appropriate organ improve – nature offering another typical example of how essential is balance, and counter-action, in the functioning of the body.

What the Ingham technique effectively achieves is the clearance of congestion which has been described as the 'only illness there is' – mental or physical! With patience, gentleness and care the Ingham compression massage technique can offer considerable relief in many conditions. When it is considered how sensitive the technique is, how dreadful to think of the callouses, corns and bunions which so often affect people's feet. Would it not be far better to look after our feet so that we can 'walk slowly, without emotion; but walk with dignity step by step, as an elephant walks in the jungle'? Surely that way would be much better than the usual headlong rush at life which so often results in both emotional and physical breakdown. Perhaps if we were more aware of the essential and intrinsic value of our feet we would tread life's path much more carefully, much more gracefully and eventually much more healthily.

Martine Faure-Alderson

BIBLIOGRAPHY, p. 250
CONTRIBUTORS, p. 222
TRAINING, pp. 231, 232

REICHIAN THERAPY

Many forms of body-therapy have originated from the work of Wilhelm Reich. Reich was a young analyst in the circle around Freud in Vienna in the 1920s when he began to focus his attention on the physical and emotional effects of repressed sexuality. His work on disturbances in the flow of pleasurable energy (libido) during orgasm led him to a very close study of ways in which undischarged energy were bound in the form of varying forms of character armouring, and in specific patterns of bodily tension, postural disturbance, and inhibited breathing.

He understood that neurosis is much more than a mental or emotional state, with 'psychic' symptoms. It was a total stress state of the body in which the overall functioning of the organism was thrown out of balance, so that the processes of intake, circulation, and outflow of biological energy were interfered with. The results of this interference appeared in a number of functional and organic illnesses which had as their common root a reduced pulsation of the tissue fluids, and a one-sided activity of the vegetative nervous system which regulates the involuntary processes (heart beat, intestinal peristalsis, muscle tone, etc.) of the body.

Reich's work was little understood at the time he developed it (during the 1930s) because it was unheard of for a psychoanalyst to be venturing so far into territory normally the preserve of purely organic medicine. Reich's focus on sexual misery as being a prime focus for the disturbance of the organism's energy economy was decades ahead of its time.

The therapy that Reich developed was first called 'vegeto-therapy' since it worked to restore the smooth and harmonious functioning of the vegetative energies of the body. He worked directly and indirectly on muscle tensions, breathing patterns and character attitudes, to bring a person in touch with the ways in which he knotted his body up to contract against the strong sensations of his own life flowing through him. There was a deep pleasure anxiety, he found, engendered by many factors in a predominantly life-negative culture-pattern, that made it difficult for people to feel deep organic satisfaction from the process of being alive. The ability to surrender fully and deeply in a loving orgasm (for Reich the loveless orgasm was a contradiction in terms) was in essence the same thing as the ability to give oneself deeply to any facet of life. People going through a course of vegeto-therapy found it put them in touch with a new vitality, and a new creativeness which became possible once they were able to relax the bodily constrictions that kept them away from deep feelings.

→**Primal therapy**, one of the offshoots from Reich's approach, has made people more familiar with the possibilities of releasing very stormy and turbulent emotions, dramatically but safely. →**Bio-energetics**, developed by Alexander Lowen, who trained with Reich, involved a number of bodily postures and expressive exercises that help people to break through some of their chronic tension-patterns and experience deeper levels of breathing. Bio-energetic analysis is a total therapy rooted in a comprehensive understanding of the bodily dynamics of character structure, and can only be carried out properly by someone trained in this approach. However, many people have found the postures and exercises introduced by Lowen a very valuable form of self-help in their own right.

In England there have been further developments in vegeto-therapy by Gerda Boyesen, who founded the Centre for Bio-energy in London. She has studied in particular the way that the intestinal peristalsis interacts with the involuntary nervous system, and functions not only as a digestive system, but as a powerful source of energy storage and discharge. To Reich's understanding of the muscular armour which can be visibly handled and observed on the body, Gerda Boyesen adds an understanding of the deepest layers of tension in what she calls the visceral armour. Her methods of dynamic relaxation and energy distribution, used in conjunction with an intuitive understanding of the nuances of fluid pressures in the tissues, enable her to work particularly sensitively with the disturbances in the energy flow in the body.

Reich was preoccupied for much of his life with the nature of this energy: was it biochemical, bio-electric, or did it involve new forms of radiation not yet discovered? In recent years a team of Soviet scientists have been researching what they call 'bio-plasma', an energy emanation from living tissues that can be recorded by high frequency discharge photograph (→**high voltage photography**). Reich did not know of this work as it was after his time, but he did claim to have discovered a biological radiation with particular effects. He studied the ways in which atmospheric energy interacted with the life-energy in the body, and came to the conclusion that both were different expressions of one fundamental energy which he called 'orgone energy'. He constructed an orgone accumulator which was designed to collect atmospheric energy and make it therapeutically available for a wide range of illnesses and ailments. Far from being a speculative device, some thirty doctors who worked with Reich were able to demonstrate and confirm his claim that it affects a wide range of conditions in the body: blood pressure, breathing rhythm, rate of healing of burns, haemoglobin level, to mention just a few. Quite independently of Reich, work in several countries on aero-ion therapy has confirmed that there are properties in the atmosphere that do indeed interact powerfully with the vegetative energies in the body, and can be used in a precisely parallel way to induce a wide range of beneficial effects on burns, asthma, hypertension, and many other illnesses, just as Reich claimed for his orgone accumulator.

The most striking results were obtained in the field of →cancer therapy. Although Reich never claimed a cancer cure as such, he did claim that cancer tumours began to regress with regular use of the accumulator. His work showed that cancer was a systemic disease caused by a deficient cell oxidation due to tissue toxification. In a low oxygen environment the weakened cells adopt fermentation as a last resort. This understanding has been confirmed by the separate cancer research of →Gerson, Warburg, and Issels. Reich's work highlighted the contributions made by emotional resignation and chronically reduced breathing to the tissue starvation state, and offered a practical therapy for re-charging the tissues by opening up the emotional and sexual lives of his patients, and building up the energetic strength of the blood through direct orgone therapy from the accumulator.

Misunderstood at the time, both vegetotherapy and orgone therapy are being taken much more seriously today. Many doctors are learning that they too have much to learn from the work of Wilhelm Reich.

David Boadella B.A., M.Ed.

ROLFING

Most of us accept a certain amount of aches and pains as a natural part of everyday life. Attempts to relieve these discomforts with exercises, sleep, hot baths, long vacations or new diets, at best seem temporary. Yet all of us sense the possibility of experiencing life more fully. The possibility of finding well-being through the physically integrated body seems to have escaped us.

Our body's contour is the dramatization of our experience, and physical expression of our personality. Our behaviour is an expression of our structure, exhibiting the relative freedom, openness and flow of our person. Our physical body is the shape of our consciousness. A structurally well organized body is a more centred and secure personality.

Dr Ida Rolf, once a biochemist with the Rockefeller Institute in the U.S.A., has dedicated forty years to the development of a technique which allows for the definition and creation of a structurally well-organized, integrated human being. A more human use of human beings begins a creative leap forward in each individual's personal evolution as well as in the evolving 'up-rightness' of the species. Visually, 'up-rightness' is evidenced by the vertical alignment of the centre of the ear, shoulder, hip, knee and ankle. A 'structurally' integrated being emerges, hence the term 'structural integration' by which rolfing is more formally known. An unintegrated or 'random' body can be guided close to this vertical alignment in ten hours of carefully designed work and can achieve significant improvement in vital function, balance and well-being.

How is it, then, that we are not vertically aligned in the field of gravity? In the course of life physical accidents, continued emotional stress, parental example, nappies (diapers), or shoes, may all distort the body into inefficient patterns of behaviour – of inefficient energy use. These are set into the body's connective tissue network as unbalanced or asymmetrical patterns of structure. This results in a less stable structure with significant loss of energy and impaired functioning, which may be sensed as 'that tired feeling'.

The whole body operates as a system; changes in one part lead to compensatory changes throughout all parts. Each of us has discovered our own unique way of surviving in the field of gravity, each achieving our own peculiar balance out of our own personal history. For example, the head may be thrust forward with the upper spine leaning back to compensate for it, which then forces the shoulders forward, giving a rounded look. The abdomen, and hence the lower spine, may be forward in turn. (This is a very common occurrence. Take a close look at the profile of the next person you see standing.) Enormous muscular effort must be expended just to prevent the whole wobbly tower from collapsing: the neck and upper back muscles must tighten to keep the head from falling to the chest, and so on down the body. This effort is using up energy which would otherwise be available for other uses. More than that, it is asking many soft parts of the body to do jobs they were not designed to do, that is, to act like bones. These parts accommodate but at a price; they stiffen and harden, thereby losing their ability to respond to the environment in a flexible and appropriate manner.

Rolfing frees and softens the connective tissue which has become frozen to support our posture, so that as the tissue is freed, the head and neck begin to fall back and ride without effort more directly above the spine. This allows the freed shoulder girdle to fall back and ride atop the rib cage, instead of in front, and so on down the body. A sense of lightness and structural support emerge, creating space and ease at the joints so they begin to open and glide smoothly. 'I feel as though my knee and hip joints have just been well oiled; the compression is gone,' was the statement of one individual after a rolfing session.

Dr Rolf's ingenious and systematic approach is based on the oft-neglected facts that (1) the human being is an energy mass organized in space and therefore subject to the laws and forces of gravity, and (2) the body is a plastic medium capable of change.

It takes effort to hold one's head in front of one's body or hold one's pelvis back. It is a bit of a struggle with gravity to find comfort in these positions. We each perceive our struggles in different ways – that sharp lower back pain, the unflattering shape of our body, constant fatigue, poor coordination in our golf game, poor circulation, or the experience of a relentless threatening environment. Those over forty may begin to refer to their symptoms as old age. Yet these may all simply be signs that we are off balance in our response to gravity.

The key to an efficient and graceful relationship to the field of gravity is a body in which the weight transmission remains close to a vertical central axis. The amount of energy required to move weight around a vertical axis decreases as the weight is moved in closer to the axis, as skaters and ballet dancers know when they achieve fast spins by pulling in their arms and legs and lengthening their bodies. If we picture the body as a stack of partially independent weight blocks, the lost energy will be used when the blocks are stacked directly above one another, such that a plumb-line dropped from the ear would pass through the shoulder, hip joint, knee and ankle.

Rolfing, then, is a process of organizing and balancing the body left to right, front to back, top to bottom, and inside to out around a vertical line, in the field of gravity, so that one is actually supported and uplifted by gravitational force rather than torn down by it.

There are many analogous ways in which we can experimentally validate the principles of rolfing. The practical aspects surround us in our everyday life. My car needs four tyres, the same size, with similar amounts of air, each one needs to be balanced, and the wheel alignment needs adjustment; all necessary for the car to run properly. When these requirements are not met, we find that it takes more energy, more petrol to reach the distance we are driving, the steering wheel may shake, the ride is bumpy, our tyres wear out more quickly, and it takes longer to reach our destination. Hence an unbalanced system is neither efficient nor comfortable. In the same fashion as we need to balance and re-align the parts of our car, we also need to balance and re-align the body.

Architects and engineers create stable structures by applying the laws of gravity. A supportive structure such as a column works because it is in vertical alignment with itself within the field of gravity. It is difficult to imagine a child's set of poorly stacked building blocks capable of supporting very much for very long. Rolfing is about stacking those blocks more neatly on top of one another so that our relationship with gravity is one that works to lengthen, balance and support us, not one which is stressful and likely to topple in on itself.

Change is possible and the process of disorganization can be reversed because the body is a plastic medium. The connective tissue bag inside which we live, called fascia, contains a chemical protein constituent known as collagen. This has similar qualities to what is known today as polymer plastics. That is, with the application of energy, the material moves and stays in the position of least stress.

In the process of living the fascial bag begins to get tense, tight, restricted, knotted and glued in areas – generally shrunken to the point of inflexibility; the joints and muscles no longer have the freedom and space to move appropriately, and certainly not efficiently. One group of muscles may stick to another, so that muscles not needed for a movement are pulled along anyway. As the bag gets tighter circulation to whole areas of the body may be shut off, re-routed or severely restricted. As this happens fewer nutrients reach that area, there is less oxygen for the production of normal body heat, and less and less toxins and impurities are eliminated. Ultimately this cycle leads to the death, or extremely low level of functioning, of that part of the body. In other words the ageing process.

Fascia should glide and slide on planes with itself. In this way the connective tissue provides for supports and free functioning of all structures. The most efficient and graceful state of the layered fascial bag we live inside is analogous to a finely spun spider's web,

balanced, even and flowing. During rolfing the tactile quality and contour of one's body changes from being like that of cotton to that of silk, from a small cluttered room to a large open space, from thickness to length, from stress and strain to freedom.

In ten sessions rolfers begin to set up an opening process in physiological as well as psychological awareness. We use our fingers, knuckles and occasionally our elbows as supporting structures, as we slowly and firmly allow our body weight to travel to deep areas within the body to provide an application of energy appropriate to the level necessary to reach and free the specific areas. Each session deals with different aspects of the body, treating them not just as isolated parts but rather as interdependent aspects of an integrated whole. This means that change in one area may be effected by working that area or another. It is like the spider's web having been pulled or pinched in one corner necessarily affecting the tensional balance and design in the rest of the web.

Fixing up the web, smoothing out places that have fallen in to support other areas, or beginning to create a movable independent layers, in other words the process of rolfing, sometimes involves what most of us have labelled as pain. Although it is not the kind of pain we experienced when we fell off our bicycles, and it is not something the rolfer creates, it does seem to be something, a sensation, the existence of which usually clues us in to 'what we are holding on to' and 'where we are holding on to it'.

A common occurrence is the recall of specific memories of physical or emotional trauma in conjunction with the physical and emotional release experienced in the rolfing process.

As one begins to trust one's rolfer, and as one begins to choose to let the pain be there when it is there, to accept it and move through the resistance, these sensations take on new meanings. The degree to which one is willing to participate in the rolfing process, to allow and assist the rolfer to move into one's own personal space, one's body influences the results of the work. Rolfing is not something that is done *to* you; it is a process two people agree to experience together. It is the context within which we can choose to hold, nurture and be aware of ourselves.

Research on rolfing has begun to flourish in many areas, bridging the physical, mental, emotional, and, if you will, spiritual disciplines (→**spiritual healing**). An over-view of the results includes:

Physiological changes in voice production.

Increased sensitivity and receptivity to environmental stimulation and significant increases in organization of the sensory information processing system.

Increased vital air capacity.

Positive attitude change, improved social intelligence, improved form perception, and fewer psychosomatic complaints.

Measurable changes in the physical structure, behaviour and subjective self-perception.

Decreased anxiety.

Postural change correlated with changes in self-esteem and self-certainty.

Psychotherapeutic benefit.

Improvement and maturation in autistic children (→**autism**).

Smoother, larger, less constrained, less random tension, more efficient patterns of energy use.

The research data may be brought into a more practical and personal point of view by quoting some of the reported experiences of those who have been rolfed. Such things as: 'lightness and ease of movement', 'I sleep less', 'more energy', 'less nervous', 'lost weight', 'clothes fit better', 'I can touch my toes', 'breathing is freer', 'no more back-ache', 'I can run longer with ease', 'more spontaneous with people', 'increased self-awareness', 'more assertive', 'more willing to participate in my own life'.

Rolfing is a process which allows you to experience your body as a changing dynamic whole. It is not psychoanalysis, it is not massage. It is letting go into one's centre. It is an attitude of being, doing and having, first from within. The process facilitates the erection of a human being able to create the space for the world to flow through.

Because of the shortage of rolfers, and due to a lack of international law, many individuals call themselves rolfers, thus taking advantage of the popularity this specific work has gained. In fact they may be using the term colloquially (to refer to any kind of deep tissue work) and have not trained at or through the Rolf Institute. Prospective clients should check a rolfer's credentials.

Darcey Ortolf

CONTRIBUTORS, p. 222

SHIATSU MASSAGE

Widely practised in Japan today, shiatsu is an ancient Japanese method of massage based on the concept of meridia connecting points (or *tsube*) just beneath the surface of the skin. These trigger points, which exist all over the body, including the hands, feet and neck, when stimulated by thumb or finger pressure have a far-reaching effect on the physiology of the body. Organs far removed from the area of stimulation can be toned or sedated.

The main therapeutic function of shiatsu massage is to correct faulty circulation, improve metabolism and treat a wide range of ailments including high blood pressure, arthritis, diabetes, rheumatism, stomach and intestinal complaints, →**migraine**, neuralgia and insomnia. Because it helps to eliminate toxic build-up and fluid retention, many women find it is effective as an aid to slimming (→**Weight Watchers**). Valuable features of shiatsu are that it can be done anywhere and that you can treat yourself. A good time for shiatsu self-massage is after a bath.

Tekujiro Namikeshi, a shiatsu specialist for more than forty years and founder of the Nippon Shiatsu School, who has treated more than 100000 patients, says that treatment can promote greater stamina, induce mental composure, cure frigidity, improve sexual performance and solve some of the problems that arise during the menopause.

John Newton

BIBLIOGRAPHY, p. 250
CONTRIBUTORS, p. 222

G

SPIRITUAL HEALING

The Aetherius Society has a simple philosophy of healing: 'Don't talk about it – give it!'

And around the British Isles and abroad at its centres or in private homes, that is exactly what members of the Society do. They give spiritual healing to hundreds of people of all ages, from all walks of life and with just about every type of condition from headaches to heart attacks.

What is spiritual healing? It is the transfer of energy from the healer to the patient. Not the healer's own energy, of course, but the charged particles of energy known to the eastern yogis as *prana*, or the Universal Life Force. This flows in abundance throughout Space and can be harnessed by the individual who sensitizes himself by certain occult practices. These include deep breathing and the use of holy mantra, or sound vibrations, chanted many times to build up the intake of energy. Prayer, too, is used to attract the Life Force to the healer.

Clad in white coats and working in spotless healing booths, the Society's healers are trained in a special technique devised by their Master and Spiritual Leader, Doctor Shri Yogiriji George King.

Doctor King relates in his book *You Too Can Heal* how he first discovered his own healing ability at the age of eleven when he gave miraculous healing to his mother who was seriously ill in their Yorkshire home. Since then, he has developed a technique which anyone – man, woman or child – can learn and use.

The technique involves the manipulation of the prana through the healer's hands into the psychic centres of the patient, which are the tiny floodgates within the aura through which energies continually pass. The healer's own magnetic properties are also used to take away the disease condition from the aura in a series of special passes.

In the book, an absent healing technique is also given for treatment when distance separates the healer and patient. This can be used over hundreds of miles (→absent healing).

Self healing is also described, and there is a lengthy section of questions and answers on healing.

What of the success of this technique?

Hundreds of case histories can be seen in which the spiritual healing technique devised by Doctor King has been successful and many are published in his book. Cases included relief from ailments such as arthritis and rheumatism, severe →migraine, post-operative illness and even tumours and →cancers.

Some of the patients have themselves recovered from near-fatal illness to become healers, thanks to the individual instruction courses in spiritual healing run by the Society, one of the few organizations to offer such training. In these courses, the student receives in-depth training in contact and absent spiritual healing under the eye of trained instructors, and is also given further information about the theory and practice of the occult practices used to become a better channel for the Universal Life Force to flow through him. These practices include advanced visualizations and personal initiations into secret rituals which have been closely guarded secrets of the highest mystery schools on earth . . . and beyond. The student is also taught about the great Law of Karma, which is a vitally important study for all healers, as it explains why all conditions can be cured . . . but not all patients.

The cosmic nature of the Society's teachings are the main aspect of this unique organization. Doctor King, through his ability to go into the deepest state of yogic trance (→yoga), samadhi, has been in contact telepathically with advanced cultures outside the Earth since 1954, and has acted as the channel for 600 amazing transmissions from these elevated beings . . . a world record for this type of trance.

These teachings can be summed up in the Society's motto, given by one of the great Masters: 'Service is the jewel in the rock of attainment.'

Through prayer and healing, the members of The Aetherius Society follow an active path towards the ultimate goal of all sentient beings, enlightenment. This path is open to all, and the spiritual healing technique can be learned and practised by all.

Other forms of healing also carried out by the Society include chromotherapy (→colour therapy) of an advanced nature; →homoeopathy – the Society maintains its own dispensary run by a qualified consultant who will give personal diagnoses; a biochemic and →health food advisory service; and a modern health food store.

Rev. Ray Nielsen

STAPLEPUNCTURE

For the smoker, compulsive eater, or alcoholic in the grip of their addiction it is possible help may only be as far away as a staple in the ear.

Lester Sacks, a Los Angeles family doctor who studied →acupuncture in the United States and London, has introduced an ear-stapling treatment for patients who want to stop smoking, overeating, drinking to excess, or taking drugs. Using a special 'gun' Dr Sacks inserts a surgical staple into the ear, near to an appropriate acupuncture point. When the craving for a cigarette, cream cake, or whisky arises the addict twiddles the staple and the desire for the craved object decreases.

Impressive results are claimed for the method by Dr Sacks. Some 60 per cent of patients treated for smoking reduced the habit from forty cigarettes or more a day to four or five, while many gave up altogether. Of 150 alcoholics who were staplepunctured nearly 40 per cent reduced their intake by half. Another 30 per cent had not taken a drink six months afterwards. Of 200 Los Angeles drug addicts who were treated, half gave up their addiction and none, according to Dr Sacks, suffered from withdrawal symptoms. Staple-

puncture is an aid; patients must be determined to achieve results.

John Newton

SWEDISH MASSAGE

Although the Swedish method is the most used and internationally known form of massage, it has only been in existence just over a hundred years. Massage, however, is one of the oldest forms of treatment referred to in history, literature and art. The early Chinese, thousands of years B.C., maintained that exercise and massage prevented stagnation and produced harmonious movements of the body fluids necessary for health. Hippocrates wrote, 'The physician must be experienced in many things, amongst others in friction.' Friction can bind a joint that is loose and loosen a joint that is rigid.

The words 'friction' and 'rubbing' are used in old literature until the end of the nineteenth century when 'massage' was introduced. The word's origin is uncertain. It could have been from the Hebrew *mashesh*, or the Arabic verb *massa* (to touch), or the Greek *massein* (to knead). France is usually credited with the introduction of the words '*massage*', '*masseur*' and '*masseuse*'.

The T'ang dynasty (A.D. 619–907) had four kinds of recognized medical practitioners: physicians, →acupuncturists, masseurs and exorcists. Priests of ancient Egypt used manipulation in the form of kneading for rheumatic pains, neuralgia and swellings. The Hindus also had some knowledge of the therapeutic value of massage. The Greeks knew its value, and priests and philosophers recommended manual treatment. Plato even divided it into active and passive movement. All classes of Greeks and Romans used massage, from the wealthy patricians to the slaves. For some it was a luxury that followed the bath, for others to hasten convalescence, and for some to render tissues more supple before and after severe tests of strength. It was used by gladiators to relieve pains as well as to invigorate the body. By the Middle Ages the use of massage had declined. Roman culture was followed by widespread decadence, a disdain for public nakedness (→naturism) and all preoccupation with body health. During the fifteenth and sixteenth centuries few physicians recommended massage. The seventeenth and eighteenth centuries brought a revival of interest, when massage was first mentioned in European literature as a treatment.

It was Per Henrik Ling (1776–1838) of Sweden who created the Swedish massage we know today. The Crown rewarded his efforts with the establishment of the Central Institute of Gymnastics in Stockholm. Although Ling's chief interest was medical gymnastics, and massage was only a small part of his system, it was massage that was popularized by his followers. The Swedish system came to London in 1838, to Paris by 1847, and later went to Germany, Austria and Russia. The Tsar's supreme medical board found that many patients treated with massage recovered from diseases which could not be cured by other remedies.

Swedish massage consists of five techniques:

1 Effleurage – a stroking movement by which the blood and lymphatic flow is accelerated.
2 Petrissage – manipulation of the muscle tissues. The deeper veins are emptied.
3 Percussion movements – hacking, clapping, beating, pounding.
4 Running vibrations – the fingertips follow the course of the nerves.
5 Friction – used over joint surfaces and over localized lesions, it produces a local hyperaemia and will help to restore mobility.

The beneficial results are that the skin and all its structures are nourished and it becomes soft and pliable. The fat cells in the subcutaneous tissue are broken down. The blood circulation is increased; the activity of the skin glands is stimulated, the muscle fibres are strengthened, the nerves are soothed and rested, body relaxed, and tension and pain are relieved.

For centuries massage has been manual but now electrical apparatuses have been introduced – heat lamps, vibrators, girators, suction units. However, most people prefer manual massage by a pair of strong, soft, skilled hands. Machinery is a poor substitute and the physical contact of a good therapist using his or her hands and powers of encouragement can give the most beneficial treatment.

Patricia Peplow

BIBLIOGRAPHY, p. 248
CONTRIBUTORS, p. 222
TRAINING, p. 233

T'AI-CHI CH'ÜAN

The T'ai-chi Ch'üan is an ancient Chinese system of exercise or an 'Art for Life'. The practice of T'ai-chi Ch'üan stimulates the nervous system, increases the blood circulation and glandular activity; it strengthens muscles, exercises the joints and retards the ageing process. It eases tension, calms the heart and coordinates the mind and the body. The movements are circular and gentle, done in an even, slow tempo synchronized with your breathing.

Although there is not much information, and what exists is often ambiguous, Chinese exercise art can be traced back to the Chou dynasty (1066–403 B.C.). The basic principles of the movements are found in the *T'ai-chi Classics*, three short treatises written from the thirteenth century onwards.

The T'ai-chi Ch'üan has both self-defence and meditative connotations. The movements have been given names, some referring to a self-defence application, others illustrating animal gestures whilst others have symbolical meanings. The T'ai-chi was used in a rugged form of combat which later developed into a sophisticated system of boxing or self-defence; but the performers were also influenced by the Taoists who attached great importance to controlled →breathing and the circulation of the Ch'i (referred to again below) or energy and these people used the T'ai-chi to improve health and as a method of meditation.

T'ai-chi means the *supreme ultimate* and is represented by a circle divided into two equal shapes called the yin and the yang, the two vital energies; yin being the receptive, feminine principle, yang the creative and masculine. The movements of the T'ai-chi illustrate the constant interplay between the yin and the yang, the passive and the active.

Ch'üan means fist or power. The fisted hand as used in the T'ai-chi Ch'üan is not an aggressive fist; it symbolizes balance and concentration. To be a 'Master of the Fist' is to have yourself within your grasp.

There is one more Chinese concept which has to be mentioned in connection with T'ai-chi and that is *Ch'i* which can be translated as breath or intrinsic energy. The movements are conceived and directed by the mind (I) and the object is to relax the body, to 'throw every bone and muscle open' so the Ch'i can flow unhindered.

Many styles of T'ai-chi are practised: the Yang, Wu, Sun and Ho. The most popular style in the West is Yang, named after one Yang Lu-ch'an who lived in Peking in the nineteenth century. There is the long and the short form of the Yang style. The former consists of 108 movements taking twenty to twenty-five minutes to perform whilst the latter has 37 movements lasting seven to ten minutes. The long form of the Yang style is divided into three parts and each part consists of several sequences.

The process of learning takes place on different levels, starting by coordinating the actions of the mind and the body, by memorizing the movements of limbs and eyes, observing how the skeleton is moved into various postures, feeling how each step and movement is related to a breath and how there is a balance between the yin and the yang, the passive (empty) and the active (full) part of the body. In this way the physical strength and awareness of the practitioner is developed. When the forms have been learned and understood, the movements will start to flow by themselves and the breath is no longer thought of as breath, but as a source of energy, Ch'i, which spreads through every part of the body.

The second level of understanding relates to the grouping of the movements, each sequence enacting a part of the archetypal story which, in Taoist terms, and on the third level of understanding, illustrates an allegorical journey by a human being from birth to death.

The Chinese say that one must practise the T'ai-chi Ch'üan for at least ten years before one becomes a Master. A transformation process takes place which cannot be hurried. Slowly your breath becomes freer and deeper, your thoughts clearer and you discover how to use the energy so there is harmony between the mind and the body.

Gerda Geddes

BIBLIOGRAPHY, p. 251
TRAINING, p. 233

THE TAO OF LOVING

The Tao of Loving or just the 'Tao' as the famous seventh-century physician Sun Ssû-Mo often so used in his book, *Priceless Recipe*, is perhaps the most important part of traditional Chinese medicine. A simple explanation of its importance is that without adequate loving a human being loses his proper purpose and will to go on living.

Perhaps no one knows exactly when the Tao of Loving was originated, but books were certainly available during the Han period 206 B.C.–A.D. 219. The ancient Chinese physicians understood that sexually women are as a rule much the stronger sex, and a man cannot hope to cope with this situation unless he learns how to conserve his energy. The Tao of Loving was created for this need. These physicians also knew that a man and a woman could live long and harmoniously by learning how to give warmth and joy to each other, and this is what is called the harmony of the yin and the yang. Without this vital harmony good health and longevity are unattainable.

The Tao considers conserving semen by regulating and controlling ejaculation as the first step towards a man's conserving his energy and vitality. A man should practise

181

for weeks or even months to achieve this. At the beginning he should seek a goal of not ejaculating more than two or three times out of ten coitions. It should be improved to an ultimate aim of one ejaculation out of a hundred. This is not quite as mechanical as it seems, because it depends on numerous other factors such as age, health and individual physical tendencies.

Does a man suffer from this régime? Far from it. When a man has truly mastered the Tao his pleasure in making love is many times more than it was before: not only because he will be able to make love much more frequently but because he will also be able to make love much longer on each occasion. Besides he will not at all suffer fatigue from making love.

A woman's pleasure is also proportionally increased if her partner has learned the Tao. After mastering the Tao a man can make love almost whenever his love-partner wishes and as often and as long as they both desire.

When a man and a woman love each other at such regular frequency their hormone balance can be more healthily maintained, which means they can stay young and vigorous longer. The result is longevity for both partners. Sun Ssû-Mo, an important authority of the Tao, was a good example. In spite of his busy professional life he lived just over a century from A.D. 581 to 682. This is well documented. A stamp issued in China fifteen years ago commemorated his many achievements.

How does the western world receive the ancient Tao of Loving? Except for Havelock Ellis, it was not even quite understood until very recently. Van de Velde confused it with Karezza which Marie Stopes advocated. But ever since Masters and Johnson published their second book, *Human Sexual Inadequacy*, in 1970, the situation slowly began to change. They are perhaps the first western research team openly to declare that a man does not have to ejaculate each time he makes love, a dogma going back almost 1800 years to Galen. But the first complete support comes from Gail Sheehy the author of a very popular

book at the moment, *Passages*, in which she clearly describes the desirability of the ancient Chinese way of love-making. This should not really be surprising because women for centuries suffered from men's sexual inadequacy. Erica Jong in her book *Fear of Flying* and Shere Hite in *The Hite Report* have both amply voiced this discontent.

The Tao does not limit its benefits to making a man more competent as a man, or by maintaining more healthy male–female hormone balance for both men and women. The Tao also promotes mental health. It is common knowledge that a lack of adequate love is the main cause of most mental disturbances. Here too the Tao can easily help. The Tao is also effective in curing the habit of smoking, in preventing drug-addiction, etc., because when a man and a woman are totally satisfied in loving and living in perfect harmony they have a much stronger wish to go on living a longer and healthier life. Thus it is much easier for such happy people to keep away from self-destructive habits. One of the most important benefits of the Tao is perhaps to divert people from the habit of eating too much. According to Stanley Robbin's recent book *Pathologic Basis of Disease* in 1967 cardio-vascular disease killed over one million Americans, well over half of U.S. total deaths of that year. Very few people today still doubt that over-eating or eating wrong food is the main cause of this killing disease. The Tao is nearly miraculous in stopping people over-eating. The simple reason that Tao could make love-making so much more pleasurable, so much more wholesome, so much more long-lasting and so much more easily available too, than the pleasure of eating.

The Tao also solved long ago the mystery whether a man can also have multiple orgasms or the extended male orgasm. For at least 2500 years the Tao has enabled a man to have as much pleasure as a woman and not only live as long as his counterpart, but also able to make both love-partners live much longer.

One more bonus of the Tao is a nearly perfect contraception method. When a man has mastered the Tao his partner's worry about which is the safest method is over. It may not be as effective as birth-control pills but it certainly has no side-effects; no bother and reduction of pleasure. Therefore on balance it could be even a better method. But I repeat that the man must learn first to be truly in control of himself.

The Tao also attaches no great importance to masturbation, neither condemning nor praising. Masturbation could be a substitute when love-partners are impossible to find. The Tao, however, certainly does not advise a substitute when love-partners are there, unlike some modern sexologists who seem enthusiastically to urge all men and women to learn better and better masturbation. The Tao would definitely suggest better and better love-making instead. The Tao considers masturbation a poor imitation of genuine love-making. In masturbation there is no exchange of human warmth, no communication of love and affection and absolutely no benefit of the harmony of the yin and the yang.

Jolan Chang

BIBLIOGRAPHY, p. 250
CONTRIBUTORS, p. 222

TRANSPERSONAL PSYCHOLOGY

Psychology today is in a state of flux. Behaviourism (or first force psychology as it is sometimes called) has lost much of its appeal, for despite its immense contribution to human understanding it persists in treating man as if he were a machine. Likewise the psychoanalytic stream (second force) is suspect. It too has had a tremendous influence, especially in opening up the whole question of unconscious factors in the psyche and in human behaviour. But many psychoanalysts persist in treating the peaks of human experience as deviant and as signs of mental imbalance. This is bound to lose them credibility in an era of the 'explosion of consciousness'.

Behaviourism and psychoanalysis have dominated psychology for nearly 100 years. But in the 1950s a new force – humanistic

psychology – began to emerge. It was pioneered by men like Abraham Maslow, who at the time was relatively unknown but who later became president of the American Psychological Association. Humanistic psychologists sought to put ordinary human beings and the full range of human experience back into the centre of the psychological stage. Since that time humanistic (third force) psychology has grown rapidly and now embraces a wide range of perspectives and techniques. It is strongly experiential and the 'growth movement' and humanistic psychology are now largely synonomous. →**Encounter** groups, T-groups, sensitivity training, →**co-counselling**, transactional analysis, →**gestalt**, and a wide range of bodytherapies and techniques are all found within its orbit. It is now well established as part of the psychological scene, accepted in a growing number of universities, and influencing large numbers of people.

But humanistic psychology failed to fulfil all the hopes of its founders. Abraham Maslow, his closest colleague Anthony Sutich and others were profoundly interested in the spiritual dimensions of consciousness, and the capacity of people to transcend their limited everyday awareness, and to explore the 'peaks and mountain tops' of the psyche. They wanted psychologists to investigate the 'farther reaches of human nature', to discover the conditions in which altered states of consciousness could be entered or induced, and to map the relationship between these transhuman states and the world of ordinary reality.

But by the middle 1960s humanistic psychology was so concerned with helping people to rediscover their feelings and their bodies, and to stop working everything out with their heads, that it seemed unlikely that the transpersonal dimensions of the psyche could receive adequate attention within the humanistic movement as it then existed in the United States. So, in 1969, after several years of preparation, Maslow, Sutich and others launched a *Journal of Transpersonal Psychology*, and eighteen months later formed an Association for Transpersonal Psychology, both based in California. Today the transpersonal movement (fourth force) in psychology is growing rapidly in North America. In the last four years it has begun to put down roots in Europe.

What then is transpersonal psychology? Definition is not easy, for transpersonal or fourth-force psychology was intended to be perspective and to provide an eclectic and informal umbrella for people who shared basic attitudes, but whose opinions on specific questions might differ widely. The factor of greatest significance is that wihin transpersonal psychology a number of major strands, woven by giants in the psychological field, are coming together to form a recognizable overall pattern and tapestry. Any selection of these strands is bound to be a personal one, and therefore arbitrary. But I give my own as a way of illustrating the new synthesis that I sense is now emerging within psychology.

First, *Abraham Maslow*, with his special interest in gifted people, in peak experiences, and his emphasis on the processes of self-actualization and self-realization, as dynamic motivating factors in human growth. Maslow began to explore these questions in the 1940s.

Second, *Roberto Assagioli*, an Italian psychiatrist, founder of a system known as psychosynthesis. Assagioli started to develop his ideas in the 1920s, and is significant for his mapping of higher consciousness states, ways of being in touch with and entering these dimensions, and his emphasis on the spiritual or transpersonal self as the essence and ultimate direction and monitor of the psychological energy system of the individual.

Third, *Victor Frankl*, founder of logotherapy. Frankl spent time as a inmate of Nazi concentration camps during the Second World War. He found that those whose lives had meaning, or those who could invest their lives or the experience with meaning, stood the best chance of survival. The will-to-meaning became the keynote of his psychological system and his methods of psychotherapy.

Fourth, and most important of all, *Carl Jung* and his immensely gifted group of followers. They have not only underlined the importance of unconscious factors, both individual and collective, in the human growth process, but have shown how individuals can become whole, and fulfil all sides of their nature, through the process they call individuation.

Note two things: how recent is the formal emergence of what we call transpersonal psychology; and how long ago the key strands from which it is being developed were started.

So far, I have mentioned only the western half of the picture. One of the most significant aspects of the transpersonal perspective is that it is beginning to relate and integrate both eastern and western approaches to psychological understanding and human growth. Down the ages mystics of all the great religions and philosophies have pioneered the exploration of transcendental states. Transpersonal psychology today embraces and applies the perspectives of religious and esoteric schools, and such eastern disciplines as →yoga in its various forms, Zen, Tao, Buddhist teachings and others.

It may be asked at this point: what practical use is all this high-flown stuff? How does it help ordinary people live better in a complex and often difficult world?

Firstly, transpersonal psychology is not for everyone. There are those for whom humanistic approaches are best. Others will be most at home and most helped within the Freudian frame. Some will fit best into the attitudes and style of behaviourist psychology. And many will not feel comfortable in psychology at all, and should turn elsewhere.

Secondly, the transpersonal perspective enlarges our understanding of life in all its aspects – higher consciousness and how it relates to ordinary life. A wider understanding is always practical.

Thirdly, there are millions of people today seeking new meanings in life. As they explore and search within, often as a result of some crisis in their lives, they become aware of unexplained impulses within the psyche, of unusual intuitions, and ideas that do not fit a rational picture. They break through into new dimensions and do not know how to handle their discovery. Such problems are now widespread. For such people transpersonal psychology can literally be a life saver.

I have said that any tight or rigid definition of transpersonal psychology is undesirable, and out of keeping with the spirit of its pioneers. But as we have seen a very real synthesis is beginning to emerge from the blending and interrelationship of the different psychological traditions. Certain key ideas provide the nucleus around which this synthesis is being built. None of them is new. What is new is that growing numbers of psychologists testify to the experiential and existential reality of these ideas and are working with them in practical ways and in terms of the psychology of quite ordinary people.

I give six ideas:

One: The idea of a field or continuum of consciousness comprising many different potential dimensions of awareness and states of being. Jung's collective unconscious (unconscious because at any one time we can only be aware of a fragment of this reality) together with oriental notions of planes of consciousness and Assagioli's concept of different levels of awareness within the psyche, provide us with the initial maps to explore and chart the consciousness field.

Two: The idea of the self, that there exists in every person a factor, energy or centre – the individual's essence – which is the core of his being. Whether we call this essence self, soul, transpersonal centre, Atman, matters not. It is the central energy of the psychological system, the key to growth, integration and expansion of awareness. Transpersonal psychology is the only branch of psychology that conceives the self in this sense.

Three: This self is not to be confused with personality, or the 'personal I'. It is something other, deeper and more profound. It is experienced in many different ways: through peak and transcendental experience: in 'big dreams'; through the activity of intuition and inspiration; at moments of crisis and desperation; in the urge to create; in the impulse to

useful action; in relationships. It can also be noted as a factor in the life patterns of those who have little conscious experience of it. The following verse of Alan Watts expresses precisely the distinction between the personal I and the self:

> There was a young man who said though
> I think that I know that I know
> What I would like to see
> Is the I that knows me
> When I know that I know that I know.

Four: The fundamental urge of the psyche towards wholeness, to become what it is, to actualize its full potential, to realize the nature of the self, the inside and the outside to become one.

Five: There are many different ways of growth to self-fulfilment. Human beings are infinitely diverse, with widely differing growth needs. What is ideal for one may be totally unsuited for another.

Six: The idea of relativity. In no sense does transpersonal psychology deny the usefulness of the many different psychologies extant today. Indeed the transpersonal psychologist will use a variety of approaches as and when appropriate. Transpersonal psychology is not in sympathy with those who assert the exclusive primacy of any single school of thought.

Finally, to give readers a flavour of the areas that are currently of interest to transpersonal psychologists, let me list topics written up in the *Journal of Transpersonal Psychology* and discussed by practitioners: altered states of consciousness; education for transcendence; mysticism and schizophrenia; cultivating intuition; states of consciousness and the chakra system in yoga; height psychology (Assagioli) and depth psychology (Jung); meditation as therapy; guided imaging; masculine and feminine principles; identity and dis-identification; myths and symbolism; archetypes; archetypal psychology; L.S.D. and experimental mysticism; voluntary control of internal states; physiology of meditation; →**biofeedback**; L.S.D.-assisted therapy; the encounter with death; →**astrology** and cycles of growth; samahdi and nirvana; synthesis and the will; paradox; actualizers and transcenders; mid-life crisis; letting 'It' do it; transpersonal counselling and psychotherapy

Ian Gordon-Brown

CONTRIBUTORS, p. 222

URINE THERAPY

Urine therapy is a method of treating disease by fasting and drinking one's own urine, together with certain quantities of plain drinking water. It is also used externally in the form of urine compresses or direct applications of urine to the skin. It was used by ancient Greeks for the treatment of wounds and is still employed by the Eskimos for this purpose. In the book *The Water of Life – A Treatise on Urine Therapy* by J. W. Armstrong (Health Science Press), the author reports a number of case histories of the successful treatment by urine therapy of jaundice, psoriasis, Bright's disease, →**cancer** and gangrene. An interesting use of the method was that of Maurice Wilson, whose courageous solo attempt to scale Mount Everest is described in the book *I'll Climb Mount Everest Alone*. Wilson attributed his remarkable stamina and freedom from minor ailments to his many urine fasts and urine skin frictions.

John Newton

BIBLIOGRAPHY, p. 251
CONTRIBUTORS, p. 223

VEGAN DIET

Veganism is a way of living on the products of the plant kingdom to the exclusion of flesh, fish, fowl, eggs, animal milk and its derivatives, and honey. It encourages the study and use of alternatives for all commodities normally derived wholly or partly from animals. It may be adopted for ethical, ecological economic, compassionate or health reasons. We are here considering it from the health point of view, bearing in mind that people at a high level of consciousness must regard the origins of their food to perfect their mental and spiritual health.

At the purely physical level there are many advantages to a vegan diet which far outweigh the one possible, and easily avoidable, disadvantage, namely that of developing Vitamin B12 deficiency.[1] This is now widely accepted among doctors and nutritionists. Moreover, orthodox medical thought leans towards this diet as a means of avoiding and mitigating against coronary artery disease which is now reaching epidemic levels in Britain, America and other areas where similar lifestyles predominate. The vegan diet has been prescribed for patients suffering from other diseases, and has been found especially helpful in the following instances, improvement generally being rapid:

Children: infantile eczema, asthma, chronic upper respiratory tract infections.
Adolescents: acne vulgaris.
Adults: maturity onset diabetes, hypertension, hyperlipidaemias, post-coronary thrombosis angina, ulcerative colitis, diverticulitis, →**migraine**, haemorrhoids, recurrent urinary infections.

Veganism should be regarded not as an adjunct to orthodox medicine but more as a superior approach as it attempts to undo situations induced by diets of animal origin and made worse by suppressive drug therapy. A therapy that goes well with a vegan diet is →**homoeopathy** where approximately 85 per cent of the remedies are of non-animal origin. Vivisection is not involved; homoeopathic practice is therefore compatible with vegan principles.

The Vegan Society was formed in 1944 by a group of →**vegetarians** who realized that there was more cruelty associated with dairy produce than in meat production. Cows, who have a strong maternal instinct, are made pregnant yearly only to be deprived of their young almost immediately after birth. They are sent to the slaughterhouse (often abroad) as soon as their yield drops. Calves are either slaughtered at birth, sent to veal units, reared for slaughter as beef or used as replacements in the dairy herd.

Some of the early vegans suffered health problems but now the properly balanced vegan diet (including a source of Vitamin B12) is widely recognized as not only healthy but as having healing properties. This is substantiated by the considerable number of clinical investigations that have been made, and by the numerous letters sent to the Society. The general health of vegans has been found to be good. They tend to weigh less than omnivores, which is good since obesity is associated with a high incidence of coronary artery disease, hypertension and diabetes mellitus. Taking no animal fats of any kind results in low cholesterol levels and lessens the chance of circulatory and heart troubles.

Megaloblastic anaemia of pregnancy does not occur in vegans as a result of their high foliate intake: it occurs in about 4 per cent of omnivores. In other respects they have normal pregnancies and their babies are healthy at birth. Vegan mothers breast-feed well and most continue to do so for nine months or more, thus giving their children the best dietary start in life. Investigation into the diet and health of life vegans by Pamela Mumford (Queen Elizabeth College, University of London) and Dr Frey Ellis (Pathology Department, Kingston General Hospital, Kingston-upon-Thames, Surrey) has confirmed that the diets appear to be perfectly satisfactory to support normal growth in children.

It has been suggested that vegans might be lacking in the long-chain fatty acids and phospholipids especially important for brain development, but adequate amounts of these nutrients have been found in the serum and red cell membrane of vegans.[2] Moreover the academic attainments of life-vegans have been generally good, sometimes very high.

Vegans have been found to be in positive nitrogen balance and there is no evidence of protein deficiency among vegans following the diet as recommended by the Society. The observation that a considerable percentage of vegans have lower blood urea levels than omnivores may indicate that they are less susceptible to renal disease than omnivores. As to Vitamin B12, the vitamin essential to the health of every cell in the body and not found in unsupplemented vegan diets, there has been little evidence of deficiency symptoms among vegans. Some vegans have lived healthily for twenty years without Vitamin B12 supplements. The vitamin is synthesized exclusively by micro-organisms living either in the intestines of animals, or in soil or water. It can possibly be obtained from contaminated plant food or water or in some cases from bacteria functioning in the alimentary canal, though normally this is not produced in the region whence it can be absorbed. To guard against the possible difficulty the Vegan Society recommends the taking of Vitamin B12 supplemented plant foods or tablets (the vitamin being obtained from bacteria grown on plant base).

Vegans may well be less susceptible to certain forms of →cancer, especially of the colon, because vegan gut bacteria are less active against bile acids; and to appendicitis and diverticulitis because of the high fibre content of most vegan diets. Recently, metabolic differences that may help to prevent the development of breast cancer have been reported in vegans. Vegans are advised to ensure adequate supplies of Vitamin D by being out of doors in the sunlight for sufficiently long to keep a slight tan (→naturism). Otherwise they need Vitamin D supplemented foods, e.g. vegan margarine and plant milks. As most food poisoning is caused by meat products or contaminated dairy products, vegans have an obvious advantage here.

Letters sent to the Society frequently refer to improved health and only rarely to difficulties. The former instance (as well as the advantages mentioned above) less catarrhal infections, fewer headaches, improvement in angina and ischaemic heart symptoms, improvement in asthmatic and eczematous conditions, greater energy and enhanced feeling of well-being. The latter instance digestive upset, flatulence, weight loss and less energy. It is advisable to make the change from an omnivorous diet slowly, to experiment among the very many plant sources of essential nutrients available, and to pay special attention to the source and form of food.

Improvements in health reported by those adopting the vegan diet may well be directly connected with the elimination of cow products but it is also undoubtedly the results of a changed attitude to diet and to life itself. Such a radical change brings with it an awareness of the hazards of the foods accepted without question by most people, of the additives and deficiencies in processed food, of the effect of preservatives, pesticides, herbicides and artificial fertilizers. Most vegans benefit from the use of whole foods, a good proportion of fresh, raw foods, where possible those that are grown veganically.

As well as the direct physical effects of the vegan diet, great benefit comes from the adoption of a disciplined way of life that has much to contribute to the solution of problems of world hunger, pollution, environmental deterioration and wastage of resources. A more positive attitude to life is engendered which, together with freedom from the guilt of dependence on the slaughterhouse, contributes to mental balance, spiritual growth and the well-being of the whole person.

Kathleen Jannaway

ASSOCIATIONS, p. 219
CONTRIBUTORS, p. 222

Notes

1. Tyson, Jon Wynne, *Food For A Future*, Davis Poynter, 1975.
2. Sanders, T. A. B., Ph.D. thesis, London University, 1977.

VEGETARIANISM

Good health depends on a multitude of factors, including heredity, environment, and one's mental and spiritual attitude to life, etc. One's diet and even how well one chews food also has an important part to play. A vegetarian is one who refrains from eating flesh foods like meat, fish, fowl and all their derivatives. Once vegetarians were regarded as fanatics by most nutritionists. Now their eating habits are increasingly being taken seriously and gaining respect from the medical profession as nutritional researchers find that more and more health benefits can come from following a meatless diet.

There are two basic kinds of vegetarians: →**vegans** who eat *no* animal foods, and lacto-ovo vegetarians who take milk, cheese, butter, cream, eggs and honey in addition to fruits, vegetables, nuts and grains. But simply eliminating flesh foods from a diet does not necessarily make it conducive to good health. To be beneficial it must be scientifically balanced to provide all the protein, fats and unrefined carbohydrates, vitamins and minerals that the body needs to function in optimum condition. It is interesting to examine the contents of mother's milk in trying to understand what an ideal diet should be.

Protein is essential, in just the *right* amount. Too little will lead to disease, as can too much in many cases. Mother's milk contains a mere 1½ per cent protein. Yet during the period of breast-feeding, normally a baby grows rapidly. Most people in the West in recent years have tended to eat too much protein, believing that the more the better. Unfortunately there are many indications that this practice has led to the onset of degenerative diseases and premature ageing. Scientists now believe we need between 25 and 50 grams a day for optimum health instead of the 75 to 150 grams they were recommending twenty-five years ago.

Mother's milk also contains 6 per cent sugar. Mankind has a natural craving for sugar but one's sugar consumption should not be excessive and however it is taken it should be unrefined. The consumption of refined sugar in this country is about 130 lb (60 kg) per person per year. Mounting evidence indicates that this has had a devitalizing effect on the health of the nation. Fats too are usually eaten in excess. And most of the fats we consume are saturated fats. Again, taking a cue from mother's milk, which contains a mere 3½ per cent fat, it is obvious we should not consume great quantities (the current average in Britain is about 42 per cent of our calories consumed in fats), particularly animal fats and other saturated fats. Most vegetarians consume considerably less fat than their flesh-eating cousins. Studies have shown that vegetarians as a group have cholesterol levels considerably lower than those of meat-eaters.

Mother's milk is insalivated in the mouth. Lack of adequate mastication leads to added strain on the digestive organs. One should always chew all foods thoroughly. Mother's milk is also raw. Many western diets contain insufficient Vitamin C, especially when too little raw food is eaten. This can lead to a lowered resistance to infection and also to scurvy. It was the lack of raw foods containing Vitamin C in the days of the sailing ship that caused scurvy. A healthy diet should contain at least 30 per cent raw food.

Vegetarians are, on the whole, more health conscious in the West than the meat-eating population. They suffer less from diseases like rheumatoid arthritis, coronary heart disease and diverticular disease. And because most vegetarians are also more health conscious in general they tend to take more exercise and do →**yoga** or →**breathing** exercises which also contribute to overall health. Many vegetarians in the West also abstain from smoking, which is an important factor in the causation of lung cancer, one of the commonest types of cancer affecting mankind. But there are other interesting facts about the health of vegetarians worth noting.

Food-poisoning is very much less common in vegetarians because four out of every five cases of food-poisoning are caused by eating meat or its derivatives. In Finland, where large quantities of fish are eaten, fish worms invade the tissue of many people causing impairment of health. Similarly, the eating of certain types of pork can lead to trichinosis. Vegetarians are not affected in this way. Diverticulitis is very much less common in vegetarians because they usually have a diet much richer in fibre than the average person, with the result that they suffer less from →**constipation** and have a quicker intestinal transit time. The incidence of coronary heart disease is also less among vegetarians. It was rare in India as in many cultures based on a

primitive diet of unrefined foods, yet Indians who have left the vegetarian way of life and have adopted the diet of western man (a diet containing an increase in animal fat, meat and more refined food, such as white flour and white sugar) have rapidly tended to develop coronary heart disease. Vegetarians usually eat less animal fat and more unrefined foods, both of which appear to be important protective factors.

Research has shown that vegetarians eat at least twice as much fibre in their meals and have a faster intestinal transit time and produce bulkier stools. Statistics show us that vegetarians suffer less than flesh-eaters from appendicitis, diverticulitis, stomach ulcer, cancer of the colon and worm diseases associated with the consumption of certain foods. Vegetarians have lower triglyceride and cholesterol levels, lower blood sugar levels and lower blood ureas. Individual health is not the only sound reason for advocating a vegetarian diet. World economics comes into it too: 85 per cent of the cultivated land in the United Kingdom, that is arable and pastoral, is used to feed animals or to grow food to feed animals. Our domestic creatures outnumber humans by three to one. Grain would be better used fed directly to people and food shortages would be greatly alleviated if livestock foraged on unused land instead of eating much of the world's grain. 50 per cent of the world cereal crop is fed to animals. In the United States of America, a remarkable and wealthy land, 90 per cent of the maize, 88 per cent of the oats, 80 per cent of wheat and 78 per cent of soya beans are fed to animals. The U.S.A. imports one million tons of protein annually, largely from the Third World, to feed its animals. For every ten tons of vegetable protein that is consumed by animals, one ton of animal protein is produced . . . a poor form of economics when one remembers that 60 per cent of human beings on this planet are underfed. So many more people could be adequately fed if this wasteful raising of animals for slaughter could be curtailed.

It is my considered opinion, and the opinion

of a growing number of my scientific colleagues, that the adoption of a balanced vegetarian diet would improve the overall way of life throughout the world in three main ways. Firstly, it would improve the health of the population. Secondly, it would help the economy by a more efficient use of land. Economists tell us that we could sustain eight times as many people on tillage, widely implemented, as we can on pasturage. Thirdly, it would improve the compassionate outlook of many people as a result of refraining from causing unnecessary suffering to the animal world. Although difficult to quantify, this benefit is too widely reported amongst meat eaters who turn vegetarian to be dismissed. So many claim turning vegetarian has brought them a deeper feeling of concern and care for all Nature's creatures and an ecological awareness that leads to greater responsibility in the preservation of the world's natural resources. One cannot help but agree with one of the world's greatest teachers of modern times, Mahatma Gandhi, who said, 'The unlimited capacity of the plant world to sustain man at his highest, is a region yet unexplored by modern science. . . . I submit the scientists have not yet explored the hidden possibilities of the innumerable seeds, leaves and fruits for giving the fullest possible nutrition to mankind.' It is time we explored them!

ASSOCIATIONS, p. 219
BIBLIOGRAPHY, p. 248

WEIGHT WATCHERS

People getting together to help each other achieve a special goal is not a new idea, but Weight Watchers was the first organization set up specifically to apply the group-therapy approach in the treatment of obesity.

Anyone who is overweight must, at some time in life, have eaten more food and/or drunk more drink than is needed to cover his or her energy output. The cure would seem to be to reverse this process: to consume less energy (food) than is used until the body achieves the desired weight. Intake can then be increased to a level that maintains a balance. However, every fat person knows that most attempts at self-discipline, whether at home or under the supervision of a doctor, are usually short-lived and the resulting weight loss (if any) tends to be temporary. As soon as the diet is discontinued, the weight goes back on.

Weight Watchers began quite simply in 1961 because one desperate fat American woman, Jean Nidetch, after dieting on and off nearly all her life, finally resolved to follow a balanced eating plan but found she could not stick to it alone. She needed someone to talk to, someone sympathetic, someone with the same problem and the same determination to beat it. From a small group of friends all following the same weight-loss programme, meeting and telephoning each other regularly, grew the world-wide organization that now offers over 13 000 weekly classes where some nine million men, women and children have already received help from, and given encouragement to, fellow-sufferers. Weight Watchers came to the United Kingdom in 1967 and there are now over 800 weekly classes, at all times of days, covering the British Isles.

Jean Nidetch lost 72 lb. (just over 5 stone or 33 kg) and found a new way of life. The eating plan that she and her friends followed was the result of many years' research by the New York City Department of Health Obesity Clinic, and became the basis of the Weight Watchers Programme, under the supervision of its own Food Research Department and regularly updated by a team of medical and nutritional experts. The informal meetings in the homes of friends became the helpful weekly classes, run along the same lines all over the world and open to any overweight person with 10 lb. or more to lose, and the desire to lose that excess weight permanently.

At each class members are weighed fully clothed except for coat and shoes and their weights recorded privately by the lecturer. If there is a slow loss, a gain or no loss in a particular week, the lecturer will discuss in confidence with the member any particular problems that may be responsible. With the member's agreement, the advice of other members may be sought in general discussion later on.

The care offered by Weight Watchers is continuous. From the first moment that the shy, self-conscious and probably unhappy fat person comes through the door, often as a last resort after years of battling with a weight problem, he or she is surrounded by a confident cheerfulness that gives new hope. In that room will be new members like himself, with ten, twenty, a hundred or more lb. to lose: slim members maintaining their goal weight and attending class for their monthly weigh in; members losing steadily and growing to like themselves more and more each week; members losing more erratically or stuck on a plateau but deriving comfort and encouragement from the weekly meeting with sympathetic friends; and perhaps visiting members from another town or another country.

Every class is led by a formerly fat person who lost weight by following the programme and then volunteered for training as a lecturer. He or she teaches the members how to follow the weight-loss programme and leads the discussions, encouraging members to contribute their own ideas and experiences. However, the lecturer never tries to usurp the function of the nutritionist or the medical adviser. All members are encouraged to consult their own doctors before joining and to have regular check-ups during the weight-loss period; anyone under a doctor's care, or a woman who is pregnant, is asked to obtain a doctor's permission to follow the programme.

Jean Nidetch and her friends discovered that an eating plan that insists on three satisfying meals a day, with plenty of scope for in-between snacks if desired, solves the problems of hunger, boredom and listlessness that so often accompany the crash or gimmick diet. The Weight Watchers Programme puts food in the right perspective; it encourages variety and enterprise in the selection and preparation of foods and guides members towards those which are nutritionally sound. The member who has reached goal weight is given the Maintenance Plan, which expands the basic programme and, building on the sensible eating habits learned during the weight-loss period, enables the member to maintain an attractive and healthy weight for life.

The behaviour patterns that influence eating habits are also examined at class and Weight Watchers offers a Personal Action Plan in support of the programme which enables members to recognize problem situations in advance and develop skills to overcome them. Dining out; shopping at the supermarket; feeling bored or depressed; there are many moments in the day when the overweight person is faced with temptation or pressure from outside and wants to turn to food for comfort, to show affection, or to conform with others. Food is also an integral part of our culture and forms the basis of many pleasurable social occasions. Discussion in class with people sharing the same problems, facing up to them and discovering solutions together can be of lasting benefit; recounting successes can also give the members a sense of personal achievement that reinforces the will to reach goal weight. The aim of the Personal Action Plan is always to encourage the member to stand on his own two feet, to help him develop a constructive approach to his own individual problems and enable him to succeed within the supportive structure of the group. Changing what are often a lifetime's habits is a very large task but by breaking this down into small manageable steps, week by week, the Personal Action Plan builds the skills necessary to establish the healthy eating habits that are the basis of permanent weight control. Once learned this positive approach need not be restricted to coping only with the problems of weight management. Members of Weight Watchers are continually discovering that these techniques can form the basis for a new outlook and a new self-awareness, leading to personal success in many other fields.

The applause that greets the reading out of

members' weight losses and the presentation of awards at the end of each Weight Watchers' class, is always warm and deeply felt and a measure of the genuine concern for one member for another; it is this personal concern that makes Weight Watchers' group-therapy approach so successful in the treatment of obesity.

Joyce Wood

ASSOCIATIONS, p. 219
BIBLIOGRAPHY, p. 249
CONTRIBUTORS, p. 223

WINE

There is no valid reason why a wine correctly chosen and prescribed by a doctor, according to the pathological case, should not be accepted one day as any other medicine.

From time immemorial the juice of the grape was considered by the disciples of Hippocrates as a first medical aid of primordial value. One only has to be reminded of the use in the French hospitals in former times of wines called 'medical wines' which bore the names of the hospital of origin. Wines of Charity – Hospital Dieu, Hospital Trousseau, etc. – gave the patients of this period (alas non-existent now) a beneficial therapy of the active principles it contained and also the pleasure to absorb a liquid with a pleasant and agreeable taste.

The grape juice, by its composition and physiological contents, may be considered on its own merit as a veritable therapeutic agent with the essential condition to be taken reasonably and with reason. It is my hope that one day, as the whisky is accepted in England, the French social security will refund the cost of a bottle of wine which a doctor has prescribed. My idea is therefore to praise the wine in a double sense, as a food and as a medicine, additional to various treatments which are classically medical.

By respecting two important principles, the excellent quality and the quantity absorbed, wine is a far cry from the drink which is often complacently written about. For human beings it is the best and healthiest drink, as Louis Pasteur proclaimed.

Apart from 80 per cent water the grape contains many minerals, for example magnesium, calcium, sodium, potassium, phosphates, glucides, proteins, phenols, tannoides, vitamins, and even anti-bacterial elements. By drinking wine, which covers a quarter of our essential calories, we indirectly draw energy from the sun. In fact, as the raisins ripen the fruit is bombarded by solar rays; furthermore they hold and metabolize in their cells the natural products of the earth in which the vine is planted. These elements will be absorbed in their turn on drinking the wine, once it has arrived at total maturity. This drink therefore plays a multiple rôle, firstly as a food, by exciting the functional mechanisms, and producing a pleasant psychic sensation, and finally according to each case, that of a medicine.

Consider the fermented juice of the vine not as a medicine capable of replacing that already prescribed by the doctor but as a cure, an addition. The wine is thus presented by its quality as an additional aid for the classical medicine, taking into consideration under this title everything which determines an improvement in general in a particular organ, be it hygienic, pharmaceutical, or surgical.

Recent chemical analysis made on the composition of grape juice has confirmed this point of view. Apart from the mineral elements it contains vitamins and organic qualities which one finds in a first-class wine, and which have a specific reaction on the lack of these substances in the invalid. The research and investigation made by Professor Rasquelier and Madame Jensen have justified the recognition of the anti-bacterial element of the wine due to the presence of oenidol, formed by the coloured pigments in the cuticle of stones in the raisin. This antibiotic quality has always been in the testimony of the surgeons in the heroic periods of history, the eighteenth century, seventeenth century, sixteenth century, and long before, when the juice of the grape was largely used to sterilize and heal infected wounds.

Wines of Champagne

By the richness of their content of tartrate of potassium, the wines of Champagne have a favourable effect on the strength and contractibility of the muscles. Champagne intervenes with this forceful element in the cardiac rhythm, which indirectly permits an important intake of oxygen in the myocardium. This wine, therefore, is indicated in all the diets for patients who have coronary troubles or those who have a tendency to infarction.

Bordeaux wines

Anaemic patients find it beneficial to take reasonable amounts of wine from the Graves hillsides. In this wine there is a high iron content which may reach 10 mg in each litre. The wines from the Médoc region also contain iron in its soluble form and oeno tanins. Because of this particular composition it is useful for patients who have lost their appetite or who are depressed, or on strict diets; it is also recommended for colitis.

The wines of the region of St Emilion with their rich content of calcium are favourable for invalids who lack this mineral, and for those who are suffering from osteoporosis (thinning of bone).

Wines of the Burgundy region

All abnormal loss of weight may be balanced by a prescription of a wine from the hills of Beaune. By their richness in iron and mineral extracts, burgundy, in particular the wines of Aloxe-Corton, is recommended for this reason for senior citizens, in which most of the cases need the addition of calories. At the same time, because these wines contain potassium, they are prescribed for patients with cardiac insufficiency and low blood pressure.

Because of its high tannin content the young beaujolais finds its place in the diet of invalids who suffer from diarrhoea, and as these wines are particularly rich in anti-bacterial elements they may replace antibiotics during simple infectious illness, for example sore throats and mild bronchial infection, etc.

Wines of the Loire valley

Their use during the illness will be in accordance with their chemical strength. To name just a few: muscadet, because of its low contents in calcium salt, would be good for patients who have arteriosclerosis, or too much cholesterol; the white wines of the Vouvray region act as a natural stimulant on the gastric juices, and therefore are recommended for dyspeptic patients.

It is not possible here to mention all the wine regions of France, but taking into account the examples given above, one realizes that wine intervenes or acts on the human being in a double rôle, as a food and as a remedy. Because of its particular qualities it is a food which economizes in the body; acts as a psychological tonic – a dynamogenetic element; a heart stimulant; excites the digestion; acts as an anti-bacterial agent; takes away toxic qualities; and gives the body minerals.

It offers so much to people in good health as well as to invalids. It is an agent of natural products, which increases the rate of health in the first instance, and completes the lack in the second.

Dr E. A. Maury

BIBLIOGRAPHY, p. 251
CONTRIBUTORS, p. 223

YOGA

Yoga is not an alternative medicine but it is self help. It goes deeper than that, for yoga is self-realization, self-awareness. Based on the understanding that knowledge is within us, yoga can parade a remarkable range of wisdom to back its claim. For all this wisdom has been gained from within, or, as we would say today, intuitively.

Yoga stems from the fundamental question:

what is life? To a high degree our ill health, even many of our accidents, result from our mental dis-ease in seeking to answer this question. As a sage once put it, 'The cause of death is birth.' Psychotherapists, and many psychiatrists too, will tell us that much of our suffering is psychosomatic in origin. Peter Blythe writes, 'Authoritative medical opinion in the United States and Britain has gone on record to the effect that up to 70 per cent of all patients currently being treated by doctors in general practice are suffering from conditions which have their origins in unrelieved stress.'[1] And stress is, of course, all too often a psychosomatic state. In many cases psychotherapists and psychiatrists are able to help patients by uncovering a particular imbalance which has set up an acute stress condition which in turn has produced identifiable physical illness (psychosomatic disorder). The yoga concept, however, goes deeper than this, relating the end-product, the illness, to the truly primary factor: the relationship between the individual and life itself. In other words, the healthy basis of life is a total acceptance of the life process, the unhealthy basis a state of alienation with life.

The very word yoga affirms this, for it stems from the Sanskrit and means the way in which the individual unit or spirit can integrate and find fulfilment with the universal spirit, or, if you prefer the phrase, 'find oneness with God'. The words are not significant in themselves. What is important is the reaction on mind and body.

If one pauses to think on the situation it will be seen that this is simple common sense. The lifestyle we have developed in mass communities has heightened a feeling of un-ease with life itself and has heightened the fear of death. Medical research now clearly shows that such a persistent state of being 'out of sync' affects the fine balance of healthy human functioning, with resulting breakdowns in the weaker areas of the system. Thus in one person mental disorder can result, while in another similar stress promotes other bodily disorders such as asthma, eczema or →migraine, etc. So the key to the problem lies in finding a personal feeling of fulfilment with life. That would seem a tall order, to many of us quite impossible if it were not for the remarkable fact that knowledge lies within us. Perhaps the best definition of the yoga approach lies in the avowal, 'Be still and know that I am God.' Not 'believe' or 'hope' or 'have faith', but 'know'. 'Be still,' of course, means calm down, quieten the mind, eliminate all the silly, stray thoughts which normally clutter our waking hours. More than 2000 years ago a great sage of yoga named Patanjali devised what has since become one of the great textbooks of yoga and he began by declaring, 'Yoga is controlling the waves of the mind.'

Such a process is more than ever important today, when the pace of life affects virtually everyone. In the same way that wars no longer are fought between opposing armies but envelop whole nations, so stressful lives are no longer merely the occupational hazards of executives but the lot of us all. A doctor in Surrey who has become convinced of the efficacy of yoga now finds that he wants to tell patients suffering from a wide variety of troubles that the successful alleviation of their illnesses depends upon taking the yoga approach. In particular he finds he has obtained remarkable results in helping arthritic patients and he begins not where the joints are affected but with the breath (→breathing). This may seem startlingly irrelevant until we begin to trace the whole action through. When sufferers from arthritis are questioned in detail about their lives and problems, a history of stress or emotional problems often emerges and these are helped along by the un-ease about life to which we have earlier referred.

As we come up against problems or sudden emotional crises which worry us severely, one instinctive reaction is to create rigidity in the abdominal area. This is brought about by the automatic reaction of the solar plexus, the great nerve centre of the body which is sometimes known as the 'second brain'. This area is directly related to our emotional reactions. If we are nervous we experience this tension and say we have 'butterflies in the stomach'.

The tension impedes the effective working of the body system, for the great piston of the body's energy is the diaphragm.

The diaphragm is a cone-shaped sheath of muscle which separates the lungs and heart from the abdominal viscera. Not only is it the primary mechanism of respiration, moving down as we breathe in, and up as we breathe out, but it also acts as a generator to the whole energy system, including the electromagnetic force with which we are charged. This regular movement of the diaphragm constantly stimulates and nourishes the visceral organs by bringing controlled pressure to bear on them, helping the blood flow and toning the neuro-muscular system. However, when the nerves in the solar plexus area are activated by tension or worry, this inhibits muscular movement and the diaphragm is dramatically reduced in its effective movement. For respiration we then come to rely on the movement of the rib cage which is only a secondary respiratory aid; and so, while we continue to absorb oxygen into the blood stream, the body's main generator is hardly working, thus running down the body's energy and, at the same time, removing the control on the visceral organs. When this persists, the overall tone of the body will be impaired. Listlessness and a feeling of enervation will follow, then illness as the weakest parts of the body give way. Thus arthritis can be caused by tension.

The Surrey doctor, therefore, concentrates first on getting the patient's diaphragm moving again. Once the energy is flowing he moves on to specific exercises to help the affected joints.

Any tense, nervous or frightened person has rigidity in the abdominal area, their breathing shallow, irregular and uncontrolled. They find it hard to hold breath in the body, impossible to breathe out slowly and carefully. A standard medical test in neurosis is to see whether the patient can breathe rhythmically, for no neurotic can control the breath. The opposite also holds true. Anyone who can breathe diaphragmatically, rhythmically and with control, cannot be badly affected by tension, fear or emotional stress.

For the beginner the full movement of the diaphragm is achieved by pulling the abdominal muscles in as one exhales, thus pushing up the diaphragm and allowing the diaphragm smoothly to expand as one inhales, thus helping it to descend. This should be achieved with little use of the rib cage. The oft-repeated injunction to 'throw the chest out' for deep breathing is nonsense, because it does not allow much air to enter the lungs and it inhibits the use of the body's generator. That gentle, rhythmical breathing has a calming influence, we all know. 'Breathe slowly and count to ten,' we are told when we find our temper rising, and we discover it works. The ancient sages of yoga were well aware of the importance of breathing and its effect upon body and mind, for they formulated precise directions for the use of respiration thousands of years ago. These exercises were intended to calm the mind and soothe the body, so that the practitioner would be able to move deeper and deeper into a state of meditation. However, it is not necessary to wish to make such progress to see the sense of using such breathing practices even in strict moderation. The exercises' calming process will reduce tension, while clearing the lungs and helping to keep them in full working order. The body will function without hindrance and the mind will lose something of the frenetic dispatch of messages which it is our normal lot to suffer.

Is this an over-simplified approach to life's fulfilment? The way to progress towards our major goal lies in using quite simple techniques at first to help us along the path. In yoga too many people seek to run before they can walk, quickly tire and drop out. One of the curses of our time is that we fritter away our energies in all directions without mastering one thing at a time. We are drowned in suggestions of all sorts of activity, all day, every day. These suggestions manipulate us rather than encourage us to think and act for ourselves. We buy some series of books to learn the secrets of the Universe, but don't read them. We over-eat or eat the wrong food, then are told tablets will put the matter right. We cannot sleep so we buy more tablets, rather than finding out the cause of our insomnia.

We have built up a society dependent on selling goods and services in the name of economic security. The *reductio ad adsurdum* is the selling of more and more goods and services to maintain a precarious economic balance, yet this pressure to buy only results in destroying the thing we seek – happy, healthy living, free from stress and tension. No political theory will solve this. Solution lies in the power of the individual to be stronger than the pressures that seek to overwhelm him. That power can be built by combining the right physical approach with the right mental attitude.

Most people know a little about the physical movements of yoga. Called *asanas* (postures) they range from sitting positions, such as the well-known lotus position, to movements which make the body supple, tone the neuro-muscular system, enhance the working of the glands and resist much illness. These *asanas* differ from any routine physical exercise; even when exercise systems seek to incorporate yoga movements, a great difference still remains.

Each posture combines mental control, respiration and bodily movement. Respiration is the catalyst, bringing the 'whole man' under control. Slowness of movement in yoga is not a quirk but has a sound physiological basis. Consider in detail just one posture, the shoulder stand. This requires standing upside down, resting on the shoulders and back of the neck, using the hands palms downward for counter-balance, the chin pressed firmly into the jugular notch. In this position the flow of blood through the body is changed, gravity pulling it to the head. This takes pressure off veins and arteries, helpful for those with venous troubles. The heart is relieved of some pressure and is thereby stimulated, while the change in the visceral organs benefits their function. Even more important, the flow of blood to the head benefits the pituitary gland, considered the great controlling gland of the body. Pressure of the chin into the jugular notch temporarily inhibits blood flow into the thyroid gland, which has bearing on the body's weight and general health. The thyroid is fed by two large arteries and is also activated by nerves running from between the fourth and fifth cervical vertebrae, just where the neck bends to take weight in the shoulder stand position. Pressures placed here are of immense benefit, for when the practitioner slowly comes down from the position, blood flushes freely through the gland and feeds the nervous system at this point. This has bearing on the healthy control of the thyroid. While holding this position and breathing gently, one thinks only about physical reactions within the body, an effective exercise in concentration and mind calming. Just one position can yield a whole range of benefits, linking control of breath and mind.

In specific illnesses the speed of the yoga remedial approach varies greatly. Sometimes success is swift; sometimes recovery comes slowly; sometimes no benefit appears to result. Where results are extremely slow or not visible, this may be due to failure to understand the basics of the approach being tried. Our lives are fractionalized and we find it hard to relate different aspects to one whole. Too often people try out a remedy on a let's-have-a go basis. So long as we prefer pills to a do-it-yourself approach, so long will this remain a real problem. There is no panacea but the successes of those who seek relief through yoga are remarkable. Great relief often comes to people who practise quite simply in a weekly group.

Many people, though, practise at home. Some dangers may be inherent in this since one is unable to check the accuracy of one's approach. Yoga should always be based primarily on group activity, supplemented by home study and practice. The number of yoga remedial groups is growing steadily, helping those suffering from nervous tension, degenerative diseases, →**multiple sclerosis**, and other problems. The *British Medical Journal*[2] has declared that yoga and meditation may become the regular form of treatment for hypertension within a few years.

After practising yoga for two or three

months, many people report, 'Everyone says I am so much easier to live with.' A society in which people are easier to live with is indeed a society transformed.

Howard Kent

Notes

1. Blythe, Peter, *Stress Disease*, Arthur Barker, 1973.
2. *British Medical Journal*, 12 June 1976.

Index

Index

Page numbers refer to the first mention of a word or subject in an article.

Part Two
Directory

Associations and Societies

The date in brackets after the name is the year founded.

The Aetherius Society
(1956). 757 Fulham Road, London
SW6 5UU. *Tel.:* 01-736 4187. *European
Secretary:* Reverend Raymond P. Nielsen.
Founder/President and Spiritual Leader: Shri
Yogiriji George King. *Members:* Several
hundreds.
Journal: Spiritual Healing Bulletin, 12
issues per year. Covers all aspects of
spiritual healing, news about new inven-
tions to help healers, case histories.
Aims: Trains spiritual healers. Runs
weekend courses, holds public healing
meetings with demonstrations. Branches
and groups in Amersham, Barnsley,
Bristol, Derby, Torquay and Warrington.
Runs a health food shop in London:
advice available on diet, herbal and
biochemic remedies and homoeopathic
treatment.
Article, p. 178

Association for Dramatherapists
(1977). 136 Oxford Street, Rugby,
Warwickshire. *Tel.:* Rugby (0788) 65809.
Secretary: Sue Jennings. *Chairman:* Roy
Shuttleworth, *Members:* 500.
Journal: Journal of Dramatherapists,
quarterly. A forum of ideas, exchange of
research and practice in creativity,
dramatherapy, remedial drama, psychodrama, rôle play etc.
Aims: To develop, stimulate and
publicize dramatherapy. Full members
(£6.50 per annum) for practising

dramatherapists through application to
the executive committee; associate
membership (£4.50 per annum) open to
all interested in the Association.
Article, p. 157

**Association for Group and Individual
Psychotherapy**
(1970). 29 St Marks Crescent, London
NW1. *Tel.:* 01-485 9141. *Secretary:* A. P.
Ormay, B.A. *Director:* D. J. Dyng M.A.,
B.SC., DIP. ED.
Aims: To provide training and treatment
in both orthodox and new methods of
psychotherapy; based on the belief that
each school has valuable contributions
to make in treatment of the
psychologically distressed.

Association for Humanistic Psychology
(1969). 62 Southwark Bridge Road,
London SE1 0AU. *Tel.:* 01-928 7102.
Membership: Secretaries: V. Milroy,
M. Charleton.
Chairperson: Hans Lobstein. *Members:*
400.
Journal: Self & Society, monthly,
subscription £4 p.a. Medium for all
new therapies.
Aims: The Association is a worldwide
network for the development of the
human sciences which recognize our
distinctly human qualities and work
towards fulfilling people's innate
capacities. Lists organizations and
therapists.

Association for Self-Help and Community Groups
(1977). 7 Chesham Terrace, Ealing, London w13. *Tel.:* 01–579 5589. *Hon Sec./ Director:* H. E. Lobstein. *Members:* 6.
Aims: To develop human resources dormant in the community.

Astrological Association
(1958). c/o Membership Secretary, 57 Woodside, Wimbledon, London sw19.
Secretary; Miss A. L. Phillips. *President:* Charles Harvey. *Members:* 1100.
Journal: Astrological Journal, quarterly. All aspects of astrology, including medical occasionally.
Article, p. 35

The Atlanteans
(1957). 42 St George's Street, Cheltenham GL50 4AF. *Founder Member:* Tony Neate. *Members:* 400.
Journal: The Atlantean, quarterly. Editor, Cynthia Kenycn B.A. Articles on mysticism, occultism, healing, U.F.O.s and New Age thought.
Aims: International society based on love and tolerance, provides understanding of man's spiritual heritage and relationship to Earth and its kingdoms and his own destiny. Meditation courses provide safe means of uplifting the consciousness and increasing sensitivity to life.

British Acupuncture Association and Register Ltd
(1962). 34 Alderney Street, London Sw1v 4EU. *Tel.:* 01–834 3352 and 01–834 1012.
Secretary: Dr Ac. Norman Willis. *Chairman* Sidney Rose-Neil.
Journal: British Acupuncture Association Register & Year Book, annual. Lists names and addresses of members, questions regarding treatments, etc.
Aims: to promote the study of acupuncture; to establish the status, regulate the conduct, and protect the interests of practitioners; to exclude malpractice and decide questions of conduct and etiquette. Minimum membership qualifications are: registered medical practitioners, osteopaths,

chiropractors, dental surgeons, physiotherapists. Minimum study is two years for Licentiate in Acupuncture; Bachelor of Acupuncture award takes a minimum of four years' postgraduate study; Doctor of Acupuncture award takes a minimum of six years.
Article, p. 21

British and European Osteopathic Association
(1976). 94 Banstead Road South, Sutton, Surrey SM2 5LH. *Tel.:* 01–642 4161.
Secretary: M. Nightingale. *President:* Denis Brookes. *Chairman:* J. Taylor.
Members: 81.
Aims: To unite all qualified osteopaths, uphold standards and provide a comprehensive register.
Article, pp. 67, 143

British Chiropractors' Association
(1925). 1 Abbotswood, Guildford, Surrey GU1 1UR. *Tel.:* Guildford (0483) 62830.
Honorary Secretary: Ian M. Hutchinson D.C. *President:* Winston Brownrigg D.C.
Members: 96.
Journal: Contact, bi-annual. Exchange of professional information and to keep British chiropractors abreast of chiropractic developments throughout the world.
Aims: Maintains a register of qualified members. Nearly all U.K. qualified chiropractors are members. Holds spring and autumn conferences, arranges post-graduate seminars. Qualified chiropractors only.
Article, p. 58

British Homoeopathic Association
(1909). 27a Devonshire Street, London W1N 1RJ. *Tel.:* 01–935 2163. *Secretary:* Mrs M. J. Munday. *Chairman:* R. J. Ede.
Members: 1500 (U.K. and worldwide).
Journal: Homoeopathy, bi-monthly. Articles, letters from members, always an application form, book list, five homoeopathic chemists who advertise regularly, information on meetings, lectures and seminars.
Aims: A registered charity. Many doctors

are members but it is primarily an association working with and for laymen. The B.H.A. exists to spread knowledge of homoeopathy and links the fully-qualified homoeopathic doctor, dentist, pharmacist and veterinary surgeon and the public. It maintains a full library of classic and modern homoeopathic books for members only. Membership open to all, though lay practitioners (those not in the British Medical Register but practising as a profession) are excluded from the Association's Medical Register.
Article, p. 113

British Hypnotherapy Association
(1958). 67 Upper Berkeley Street, London W1H 7DH. *Tel.:* 01–723 4443. *Secretary:* Alison Wookey. *Chairman:* R. K. Brian. *Members:* 31.
Aims: Maintains a register of qualified practitioners in England and Wales. Arranges lectures and seminars, and publishes papers. Membership confined to the fully-trained.
Article, p. 122

British Mazdaznan Association
(1910) 19 Hillbrow Road, Withdean, Brighton BN1 5JP. *Tel.:* Brighton (0273) 500114. *Hon. Secretary:* Mrs Violet Hammerton. *Co-Leaders:* Mr Rex and Mrs Evelyn Allen. *Members:* 250.
Journal: British Mazdaznan, monthly. Excerpts from lectures, articles, season hints, notices of meetings and courses in the U.K. and on the Continent.
Aims: The Association acknowledges that Infinite Intelligence (the true meaning of God, Mazda, Allah, etc.) is imminent in all creative and evolutionary processes. Therefore it works with this Power (1) to maintain wholeness of body, mind and spirit, (2) to use our abilities constructively, (3) in family life to uphold the rôle of the mother as the primary educator. Ultimate purposes is a World Order where Nature's laws are observed – mutual respect; co-operation and harmony in all human relationships.
Article, p. 128

British Natural Hygiene Society
(1957). 'Shalimar', First Avenue, Frinton-on-Sea, Essex. *Tel.:* Frinton-on-Sea (02556) 2823. *Hon. Secretary:* K. R. Sidhwa N.D., D.O. *President:* K. R. Sidhwa N.D., D.O. *Members:* 200.
Journal: The Hygienist, quarterly. Devoted to health – rest, sleep, exercise, fresh air, nutrition through vegetarian food, mental and emotional poise, fasting and loving care.
Aims: Maintains a register of hygienic practitioners, provides training in natural hygiene, encourages and assists clinics and health schools. Associate membership open to all, professional membership exclusive to qualified practitioners.

British Osteopathic Association
(1911). 8–10 Boston Place, London NW1. *Tel.:* 01–262 1128. *Hon. Secretary:* Dr N. J. Healey. *Chairman:* Dr S. S. Ball. *Members:* 100.
Journal: Newsletter, quarterly.
Aims: Upholds professional ethical standards, maintains list of qualified osteopaths. Practitioners only.
Article, pp, 67, 143

British Society for Music Therapy
(1958). 48 Lanchester Road, London N6 4TA. *Organizing Secretary:* Mrs Denize Christopher. *Chairman:* Miss Juliette Alvin F.G.S.M., M.T. *President:* Malcolm Williamson, Master of the Queen's Music. *Vice President:* Dr Donald Blair, Consultant Psychiatrist. *Members:* 500.
Journal: British Journal of Music Therapy, quarterly. Learned articles, book reviews, events and meetings in the U.K. and overseas, reports of meetings, letters, international contacts, regional activities.
Aims: To promote music therapy in the treatment, education, rehabilitation and training of children and adults suffering from emotional, physical or mental handicap. Registered as a charity. Members include musicians, physicians, psychologists, psychiatrists, social workers, teachers, educationists, nurses.
Article, p. 133

British Wheel of Yoga
(1965). Glyn Galleries, Glyn Ceiriog,
Llangollen, Clwyd. *Tel.:* Glen Ceiriog
(069 172) 564. *Secretary:* Vivian
Worthington. *Chairman:* Bill File.
Members: 3000.
Journal: Yoga, quarterly. World-wide
yoga events, articles, poems.
Aims: Co-ordinating body mainly in the
U.K. but with members throughout the
world. Public meetings, instructional
seminars. Co-operates with local education
authorities in yoga tuition and publication
of literature. Registered charitable trust.
Article, p. 193

Central Council for British Naturism
(1964, by amalgamation with two previous
organizations). Sheepcote, Orpington,
Kent BR5 4ET. *Tel.:* Orpington (0689)
33390. *Hon. Secretary:* Roy Lambert.
President: G. W. Ryland. *Members:* 15000.
Journal: British Naturism, quarterly.
National and international naturism news,
free to members of the C.C.B.N.
Supporters' Section.
Aims: Furtherance of the physical, moral
and mental well-being of the community
through naturism; to ensure the continuing
co-operation of bona-fide sun clubs for their
mutual assistance and encouragement.
Article, p. 137

Church of Scientology
(Early 1950s). St Hill Manor, East
Grinstead, West Sussex. *Tel.:* East
Grinstead (0342) 24571. *Resident Agent:*
Mrs Judy Tampion. *Founder:* L. Ron
Hubbard. *Members:* Internationally
3000000.
Journal: Freedom, quarterly. A human
rights newspaper in which the
campaigning Church takes up issues.
Aims: Believes one must apply to this life
those principles in which he believes.
Hence deep involvement with social
reform, mental health, reform of
psychiatric abuse, education, drug
rehabilitation, criminal rehabilitation and
other areas.
Article, p. 70

**College of Osteopathy & Manipulative
Therapy Ltd**
(1948). 21 Manor Road North,
Wallington, Surrey SM6 7NS. *Tel.:*
01–647 2452. *Secretary:* Hugh Hellon-
Harris B.SC., D.O., D.N.Th., F.C.O.
President: Donald Upton D.O., D.N.Th.,
LIC.AC., M.AC.A., F.C.O. *Members:* 64.
Aims: To promote study and practice of
natural therapeutics with emphasis on
osteopathy. To establish the status,
regulate the conduct, and protect the
interests of members.
Article, pp. 67, 143

Community Health Foundation
(1976). 188–94 Old Street, London EC1V
9BP. *Tel.:* 01–251 4076. *Liaison Officer:*
Neil Gulliver. *Programme Director:*
William Tara. *Members:* 200.
Journal: Spiral, quarterly. In its context
of macrobiotic philosophy, it proposes a
holistic view of life, man and society,
past, present and future in terms of the
creative processes of the Universe. Health
and healing, wholefood cooking,
cosmology, natural agriculture.
Aims: To promote self-help in health care
by providing an educational services to
members and public. Faculties include
East West Centre (classes and tuition),
Earth Mother Playschool, East West
Natural Food Shop, Seven Sheaves
Restaurant, Natural Birth Centre, School
of Oriental Medicine & Philosophy.
Membership open to public.

Counselling International
(1975). 5 Victoria Road, Sheffield,
Yorkshire S10 ZDJ. *Tel.:* Sheffield
(0742) 686371. *Communications
Coordinators:* Richard Horobin and Rose
Evison. *London contact:* Anne Dickson,
83 Fordwych Road, London NW2
(*Tel.:* 01–452 9261). *Members:* 1200.
*Journal: Counselling International
Newsletter*, twice a year. Details of national
and international workshops, classes
and groups; local contact persons in
Europe and U.S.A.; articles on theory
and practice.

Aims: Shares address lists and enables people to co-counsel when abroad or otherwise away from home. Holds national and international workshops.
Article, p. 61

European Osteopathic Register
(1977). 21 Bingham Place, London W1M 3FH. *Tel.:* 01–935 6933. *Secretary:* Mrs Margery J. Dummer. *Members:* 120.
Aims: To provide within Europe a register of qualified osteopaths, promote and maintain standards in Europe. Qualified practitioners only.
Article, pp. 67, 143

General Council and Register of Osteopaths Ltd
(1936). 16 Buckingham Gate, London SW1E 6LB. *Tel.:* 01–828 0601. *Secretary:* Barrie Darewski M.A. *Chairman:* Arthur J. Smith D.O., M.R.O. *Members:* 300.
Aims: To establish and maintain standards of education for practitioners for the protection and benefit of the public; to assist, approve or co-operate with any osteopathic institutions which conform with the standards of the Register. Members drawn from The British School of Osteopathy and The London College of Osteopathy.
Article, pp. 67, 143

Guild of Natural Medicine Practitioners
(1972). Thornton House, Northiam, Rye, East Sussex TN31 6LP. *Tel.:* Rye (079 73) 2210. *Hon. Secretary:* Peter J. Hudson D.SC., N.D., D.O. *President:* James Taylor N.D., D.O. *Members:* 50.

Hahnemann Society
(1958). Humane Education Centre, Avenue Lodge, Bounds Green Road, London N22 4EU. *Tel.:* 01–889 1595. *Acting Hon. Secretary:* Miss H. M. Lishman. *Chairman:* Michael Fryer. *President:* Yehudi Menuhin K.B.E. *Members:* 500.
Journal: The Hahnemann Newsletter, quarterly.
Aims: To encourage homoeopathy and to inform the public. Membership £2.10 p.a. inclusive of journal.
Article, p. 113

Healing Research Trust
(1967). Field House, Peaslake, Guildford, Surrey GU5 9SS. *Tel.:* Dorking (0306) 730080. *Secretary:* J. O. Wilcox M.A. *Chairman:* Dr H. A. W. Forbes M.A., D.M., F.R.C.P. *Members:* None – the Trust is not a membership body.
Aims: To secure the recognition of natural therapeutics as standard forms of treatment by the public, Parliament and medical profession.

Health for the New Age
(1972). 1a Addison Crescent, London W14 8JP. *Tel.:* 01–603 7751. *Company Secretary:* Marika McCausland. *Director:* Marcus McCausland. *Members:* 95.
Journal: Health for the New Age, quarterly. Circulates free to members and non-members globally. Articles on research, self-understanding, healing, book reviews, conferences and seminars.
Aims: Advocates holistic medicine within a caring community.

Herb Society
(1927). 34 Boscobel Place, London SW1. *Tel.:* 01–235 1023. *Secretary:* Mrs M. Shanahan. *Director:* Dr M. Stuart PH.D. *Chairman:* John Meade. *President:* Lady Meade Featherstonhaugh.
Journal: The Herbal Review, quarterly. Articles, diary of events, held by the Society, reviews, services lists.
Aims: To promote, improve and increase knowledge of herbs particularly in the preservation of health and prevention of disease.
Article, pp. 98, 101

Independent Register of Manipulative Therapists Ltd
(1963). 106 Crowstone Road, Westcliff-on-Sea, Essex SS0 8LQ. *Tel.:* Southend-on-Sea (0702) 48820. *Secretary:* Mrs J. M. Green. *President:* D. C. D. Kemp. *Members:* 144.

Institute of Biodynamic Psychology
(1964). Acacia House, Centre Avenue, The Vale, Acton Park, London W3 7JX. *Tel.:* 01–743 2437. *Director:* Ms Mona Lisa Boyesen. *Chairman:* Ms Gerda

Boyesen. *Members:* 250.
Aims: To promote the practice, training
and development of biodynamic
psychology.
Article. p. 45

**International Federation of Practitioners
of Natural Therapeutics Ltd**
(1963). 21 Bingham Place, London
W1M 3FH. *Tel.:* 01-935 6933. *Hon.
Secretary-General:* Thomas G. Dummer.
President: Pierre Corriat. *Members:* 40
associations with 5000 practitioners in
14 countries.
Journal: I.F.P.N.T. Newsletter, bi-monthly.
Mainly of interest only to members but
available at £10 p.a. to sympathizers of
natural therapeutics.
Aims: To provide a central organization
for all bona fide associations of
practitioners of natural therapeutics. Most
member bodies have stringent educational
standards, many a four-year full time
course.

**London and Counties Society of
Physiologists**
(1919). 100 Waterloo Road, Blackpool,
Lancashire FY4 1AW. *Tel.:* Blackpool
(0253) 403548. *Organizing Secretary:*
Kenneth Woodward. *President:* Thomas
H. Hawes. *Members:* 650.
Journal: Skill Bulletin, bi-monthly. Over
2000 circulation to past and present
students of the Northern Institute of
Massage and the Society. News relating
to manipulative therapy skills.
Aims: To raise the professional status of
the practitioner in massage and
manipulative therapies. Holds congresses,
lectures, demonstrations and social events.
Publishes a list of practitioner-members,
offers a choice of two professional
indemnity insurance policies for members.
Membership exclusive to practitioners of
manipulative and remedial massage,
osteopaths, chiropractors, health and
beauty therapists, chiropodists, etc.

Martindale Trust Ltd
(1967). 'Moorlands', 24 South Road,
Newton Abbot, Devon TQ12 1HQ. *Tel.:*

Newton Abbot (0626) 5493. *Secretary:*
James Bruce A.M.C.T. *Members:* None –
charity rules by company limited by
guarantee.
Aims: To encourage natural healing
therapies principally by means of
acupuncture, homoeopathy, osteopathy,
etc. Assists in developing private
consultative practice; assists professional
organizations and practitioners.
Scholarships available to students of
approved teaching colleges and
organizations.

National Association for Health
(1967). Tremaine, 21 Milbourne Lane,
Esher, Surrey KT10 9EB. *Tel.:* Esher
(0372) 62588. *Chairman:* Maurice Hanssen.
Members: 620.
Journal: N.A.F.H. Newsletter, three times
a year.
Aims: The consumer's watchdog on
medicine and food. Keeps a keen eye on
proposed changes in legislation at
Westminster and Brussels. The Academic
Committee is composed of distinguished
scientists and medical men. Open to
public.
Article, p. 92

National Association of Health Stores
(1931). St Annes, Lower North Street,
Exeter, Devon. *Tel.:* Exeter (0392) 79621.
Secretary: F. B. Wilson. *Chairman:*
G. Wright. *Members:* 350.
Journal: N.A.H.S. Newsheet, quarterly.
Aims: To provide a common bond between
health food store retailers, a source of
information on wages, legislation and
other matters. Takes responsibility for
educational programmes. Provides link
between retail side of the health food
industry and manufacturers.
Article, p. 92

National Childbirth Trust
(1956). 9 Queensborough Terrace,
Bayswater, London W2 3TB. *Tel.:*
01-229 9319. *Secretary:* Margaret B.
Duncan Shearer. *President:* Lady
Micklethwait. *Members:* 5000.
Journals: N.C.T. Journal, annual: *N.C.T.*

Bulletin, three times a year.

Aims: To widen understanding of childbirth as a normal physiological event which need not be feared, and to give practical help on those lines to expectant mothers through antenatal classes. Activities include antenatal classes, breastfeeding counselling, and postnatal support organized through 100 U.K. branches. Registered educational charity. Open to any U.K. resident over sixteen.
Article, pp. 135, 149

National Federation of Spiritual Healers
(1955). Shortacres, Church Hill, Loughton, Essex. *Tel.:* 01–508 8218. *Administrator:* Michael Endacott. *President:* Dennis Fare. *Members:* 5000.
Journal: The Review, twice yearly. Information on activities, functions, viewpoints, sanctuaries, research developments.
Aims: A charity to promote the study of spiritual healing. Protects healers and their patients. Inter-denominational, open to members of all religions. Holds lectures and demonstrations. Postal study courses and cassettes available dealing with healing and meditation. Annual Spring School held at a popular coastal resort.
Articles: pp. 19, 178

National Institute of Medical Herbalists
(1864). 50 Sandygate Road, Crosspool, Sheffield s10 5RY. *Hon. Secretary:* H. H. Zeylstra M.N.I.M.H. (Tidebrook Manor Farm, Wadhurst, Sussex). *President:* Mrs N. Gosling F.N.I.M.H. *Members:* 100.
Journal: New Herbal Practitioner, three to four times a year. Technical articles of interest to the profession.
Aims: Founded in 1864, incorporated in 1895, received a grant of Arms in 1958, the Institute played a major part in retaining as a statutory right the freedom to practise herbal medicine contained in the Medicines Act 1968. Members receive a certificate, adopt a strict ethical code. Professionals only.
Articles, pp. 98, 101

Prenatal Therapy Association
(1977). 17 Bereweeke Road, Winchester, Hants. *Tel.:* Winchester (0962) 4080. *Secretary:* R. St John. *Members:* 10.
Journal: Prenatal Therapy Association Newsletter, quarterly. List of accredited practitioners; gives practitioners chance to air views.
Aims: Promotes prenatal therapy, provide seminars and lectures, gives some financial support for indigent students, and provides premises. Open to all with genuine interest.
Article, p. 149

Psionic Medical Society/Institute of Psionic Medicine
(1968/70). Beacon Hill Park, Hindhead, Surrey. *Secretary:* Carl Upton L.D.S. (Birm.), M.I.PSi.Med. *President:* George Laurence F.R.C.S. (Edin.), M.R.C.S., L.R.C.P., F.I.PSi.Med. *Members:* 200.
Journal: Psionic Medicine, twice yearly. Contributions welcomed by editor, Aubrey Westlake B.A., M.B., Sandy Balls House, Godshill, Fordingbridge, Hants.
Aims: Promotes research into cause of chronic and apparently incurable disease to advance methods of treatment, particularly the homoeopathic which are known to be free from toxic risk. Provides psionic medical training for medical and dental practitioners. Holds examinations, maintains register. A registered charity, invites donations. Membership open to professionals only; associate membership open to others.
Article, p. 153

Radionic Association
(1943). 16a North Barr, Banbury, Oxon OX1 0GF. *Tel.:* Banbury 3138. *Chairman:* D. Upton D.O., Lic.AC., M.AC.A., M.Rad.A. *Members:* 98 qualified, 428 associates.
Journal: Radionic Quarterly, quarterly. News, articles, transcripts of lectures, book reviews. Free to all members. Non-members, £2.50 annually in Europe, U.S. $7.50 elsewhere.
Aims: Promotes radionics as an honourable and skilled profession, fosters research,

encourages study of subjects having a bearing on radionics, provides a world clearing house for information. Annually holds several meetings in London on radionics, natural therapeutics, healing and parascience generally. Maintains a library; members may borrow by post. Lists practising members and advises on fees. For professionals and laypersons.
Article, p. 164

Relaxation for Living
(1972). Dulnesk, 29 Burwood Park Road, Walton-on-Thames, Surrey. *Tel.:* Walton-on-Thames (093 22) 27826. *Hon. Secretary:* Mrs Amber Lloyd A.M.R.S.H., M.I.H.E. *Chairman:* Mrs Jane Madders DP.P.E., M.C.S.P. *Members:* 35.
Journal: Relaxation for Living News Letter, quarterly. Primarily for teachers but several doctor readers. Annually £1.50.
Aims: Promotes the teaching of physical relaxation to combat stress, strain, tension of modern life. As a preventative therapy it can ease the over-burdened National Health Service. Correspondence course for those unable to reach a teacher. Custom-designed seminars arranged for businesses, colleges, etc.

Release
(1967). 1 Elgin Avenue, London w9. *Tel.:* 01–289 1123, 01–603 8654.
Journal: News Release, quarterly, 30p.
Aims: Provides 24-hour phone service for people with drug problems. Sympathetic counselling and referrals to other organizations; does not moralize. Doctor available at London H.Q. Monday and Thursday evenings.

Research Society for Natural Therapeutics
(1959). 8 Stokewood Road, Bournemouth BH3 7NA. *Tel.:* Bournemouth (0202) 25997. *Hon. Secretary:* Martin L. Budd. *President:* A. L. Winer N.D., D.O., D.C., M.B.N.O.A. *Members:* 140.
Journal: Journal of the R.S.N.T., annually. Research carried out by members, selected lectures, comments, reviews of national and international publications.

Aims: Inaugurates and carries out original research, investigates new or neglected therapeutic and diagnostic techniques, brings such knowledge to the notice of practitioners through post-graduate courses and seminars and publications. When possible the Society makes grants towards specific research projects. Associate and full membership.

Schizophrenia Association of Great Britain
(1970). Tyrtwr, Llanfairhall, Caernarvon, Gwynedd LL55 1TT. *Tel.:* Bangor (024 875) 379. *Secretary:* Mrs Gwynneth Hemmings. *Chairman:* Basil Moore. *Members:* 2000–3000.
Journal: Newsletter, twice yearly.
Aims: Annual conference.

Society of Metaphysicians Ltd
Archers' Court, Stonestile Lane, The Ridge, Hastings, East Sussex. *Tel.:* Hastings (0424) 751577. *General Secretary:* Miss M. Ross. *Founder-President:* John J. Williamson. *Members:* 1750, plus 1750 students, 2500 scientists, 800 associated groups.
Journal: Neo-Meaphysical Digest, annually. Also newsletter issued from time to time.
Aims: Seeks to develop study of fundamental laws and to apply the resulting science in all human affairs. Publishes, imports, exports, researches. Concerned with induction of esoteric, psychic, parapsychological and other transcendental abilities and from empirical data gained to derive theoretical systems. Student, provisional, graduate and full memberships.
Articles, pp. 111, 120, 141, 161

Society of Osteopaths
(1971). Slaters, 5 Guildford Road, Broadbridge Heath, Horsham, West Sussex RH12 3JT. *Tel.:* Horsham (0403) 65087. *Hon. Secretary:* John Barkworth. *President:* Barry Savory. *Members:* 80.
Journal: The Journal of the Society of Osteopaths, twice yearly. Primarily technical. Domestic matter carried in a newsletter.

Aims: Primary object is to preserve the identity of osteopathy as laid down by the founder of osteopathy, Andrew Taylor Still, but encouraging members of progressively higher standards through postgraduate study and research. Members bound by strict ethical code. Full, associate and student memberships.
Article, pp. 67, 143

Society to Support Home Confinements
(1972). *Headquarters:* Margaret Whyte, 17 Laburnam Avenue, Durham. *Tel.:* Durham (0385) 61325. *London:* Pauline Stevens, 274 Merton Road, London sw18 (*Tel.:* 01–874 7940).
Aims: Advises on home confinements, helps women find G.P.s and midwives sympathetic to home confinements. Campaigns against the deterioration of the domiciliary midwives service. Fights for right of continuity of care throughout pregnancy.
Articles, pp. 135, 149

Society of Teachers of the Alexander Technique
3 Albert Court, Kensington Gore, London sw7. *Tel.:* 01–589 3834.
Secretary: Mrs S. Langley. *Chairman:* Eric de Peyer (7 Wellington Square, London sw3). *Members:* 130.
Journal: The Alexander Journal. Articles by teachers and pupils.
Aims: Maintains standards of teachers, safeguards them against unqualified teachers, promotes the principles of the Alexander technique.
Article, p. 22

Vegan Society
(1944). 47 Highlands Road, Leatherhead, Surrey. *Tel.:* Leatherhead (03723) 72389.
Hon. Secretary: Kathleen Jannaway.
President: Frey Ellis M.D., F.R.C.path.
Members: 2000.
Journal: The Vegan, quarterly. Deals with health, ecological, economic, compassionate and ethical aspects of veganism, plus recipes and practical hints to help practise and propagate the vegan way of life. 25p post free.

Aims: Formed by vegetarians who, realizing more cruelty is involved in dairy produce than in meat production, decide to exclude all animal ingredients from their diet. Registered charity. Annual general meeting held in different parts of Britain each autumn; garden party each June in Surrey and growing number of local meetings. Speakers go to great variety of groups in return for expenses. Publishes leaflets, booklets and a cookery book.
Article, p. 186

Vegetarian Society (U.K.) Ltd
(1847). Parkdale, Dunham Road, Altrincham, Cheshire WA14 4QG. *Tel.:* Altrincham (061 928) 0793. *General Secretary:* David Knowles. *President:* Dr G. Latto. *Journal: The New Vegetarian,* monthly. Articles on nutrition, ethics, ecology and health. Annually £3.
Aims: Promotes knowledge of vegetarianism, publishes leaflets and recipe books, operates an information service, provides speakers and cookery demonstrations nationwide, sponsors scientific research on nutrition, stages exhibitions.
Article, p. 188

Weight Watchers (U.K.) Ltd
(1967). 1 Thames Street, Windsor, Berks SL4 1sw. *Tel.:* Windsor (07535) 69131.
Directors: Derek Batha, Mrs Barbara Hardwick. *Members:* 40000
Journal: Weight Watchers Magazine, monthly. 35p. Editor, Audrey Slaughter. Also free paper for members, *Countdown,* five issues per year.
Aims: Every Weight Watchers lecturer has lost weight by following the Programme of Eating, maintained that weight loss and been trained to help others. Runs classes to help members lose excess weight and learn how to keep it off for life. To join, new member must have 10 lb. or more to lose. 800 weekly classes all over U.K. Registration fee £1.50, weekly class £1.30.
Article, p. 190

Contributors

Not all contributors wished to be listed. In some instances contributors preferred to have the name and address of a clinic or association listed, so that readers requiring treatment or further details could make contact.

Absent healing (p. 19)
Phil and Kath Wyndham, Canberra, Dropwell Meadow, Torrington, Devon EX38 7BE

Acupuncture (p. 21)
John Newton, Journalist, 2 Spencer Gardens, London SW14 7AH (01–876 0856)

Alexander Technique (p. 22)
Eric de Peyer, 7 Wellington Square, London SW3 4NJ (01–730 3141)

Applied kinesiology (p. 29)
Brian H. Butler, Personal Development Seminars, 42 Worthington Road, Surbiton, Surrey KT6 7RX (01–399 7377)

Aromathérapie (p. 33)
Danièle Ryman, Marguerite Maury Aromathérapie, Park Lane Hotel, Piccadilly, London W1A 4UA (01–493 6630)

Autism (p. 40)
Barbara Roberts S.R.N., A.F.phys., Hillside, 78 Park Road, Kingston-upon-Thames, KT2 5JZ

Baldness (p. 42)
See **acupuncture**.

Bates method (p. 43)
Evelyn B. Sage, 76 Twyford Avenue, Fortis Green, London N2 9NN (01–883 4776)

Belly dancing (p. 44)
See **acupuncture**.

Bioenergy and Biodynamics (p. 45)
Gerda Boyesen, Centre of Bioenergy,

Acacia House, Centre Avenue, The Vale, Acton Park, London W3 7JX (01–743 2437)

Biofeedback (p. 46)
Geoffrey Blundell, Audio Limited, 26 Wendell Road, London W12 9RT (01–743 1518)

Biorhythms (p. 49)
Michael McDonald B.SC., C.Eng., M.I.E.E., Bio-Cal Limited, 27 Church Road, Tunbridge Wells, Kent TN1 1HU (Tunbridge Wells (0892) 38919)

Breathing (p. 52)
Capt. William P. Knowles M.C., Ingleby, Cherry Rise, Chalfont St Giles, Bucks HP8 4HL (Chalfont St Giles (02407) 2697)

Cancer (p. 53)
See **acupuncture**.

Chiropractic (p. 58)
R. Gerald Cooper D.C., 5/ 120 Wigmore Street, Portman Square, London W1H 9FD (01–935 8117)
and
76 Woodside, Leigh-on-Sea, Essex SS9 4RB (Southend-on-Sea (0702) 525627)

Co-counselling (p. 61)
John Heron, Assistant Director (Medical Education), British Postgraduate Medical Federation, 33 Millman Street, London WC1N 3EJ (01–831 6222)

Colour therapy (p. 63)
Theo Gimbel D.C.E., Hygeia Studios, Brook House, Avening, Tetbury, Glos., GL8 8NS (Nailsworth (045 383) 2150)

Copper (p. 65)
Lt. Col. A. Forbes, Coln Farm,
Sevenhampton, Cheltenham GL54 5SN
(Cheltenham (0242) 82491)

Cosmetics (p. 66)
Rona Batson, Faith Products Natural
Cosmetics, 17 Bellevue Crescent, Edinburgh
EH3 6NE (031–556 0312)

'Cranial' osteopathy (p. 67)
D. E. Gilhooley D.O., M.R.O., c/o The
General Council & Register of
Osteopaths, 16 Buckingham Gate, London
SW1E 6LB (01–828 0601)

Cupping (p. 69)
See acupuncture.

Dianetics (p. 70)
Tom Shuster B.A., The Church of
Scientology, The Guardian Office U.K.,
Saint Hill Manor, East Grinstead,
West Sussex (East Grinstead (0342)
24571)

Encounter (p. 72)
Margi Robinson, 25 Lena Gardens,
London W6 7PY (01–603 3260)

Endogenous endocrinotherapy (p. 74)
Michael Nightingale D.O., M.AC.A., 94
Banstead Road South, Sutton, Surrey
SM2 5LH (01–642 4161)
Denis Brookes D.O., M.R.O., Sidney House,
School Court, Castle Street, Shrewsbury
SY1 2AJ (Shrewsbury (0743) 62323)

Flower healing (p. 77)
Elizabeth Bellhouse, Vita Florum
Products Limited, Lydeard St Lawrence,
Taunton, Somerset TA4 3QA (Lydeard
St Lawrence 098 47 7329)

Gerson therapy (p. 79)
Margaret Straus, 97 Bedford Court
Mansions, Bedford Avenue, London
WC1B 3AE (01–637 4648)

Gestalt therapy (p. 82)
Dr G. Seaborn Jones B.A. (Oxon.), PH.D.
(Lond.), Director, Bodymind Centre,
8 Princes Avenue, London N10 3LR
(01–444 5077)

Ginseng (p. 85)
Lee Harris, Emperor Ginseng Company
Limited, 43 All Saints Road, London
W11 1HE (01–221 4331)

Hand healing (p. 88)
Elizabeth Baerlein, Swinbrook Cottage,
Swinbrook, Oxford OX8 4DZ

Health farms (p. 91)
Rita Carter, Journalist, 28 Beverley Court,
Wellesley Road, London W4 (01–995–6162)

Health foods (p. 92)
Maurice Hanssen, Tremaine, 21 Milbourne
Lane, Esher, Surrey KT10 9EB (Esher
(0372) 62588)

Hebraic name changing (p. 98)
Adam Joseph, Journalist, 266 The
Colonnades, Porchester Square,
London W2 (01–402 3929)

Herbalism (p. 98)
E. F. Didcott, Medical Herbalist, 117
Landseer Avenue, Bristol BS7 9YP
(Bristol (0272) 697798)

High colonic irrigation (p. 110)
Mrs P. Haering D.O., D.Phys., M.I.O.P.,
Ingleby Hydro Clinic, 13 Ranulf Road,
Hampstead, London NW2 2BT
(01–435 9781)

High voltage photography (p.111)
John J. Williamson D.SC.(H.C.), F.S.M.,
M.Brit.I.R.E., F.C.G.L.I., The Society of
Metaphysicians Limited, Archers' Court,
Hastings, Sussex (Hastings (0424) 751577)

Homoeopathy (p. 113)
J. B. L. Ainsworth M.P.S., A. Nelson &
Company Limited, 73 Duke Street,
Grosvenor Square, London W1M 6BY
(01–629 3118)

Human aura (p. 120)
See high voltage photography.

Hypnotherapy (p. 122)
Contact: British Hypnotherapy
Association, 67 Upper Berkeley Street,
London W1 (01–723 4443)

Jogging (p. 125)
See acupuncture.

Mazdaznan – master thought (p. 128)
Violet Hammerton B.SC., L.T.C.L., British
Mazdaznan Association, 19 Hillbrow
Road, Withdean, Brighton BN1 5JP
(Brighton (0273) 500114)

Medicated bee venom therapy (p. 130)
Julia Owen, P.O. Box 91, Bromley, Kent
BR1 2PP

Migraine and tension headache (p. 131)
Charles Bentley M.A., Consultant
Psychotherapist, 194a Ebury Street,
London SW1 8UP (01–730 6314)

Multiple sclerosis (p. 133)
See **acupuncture**.

Music therapy (p. 133)
Juliette Alvin F.G.S.M., M.T., Music
Therapist, British Society for Music
Therapy, 48 Lanchester Road, London
N6 4TA (01–883 1331)

Natural childbirth (p. 135)
Margo Hogan S.R.N., S.C.M., 10 Burnham
Court, Moscow Road, London W2 (01–229
5447)

Naturopathy (p. 138)
Nigel P. Castle, Naturopath and Osteopath.
19 Bristol Gardens, London W9
(01–286 8921)

Neometaphysical concepts of psychology
(p. 141)
See **high voltage photography**.

Orthomolecular psychiatry (p. 143)
See **acupuncture**.

Osteopathy (p. 143)
Thomas G. Dummer D.O., M.S.O., Principal,
École Européenne d'Ostéopathie, 28/30
Tonbridge Road, Maidstone, Kent
ME16 8RT

Prenatal therapy (p. 149)
Robert St John, Prenatal Therapy
Association and School, 17 Bereweeke
Road, Winchester, Hants. (Winchester
(0962) 4080)

Primal therapy (p. 150)
See **gestalt therapy**.

Psionic medicine (p. 153)
Contact: The Secretary, The Institute of
Psionic Medicine, Beacon Hill Park,
Hindhead, Surrey GU26 6HU

Psychic surgery (p. 155)
George Chapman, St Brides, 149
Wendover Road, Aylesbury, Bucks
HP21 7NN

Psychodrama (p. 157)
Dr Joel Badaines PH.D., 83a Oxford
Gardens, London W10 5UL (01–969
7766)

Pulsed high frequency (p. 160)
Kay Kiernan L.C.S.P.(phys.), M.F.Phys.,
I.R.M.T., Bluestone Clinic, 99 Harley
House, Marylebone Road, London NW1
(01–935 7933)

Radiesthesia (p. 161)
See **high voltage photography**

Radionics (p. 164)
John Wilcox, The Radionics Association,
Field House, Peaslake, Guildford GU5
9SS (Dorking (0306) 730080)

Recessed heel footwear (p. 168)
Alan K. Jackson, Roots Natural Wear
Limited, 4 Conduit Street, London W1
(01–493 4555)

Reflexology (p. 170)
Martine L. Faure-Alderson D.O., N.D.,
M.B.N.O.A., 'Compton House', 87 High
Street, Hampton, Middlesex (01–979 3119)

Reichian therapy (p. 172)
Contact: Centre of Bioenergy, Acacia
House, The Vale, Centre Avenue, Acton
Park, London W3 7JX (01–743 2437)

Rolfing (p. 174)
Darcey Ortolf, Quaesitor, 187 Walm
Lane, London NW2
Contact: Rolf Institute, P.O. Box 1868,
Boulder, Colorado 80306, U.S.A.

Shiatsu massage (p. 177)
See **acupuncture**.

Spiritual healing (p. 178)
Rev. Ray Nielsen, Secretary – European
Headquarters, The Aetherius Society,
757 Fulham Road, London SW6 5UU
(01–736 4187)

Staplepuncture (p. 179)
See **acupuncture** *and*
Treatment: Acupuncture Centre, 34
Alderney Street, London SW1

Swedish massage (p. 791)
Patricia Peplow, 14 Bedford Park
Mansions, The Orchard, London W4
(01–994 2654)

The Tao of loving (p. 181)
Jolan Chang, Grevg. 9, 11453 Stockholm,
Sweden.

Transpersonal psychology (p. 183)
Ian Gordon-Brown, Centre for

Transpersonal Psychology, 26a Gilston Road, London sw10 9ss

Urine therapy (p. 186)
See **acupuncture.**

Vegan diet (p. 186)
Kathleen Jannaway, Honorary Secretary, The Vegan Society, 47 Highlands Road, Leatherhead, Surrey (Leatherhead (03723) 72389)

Weight Watchers (p. 190)
Joyce Wood, Weight Watchers (U.K.) Limited, 1 Thames Street, Windsor, Berkshire sL4 1sw (Windsor (07535) 69131)

Wine (p. 192)
Docteur E. A. Maury, L'Esteral, Boulevard Maréchal Leclerc, 06130 – Grasse, France

Yoga (p. 193)
Howard Kent, Yoga for Health Foundation, 9 Old Bond Street, London w1x 3TA (01–493 0165)

Products

The prices, given here for comparison purposes only, were correct when this directory was compiled. These prices are not necessarily binding on any of the manufacturers and suppliers listed here. Arrangement is by alphabetical order of the names of the suppliers or supplying agents.

THE AETHERIUS SOCIETY
757 Fulham Road, London sw6
5uu

Auric Energy Harmonizer/TM. Two copper loops that go round body from head to foot and round chest, plus two 24-carat gold-plated discs to fit over heart centre, plus sixty-minute explanatory cassette tape and complete Aura Charging Practice. Increases balance and harmony, enhancing spiritual development and healing abilities. £65.50 inc. v.a.t. p.&p.

Radionic Pendulum. Hand-crafted beechwood pendulum with pure silk cord. Aids all forms of healing diagnosis, character analysis, psychic experiment, etc. £3.05 inc. v.a.t., p. & p. Explanatory cassette tape (lecture, *The Pendulum – How Does it Work?*, by Dr George King) £4.45 inc. v.a.t., p. & p.
(See articles, pp. 164 and 177)

AUDIO LTD
26 Wendell Rd, London W12 9rt

Omega 1. Electrical skin resistance meter. Measures arousal or relaxation of autonomic nervous system by indication from palm of hand. £20.

Omega 2. Electrical skin resistance meter. Similar to Omega 1 but has greater sensitivity to indicate emotional responses. £75.

Temperature Meter. Reads 1°C change of temperature. Useful aid in reduction of tension. £25.

Moniter-M EEG. Meter. Indicates beta, alpha, theta, and delta brain rhythms. There is also a myograph facility to aid muscular relaxation. £165.
(See article, p. 46)

BIO-CAL LTD
27 Church Rd, Tunbridge Wells, Kent
TN1 1HU

Biocalendar. Computer-produced display of twelve months' biorhythms. You relate your pattern of behaviour to the pattern of your biorhythmic energies; tells how to use this knowledge in advance. £1.75 basic, £3.50 de luxe.
(See article, p. 49)

BIOMATE (U.K.) LTD
20 Bride Lane, Ludgate Circus, London
EC4Y 8DX

Astro-Guide. Astrological indicator. Shows the characteristics (under eleven different headings) of every person and enables you to analyse at-a-glance the character of any individual and to ascertain the compatibility of any number of people. 95p inc. v.a.t., p. & p.
(See article, p. 35)

Biomate. Four-gear calculator, with instructions and application guide, chart forms and calendars. Shows anyone's biorhythms; enables you to ascertain your emotional, intellectual and physical condition – past, present and future – at a glance. £5.45 inc. V.A.T., p. & p. (*See article, p. 49*)

OMNI-Detectors. Four different dowsing (divining) instruments and forty-page manual. Test food, soil, water, etc, for pollution. Locate lost objects, people, treasure. Examine the aura of living objects. Select a personal diet. £5.50 inc. V.A.T., p. & p.

Pyramid. Scale-size model of the ancient pyramids. Preserves foods, enhances flavour of food and beverages, stimulates health and growth of plants, aids vitality of humans and animals, helps in meditation and also sleep, extends life expectancy. Hundreds of applications. From £3 upwards depending on size.

EMPEROR GINSENG CO LTD
43 All Saints Road, London W11 1HE
Emperor Ginseng. Root, tablets, capsules, chipped root pieces. Herbal tonic with long-term beneficial effects. Send S.A.E. for price list.
(*See article, p. 85*)

FAITH PRODUCTS
17 Bellevue Crescent, Edinburgh EH3 6NE
Honey and Almond Moisturiser. For dry skin, blended with pure honey, rose, almond and soya oils, enriched with beeswax to penetrate and diminish wrinkles and improve skin texture. £1.20.

Marigold Cleansing Cream. For normal, dry and sensitive skin, blended from the herbal extract of marigold petals, soya and geranium oils; enriched with beeswax to cleanse and soften your skin. £1.20.

Marigold Sunshine Shampoo. For dry, damaged or split hair. Herbal extracts of marigold combined with a natural vegetable base. 60p.

Oatmeal Cleansing Cream. For oily and combination skin; blended with plant extract of pure oatmeal, soya oil and

beeswax; an astringent cleanser without any drying effect. £1.20.

Organic Seaweed Shampoo. Suitable as family shampoo. Made from freshly gathered seaweed. 50p.

Rose and Wheatgerm Moisturiser. For normal and dry skin. Blended from rose and wheatgerm oils, beeswax and soya oil, enriched with natural Vitamin E. £1.20.

Rosemary and Chamomile Moisturiser. For oily and combination skin; blended with herbal extracts of rosemary leaves and chamomile flowers, soya and wheatgerm oils, enriched with the stimulating oil of rosemary. £1.20.

Sunflower and Wheatgerm Scrub. Masque cum deep pore cleanser. Does not harden on face or pull at skin. Blended from sunflower, wheatgerm and lilac oils, rich in natural Vitamin E. Will gently remove top layer of dead skin from face. £1.20. (*See article, p. 66*)

LT. COL. A. FORBES
Coln Farm, Sevenhampton, Cheltenham GL54 5SN
Forbes Copper. Bracelets, watch straps, bangles, necklaces, dog collars, etc., of copper. Worn next to skin may relieve pain in nearly all types of rheumatism, lumbago, sciatica, possibly arthritis. From 20p.
(*See article, p. 65*)

GREAT EARTH HEALING LTD
P.O. Box 24, London SW11 5QF
MA Roller. Wooden lie-on self-massage roller. Stretches spine, puts pressure on acupuncture points, stimulates bloodflow to internal organs, gives depth massage. £5.45 plus 70p p. & p.

HARMONY FOODS
1–19 Earl Cottages, Earl Road, London SE1
U.S. Ginseng Roots. Wild per ½ oz. £4.35 plus V.A.T., cultivated per 1 oz. £4.35 plus V.A.T.
(*See article, p. 85*)

I

PRODUCTS

HOFELS PURE FOODS LTD
Woolpit, Bury St Edmunds,
Suffolk

Hofels Garlic Pearles. Capsules containing the essential oil of garlic. Internal purifier, reduces cholesteron serum levels. Tasteless and odourless. Prices range from 75 Pearles for 47p to 1000 Pearles for £4.15.

Hofels Vitamins and Minerals. Tablets. Supplements acceptable to vegetarians. Four weeks' supply 59p, nine weeks £1.26, both plus 15p p. & p.

Protat. Herbal mixture of fluid extracts and tinctures. Ingredients: tansy, thuja, avena sativa, pulsatilla and sabal. Beneficial to genito-urinary system. Six weeks' supply 96p plus 12p p. & p.

HONEYROSE PRODUCTS LTD
P.O. Box 4, Greetings Rd, Stowmarket, Suffolk

Honeyrose De Luxe Cigarettes. Herbal cigarettes. Nicotine-free, help you reduce or quit smoking; non addictive. Twenty cigarettes 33p.

Honeyrose Special Smoking Mixture. Herbal smoking mixture. Non-addictive. Suitable for pipe or hand rolling. 50 gm 37p.

CAPT. WILLIAM P. KNOWLES M.C.
Ingleby, Cherry Rise, Chalfont St Giles, Bucks HP8 4HL

Knowles Method of Breath Training. Postal course. Helps combat bronchitis, asthma, emphysema, catarrh, nerves, fatigue, respiratory problems; can reduce smoking. £12.50.
(*See article, p. 52*)

LITTLE MISS MUFFET LTD
Nutrition House, 64 Sedlescombe Road North, St Leonards-on-Sea, Sussex

Little Miss Muffet Junket. Tablets or liquid. Mixed with milk, breaks down the tough curd to make junket. Ideal dessert for invalids, young children. Six tablets 17p, bottle 19p.

THE MALTINGS
Horsecroft Road, Bury St Edmunds, Suffolk IP33 2PS

Country Hop Pillows. Pillows filled with selected dried, purified English hops and quality feathers, down or non-allergic dacron. Old country remedy for insomnia and nervous tension. £3.50 to £20.50.

MARGUERITE MAURY
Park Lane Hotel, 1st Floor (Suite 101), Piccadilly, London W1

Marguerite Maury – Aromathérapie. Oils and creams containing pure essence from flowers, plants and tree resins. Preparations have therapeutic properties, help cure acne, wrinkles, broken capillaries, poor circulation, rheumatism, sinusitis, depression. Prices from £1.95 to £15.80. Send for extensive price list. (*See article, p. 33*)

MARY BARFIELD
2 Toot Rock Coastguards, Pett Level, East Sussex TN35 4EW

Relaxation for Everyday Living. Cassette tape. Explains the Mary Barfield method of deep relaxation. An alternative to fight/flight situations with formula for dealing with on-the-spot stress situations. Helps in childbirth, migraine, multiple sclerosis, etc. £3.20 inc. p. & p.

MELFOODS
225 High St, Aldershot, Hants GU11 1TJ

Ginseng – Korean panax. Herb. Taken to restore health, for extra vitality, strength and vigour. 25 500mg capsules £1, 100 200mg capsules £2, all inc. p. & p. (*See article, p. 85*)

METAPHYSICAL RESEARCH GROUP
Archers' Court, Stonestile Lane, The Ridge, Hastings (Hastings (0424) 751577) Add 8 per cent V.A.T. plus p. & p. to all these prices.

Aura Goggles. Fitted with standard aura filters; sensitize eyes to near ultra-violet for direct aura seeing. Diagnosis, prognosis, research. £4.75.

Complementary Colour Filters. Set of six. Different colours. Fit to standard goggles. Use similar to aura goggles. Also use in chromotherapy. £5.50 per set of six pairs.

Empty Goggle Frames. Use with aura and colour filters. £1.50.

Inner Aura Filters. Composite filter of near infra-red/near ultra-violet material and blue laminated protective glass. Prognosis, diagnosis, research. £1.50.

Outer Aura Filters. Carmine laminated. Enhance complementary colour response of eyes to outer aural light. Determine psychological states. £1.50.

Complete Aura Research Kit. Goggles, various aura filters, spare goggle frames, instruction booklet. Research and medical application. £20.
(*See article, p. 120*)

High Voltage Camera. For use on 200–250V A.C., 40–60 Hz with film-plate size 7 x 5 in. (770 mm x 270 mm). High voltage discharge from 10 000–36 000 volts approximately. Full instructions in English and Spanish. Research into mental states and images. £85.

Set of Kirlian Slides. Twenty slides showing inorganic and organic objects photographed by high voltage corona discharge method. Lecture report, plastic holder. Believed to evidence life after death. £17.
(*See article, p. 111*)

Beechwood Pendulums. Pair. Both corded, have cavities for samples or 'witnesses'. Determination of illness and cures by radiesthetic methods. £1.75.

Mermet Type Pendulums. Heavy brass, chromed on nickel. Corded. Drop shapes. For intense responses; stabilize rapid fluctuations. £7.50.

Various Pendulums. Many types: wood waxed, black wood, clear perspex, ivorine torpedo shape. Solid and cavity, corded and boxed. From £1.75 to £3.50.

Divining Rods. Rods of two strips of whalebone. Round, square or flat. For all radiesthetic analyses requiring large-scale indications. 12 in. (30m) £5, 18 in. (45cm) £6.
(*See article, p. 161*)

Mager Rosettes. Circular disc with colour segments. Use to set up table of radiesthetic correspondence for chromotherapeutic and other forms of medical radiesthesia. £2.50.

Pasquini Amplifying Pendulum or Wand. Beechwood cavity handle. For radiesthetic work including diagnosis. £2.50.

Full-Range Pasquini Kit. Research kit – two types of pendulum, bead weights, etc. £6.

Cameron Aurameter. Precision instrument. Countered spring and balanced pointing-weight system. Use as pointing wand. Believed the most sensitive radiesthetic instrument known. Diagnosis, prognosis. £15.

Mnemonic Charts. Circuit printed on hardboard base with felted undersurface. Input and output plates, eight dials and knobs indicating in decimal system. Interconnectable with other test equipment. For discovery of 'rate' signature of any substance, illness, etc. Paraphysical instrument for radionic therapy. Price on request. Made to order.

Vertical Magnetic Tuner. Mounted magnet on spindle. Aid to tuning and identification for therapeutic instruments. £25.

Biomate. Geared plastic calculator. Personal biorhythms at any time. £5.

Bio-Rhythm Service. *Pre-calculated* cards showing cycles in colour form for each day of month. Easier to use than Biomate. 12 months £7.

Seven Cycle Biorhythm Calculator. Disk calculator. Introduces Eastern mysticism to biorhythmic study. Instructions. Spiritual and mental characteristics. £4.
(*See article, p. 49*)

Ouija-Planchette. Heart-shaped beechwood board, three castors, holder for pencil or Biro. Use to assess automatism. £4.50.

Ouija-Table. Hardboard base with printed letters and numbers. Better than ouija-planchette in elementary psychic research. £5.

Planchette. Heart-shaped platform, two castors and metal pencil holder. For analysis of automatic writing processes. £3.50.

Biometer. Plated scale mounted on felted beechwood base. Metal tipped glass probe, tilting block. Enables position of aura bands surrounding any object to be located in millimetric distances from zero point. Data indicates life, intelligence, illness, efficacious treatment, etc. Price on request. Made to order.

MING GINSENG CO
11 Woodland Drive, Burton Latimer, Northants.

Ginseng (Whole Red Root). Herb. Regulates central nervous system, blood pressure, metabolic rate, increases energy, concentration, appetite. Approx. 50p per gram.
(*See article, p. 85*)

NUTRITION HOUSE PRODUCTS (U.K.) LTD
Nutrition House, 64 Sedlescombe Road North, St Leonards-on-Sea, East Sussex

Healthrite B. & C. Vitamin Formula. Food supplement in tablet form. Helps people feeling below par. 100 tablets (50 day supply) £1.95.

Healthrite Calcium Pantothenate. Food supplement in capsule form. Recommended in treatment of arthritis. 50 capsules 95p.

Healthrite Vitamin E 400 i.u. Food supplement in capsule form. Believed to oxygenate the body's tissue and assists in the utilization of carbohydrates and proteins. 50 capsules £1.99.

Iodo-Bromic Salt. Salt from Poland. A hospital has been constructed deep in a Polish salt mine; sufferers from rheumatism and asthma have gained relief from inhaling and bathing in the salt. 1 lb. bag 54p.

PARAGON ENTERPRISES
17 Arlington Road, Eastbourne, East Sussex BN21 1DJ

Paragon Truss. No belts, no straps, highly corrective. Maximum hernia control by frame on cantilever. £7.50 for single support, £12 for double.

POWER HEALTH FOODS LTD
4 Kirkland St, Pocklington, York YO4 2DE

Gamma Copper Bracelet. Copper bracelet with gold plating. By conducting static electricity out of body found to help in some cases of nerves, over-excitability, and insomnia. £5.99.

PURLVALE LTD
71 Ardmore Lane, Buckhurst Hill, Essex

Country Air Hop Pillow. Pillow filled with hops and other sleep-inducing herbs. £2.70.

Herby Cat Cushion. Flea-dispellent pillow. Cushion is laid on cat's bed; contents keep cat smelling fresh and completely free of fleas. £3.40.

Herby Dog Cushion. Same as Herby Cat Cushion but for dogs. £3.70.

Sleepy Time Doll. Sleep-inducing doll. A pretty rag doll filled with sleep-inducing herbs. Completely safe for young children. Natural sleep without side effects. £2.50.

Victorian Love Bath. Bath additive. A relaxing, perfumed bath is created from herbs. Three sachets 80p.

Victorian Mustard Bath. Bath additive. Makes you feel refreshed, invigorated, aches and pains soothed away. Two drums (enough for eight baths) £1.

Victorian Seaweed Bath. Bath additive. Creates refreshing bath with properties of the sea. Three sachets 50p.

RAYNER & PENNYCOOK LTD
Rayvit House, Govett Avenue, Shepperton, Middlesex.

Rayvit Dietary Supplements. Vitamins, minerals, herbs, honey, natural foods and ointments. Comprehensive range of products formulated for balanced nutrition and good health. Write to supplier for mail order price list.

J. I. RODALE & CO. LTD
91/2 Akeman Street, Tring, Herts HP23 6AA

Fontana 500 Humidifer. Air humidifer. Restores relative humidity. Helps bronchial and asthmatic sufferers, eases dry throats, sinus caused by dry air from central heating. Portable. Runs from domestic electricity supply. £32.45.

Mayrei Water Filter. Fits most domestic taps. Removes chlorine, lead, mercury and other impurities. Standard model £2.55, Model 2000. £3.72.

Relaxator Chair. Scientifically designed to provide complete relaxation, reduces tension and fatigue. Adjusts to give choice of recline and incline positions. Standard £50.50, de-luxe £62 (both with mattress and head pillow).

Yogamagic. Yogurt maker. Heated container, removable inner container, ferment, full instructions and guarantee. £8.83.

ROOTS NATURAL WEAR LTD
4 Conduit St, London w1

Roots Natural Wear. Footwear. Special recessed heels that spread the weight of the body evenly, better for posture. £20 to £25.
(*See article, p. 168*)

SABENEX LTD
622 Finchley Road, London NW11

Bee Venom. Produced by bees. Powerful antiseptic against arthritis, rheumatism, disorders of nervous system, sciatica, asthma and migraines. 50 enteric pills £11.50.
(*See article, p. 130*)

Pollen. Helps restore energy, regulates intestinal functions, sedative, improves blood pressure. 50 enteric pills of dehydrated pollen £4.60.
(*See article, p. 77*)

Propolis. Produced by bees. Regulates whole digestive system, has antibiotic and healing powers. 50 enteric pills £11.50.
(*See article, p. 130*)

Royal Jelly. Natural food product mixed with honey or frozen dried in enteric pills. Regulates appetite, stimulant on human body, facilitates sexual activity. 50 enteric pills £10.50.

SPEAKERS INTERNATIONAL AGENCY LTD., 77 New Bond Street, London w1Y 0BP

Recorded Talks. Cassette tapes.

No.	Speaker	Subject
F.M.B.2	Torben Nordal M.N.I.M.H.	Herbal medicine in the twentieth century (*See articles, pp. 98, 101*)
	Dr Chandra Sharma	Homoeopathy today (*See article, p. 113*)
F.M.B.5	Barbara Cartland D.StJ.	You and your health
F.M.B.8	Marcus McCausland B.A.	Health care and the healing method
	Rose Gladden	The power of healing
	Elizabeth Bellhouse	Vita florum (flower potencies) (*See article, p. 77*)
F.M.B.12	Charlotte Gerson Straus	The Gerson therapy – healing of cancer and other diseases (*See article, p. 79*)
F.M.B.13	Eva Reich M.D. and Myron Sharaf PH.D.	The energy of life – work of Wilhelm Reich (*See article, p. 172*)
V.S.A.3	Vera Stanley Alder	Diet and evolution, meditation made simple
V.S.A.5	Vera Stanley Alder	Advance knowledge of the ethers Breathing your way to success (*See article, p. 52*)

£3 each inc. V.A.T., plus 20p p. & p. (Overseas £3.30 each inc. p. & p.)

PRODUCTS

STRESSWATCH

P.O. Box 4AR, London W1A 4AR

Anxiety Control Cassette Course. Two cassette tapes, *Relaxation* and *Stress Control.* Relieves tension, anxiety, headaches, insomnia, digestion problems, fear of flying and other phobias; reduces sexual, social and executive tensions. £3.50 each or £6.00 for the two.

'Stress Watch' Stress Control Meter. Small hand-held electronic biofeedback device. Light-display meter shows how tense user is. £9.95.

VITA FLORUM PRODUCTS LTD

Lydeard St Lawrence, Taunton, Somerset TA4 3QA

Vita Florum. A self-adjusting homoeovitic blend of flower potencies (water, lotion, ointment). Tonic for all living things. Used for all disorders of mind or body. For humans, animals, gardens. Introductory pack with water, lotion and ointment enough for three months, £4.50. The same for pets, £3.85. Enough soil conditioner and foliar spray for average garden for a year, £2.90. All prices inc. p. & p. and V.A.T.

(See article, p. 77)

Training Centres

Places and people where you may learn to become a practitioner.

The Aetherius Society
757 Fulham Road, London SW6 5UU.
Tel.: 01–736 4187. *Principal:* Dr Shri
Yogiriji George King.
Courses: Spiritual healing (full weekend
course), metaphysical education (evening
lectures).

The Alexander Institute
3 Albert Court, Kensington Gore, London
SW7. *Tel.:* 01–589 3834. *Principal:*
Marjory Alexander Barlow.
Courses: Alexander technique.

Anglo-European College of Chiropractic Ltd
Cavendish Road, Bournemouth, Dorset
BH1 1RA. *Tel.:* Bournemouth (0202)
24777. *Principal:* Dr Stanley R. Lord.
Courses: Chiropractic manipulation
(adjustments) of all joints especially the
spine (four years full time).

Arnould-Taylor Organisation Ltd
Education Division, 22 Montagu Street,
Portman Square, London W1H 2BR. *Tel.:*
01–262 1458. *Principal:* W. R. Arnould-
Taylor.
Courses: Anatomy, physiology and
massage (four months).

Arthur Findlay College
Stansted Hall, Stansted, Essex. *Tel.:*
Bishop's Stortford (0279) 813636. *Principal:*
Charles Sherratt.
Courses: Psychic study, weekly courses
(residential).

Bayly, Doreen E.
107 West Kensington Court, London
W14 9AB. *Tel.:* 01–603 2722.
Courses: Reflexology (weekend seminars).

Blythe Tutorial College of Hypnosis and Psychotherapy
Warwick House, 4 Stanley Place, Chester.
Tel.: Chester (0244) 311414. *Principal:*
Peter Blythe M.A.H.P.
Courses: Hypnosis and psychotherapy
(weekends).

Bodymind
10 Steeles Mews South, London NW3.
Tel.: 01–586 4109. *Principal:* G. Seaborn
Jones PH.D.
Courses: Reciport (reciprocal non-
professional support in groups and in
pairs) (6 months); Primal release and
reintegration (2 years).

Brantridge Forest School
Highfield, Danehill, Sussex RH17 7EX.
Tel.: Danehill (082 573) 214. *Principal:*
Professor Bruce Copen PH.D., D.Litt.
Courses: Homoeopathy (3 years),
naturopathy (2 years), dietetics (1 year),
botanic medicine (3 years), psychology
(2 years), chromotherapy (1 year).

British College of Naturopathy and Osteopathy
'Frazer House', 6 Netherhall Gardens,
Finchley Road, London NW3. *Tel.:*
01–435 7830.
Principal: Denis J. Kiely N.D., D.O.,
M.B.N.O.A.
Courses: Naturopathy, osteopathy (four
years full time).

British School of Osteopathy
16 Buckingham Gate, London sw1e 6lb.
Tel.: 01–828 9479. *Principal:* S. F. G.
Bradford b.sc.
Courses: Diploma in osteopathy (four
years full time).

British Wheel of Yoga
Glyn Galleries, Glyn Ceiriog, Llangollen,
Clwyd. *Tel.:* Glen Ceiriog (069 172) 564.
Courses: Yoga.

**Centre for Group Work and Sensitivity
Training**
7 Chesham Terrace, Ealing, London w13
Tel.: 01–579 5589. *Principal:* H. E.
Lobstein.
Courses: Group work and leadership,
group therapy, massage, hypnotherapy,
self-help groups.

Church of Scientology of Manchester
48 Faulkner Street, Manchester.
Courses: Dianetics and scientology.

Churchill Centre
22 Montagu Street, Marble Arch, London
w1h 1tb. *Tel.:* 01–402 9475. *Principal:*
K. Holme.
Courses: Reichian therapy, gestalt,
hypnosis and deep relaxation, massage,
acupressure, postural integration.

College of Acupuncture
118 Foley Road, Claygate, Esher, Surrey.
Tel.: Esher (0372) 64171. *Principal:* Dr
Ac. K. Lamont.
Courses: Acupuncture (two years
postgraduate).

**College of Alternative Medicine and Science
(C.A.M.S.)**
St Joseph's Centre, Crackington Haven,
Bude, Cornwall. *Tel.:* St Gennys (084 03)
440. *Principal:* Dr A. E. M. Ash m.r.c.s.,
l.r.c.p., m.a.
Courses: Introductory short courses in
alternative medicine and science (one week).

**College of Osteopathy and Manipulative
Therapy Limited**
21 Manor Road North, Wallington,
Surrey. *Tel.:* 01–647 2452. *Principal:*
Hubert John Cooper d.d., f.c.o.
Courses: Osteopathy (four years), natural
therapeutics (ad hoc basis).

Constructive Teaching Centre Limited
18 Lansdowne Road, London w11.
Tel.: 01–727 7222. *Principal:* Walter
Carrington.
Courses: Alexander technique (three years).

École Européenne d'Ostéopathie
28/30 Tonbridge Road, Maidstone, Kent
me16 8rt. *Tel.:* Maidstone (0622)
671558. *Principal:* Thomas G. Dummer
d.o., m.s.o.
Courses: Osteopathy, basic sciences,
general medicine (four years full time and
five years postgraduate part time).

Guildhall School of Music and Drama
Barbican, London ec2y 8dt. *Tel.:*
01–628 2571. *Principal:* Allen Percival
c.b.e. *Head of Music Therapy Department:*
Juliette Alvin.
Courses: Full one year postgraduate
diploma course in music therapy, in
association with the British Society for
Music Therapy, leading to the diploma
in Music Therapy L.G.S.M. (Music
Therapy).

Healing Research Trust
16a North Barr, Banbury, Oxn. ox1 0gf.
Tel: Banbury 3138.
Courses: Hand healing (usually three
weeks).

Hubbard Academy of Personal Independence
20 South Bridge, Edinburgh.
Courses: Dianetics and scientology.

Hubbard Scientology Organization
68 Tottenham Court Road, London w1.
Courses: Dianetics and scientology.

Human Potential Research Project
Department of Adult Education,
University of Surrey, Guildford, Surrey.
Tel.: Guildford (0483) 71281, ext. 768.
Principal: John Heron.
Courses: Co-counselling (five-day work-
shops, weekly evening classes over twenty
weeks).

Institute of Biodynamic Psychology
Acacia House, Centre Avenue, The Vale,
Acton Park, London w3 7jx. *Tel.:*
01–743 2437. *Principal:* Gerda Boyesen.
Courses: Biodynamic massage and
therapy (nine months).

Institute of Psychosynthesis
Highwood Park, Nan Clarke's Lane,
Mill Hill, London NW7. *Tel.:* 01–959
3372.
Principals: Roger Evans and Joan
Wasserman.
Courses: Psychotherapy (duration
according to individual).

International College of Radionics
Highfield, Danehill, Sussex RH17 7EX.
Tel.: Danehill (082 573) 214. *Principal:*
Professor Bruce Copen PH.D., D. Litt.
Courses: Radionics, radiesthesia and
dowsing sciences (six months to 3
years).

International Tai Chi Chuan Association
40 Hillcroft Crescent, Wembley Park,
Middlesex. *Tel.:* 01–902 2351. *Principal:*
Master K. H. Chu.
Courses: Tai Chi Ch'uan (Yang style)
(5 months); h'sing I (eight months);
pa ku (twelve months); ta lu (pushing
hands) (twelve months); taoist health
massage, meditation, exercises, diet and
health (one year).

Liu School of Taoist Therapeutics
13 Gunnersbury Avenue, Ealing Common,
London W5. *Tel.:* 01–993 2549. *Principal:*
Master Liu Hsiu-Ch'i.
Courses: Acupuncture and moxibustion
(three years), pa kuan and massage (three
years), herbal remedies (three years),
therapeutic exercises (three years), dietetics
(one year), dental acupuncture (four
intensive weekends), acupuncture
anaesthesia (four intensive weekends),
acupuncture in dentistry and anaesthesia
(introductory course) (one intensive
weekend).

Macdonald, P.
50a Belgrave Road, London SW1. *Tel.:*
01–821 7916.
Courses: Alexander technique (three
years).

Maitreya School of Healing
10 Gunterstone Road, London W14.
Courses: Colour healing (twelve
weeks).

Northern Institute of Massage and Northern

College of Physical Therapies
100 Waterloo Road, Blackpool, Lancs
FY4 1AW. *Tel.:* Blackpool (0253)
403548.
Principal: K. Woodward F.L.C.S.P.(phys.).
Courses: Swedish (Remedial) massage,
body massage and physical culture, health
and beauty therapy. Full-time training,
short-period practical classes, and
correspondence courses.

Nottingham College
Mortimer House, 1 Castle Road,
Nottingham NG1 6AA. *Tel.:* Nottingham
(0602) 47874. *Principal:* K. H.
Sainsbury.
Courses: National Association of Health
Stores training course; diploma of the
Society of Nutrition and Health.

Prenatal Therapy Association
17 Bereweeke Road, Winchester, Hants.
Tel.: Winchester (0962) 4080. *Principal:*
Robert St John.
Courses: Prenatal therapy (weekend
introductory course; ten-week course for
professionals).

Psychotherapy Centre
67 Upper Berkeley Street, London W1.
Tel.: 01–262 8852. *Principal:* R. K.
Brian.
Courses: Psychotherapy (two years).

Saint Hill Foundation
Saint Hill Manor, East Grinstead,
Sussex. *Tel.:* East Grinstead (0342)
24571.
Principal: Judy Tampion.
Courses: Dianetics and scientology.

School of Alexander Studies
61a Onslow Gardens, London N6. *Tel.:*
01–883 7659. *Principal:* Miss E. F. B.
Rajna.
Courses: Alexander technique (three
years).

School of Herbal Medicine
National Institute of Medical Herbalists
65 Frant Road, Tunbridge Wells, Kent.
Tel.: Tunbridge Wells (0892) 27439. *Dean:*
F. Fletcher Hyde B.SC., F.N.I.M.H.
Principal: Hein H. Zeylstra M.N.I.M.H.
Courses: Herbal medicine (four years).

I*

School of Radionics
16a North Barr, Banbury, Oxon. OX1 0GF.
Tel.: Banbury 3138.
Registrar: Miss E. A. Eden,
Sycamore Farm, Chadlington, Oxon.

Scott, P.
25 Corfton Road, Ealing, London W5.
Tel.: 01–997 2667.
Courses: Alexander technique (three years).

Health Farms

Prices quoted were correct at the time of going to press. They are given only for comparison.

Champneys at Tring Health Resort
Tring, Hertfordshire HP23 6HY.
Directors: Allan and Tanya Wheway.
Tel.: Administrative and guests, Lindfield
(04427) 3351; reservations, Lindfield
(04427) 73155/6. *Capacity:* 95. *Fees:*
£129.50 to £280 per week.
Treatment: Various massage, heat and
hydrotherapy treatments are given each
morning for relaxing, toning and cleansing.
A range of physiotherapy treatments are
available and osteopathy is given by a
qualified doctor. Facials, cathiodermie,
Slendertone, depilatory waxing, bio
peeling, manicure and pedicure, and other
beauty treatments are available, including
solarium. Fully equipped hairdressing
salon. All kinds of exercises: jogging,
gymnast trail, indoor swimming pool,
tennis, badminton, golf driving net,
American swing ball; golfing, horseriding
and squash can be arranged. Weight-
losing and special medical diets. Vegetarian meals available. Lectures on health,
fitness and beauty. Guests can be energetic
or lazy, as they wish. Games room,
library, leisure craft centre with tuition
in painting, pottery and flower arranging.
Film shows and musical evenings.
Fashion shows, casino nights, dancing.
Location: Set in beautiful 170-acre
parkland estate in Chiltern hills, one hour
from London. Elegant country mansion
built in 1874. All bedrooms have phone,
radio, colour television, electric blankets,
central heating; the majority have toilet
and shower en suite. Each year guests
come from about fifty different countries.

Chevin Hall Health and Beauty Hotel
Otley, West Yorkshire. *Tel.:* Otley
(094 34) 2526.
Treatment: All types of massage, faradism,
G.5 facials, manicure, pedicure, hand and
foot waxing, short wave diathermy,
hairdressing, steam, bubble and sauna
baths, solarium and infra-red ray.
Amenities include outdoor swimming
pool, tennis court, table tennis, gym and
Roman Spa Bath.
Location: Stands in secluded grounds,
750 feet above sea level with glorious
views of the Wharfe valley.

Craig End Lodge Guest House
Cowpasture Road, Ilkley, West Yorkshire
LS29 8RS. *Principal:* Mrs Enid Hunter.
Tel.: Ilkley (0943) 609897. *Capacity:* 24.
Fees: £23.10 to £54.60 per week.
Treatment: No special treatment given,
but all food is chosen for health-giving
properties and vegetarian and special
diets are available.
Location: Moorland setting with rural
views all round. Special facilities for
disabled people, or those recovering from
illness.

Enton Hall Health Centre
Near Godalming, Surrey GU8 5AL.
Principal: Peter Lief. *Tel.:* Administrative,

Wormley (042879) 2233; guests, Wormley 2233. *Capacity:* 81. *Fees:* £82.60 to £136.85 per week.

Treatment: On arrival each patient is given a consultation and prescribed a suitable diet. Treatment includes osteopathy, naturopathy, hydrotherapy, massage, sauna, steam-cabinets and pyretic blanket baths. A well-equipped physiotherapy department includes ultrasonic, faradism, traction, ultra-violet, infra red, wax baths and depolaray. Remedial exercise and relaxation classes are available daily to all patients, and lectures on health and disease are arranged weekly, along with yoga for beginners. Additional optional facilities include Slendertone, hairdressing, nature-cure facials and vitamin injections. There is a fully qualified nursing staff. Local facilities include a golf course, and during winter classical music recitals and theatre outings are arranged. Much of the food provided comes from the Hall's own organic garden.

Location: Guests are accommodated in the Hall, or in chalets, or in near-by Oak House. All rooms include telephone, radio, wash-basin and electric blanket. The Hall and Oak House have central heating and each chalet is provided with an electric fire. Situated in the heart of Surrey, surrounded by woods and fields, Enton Hall is 38 miles from London.

Forest Mere Health Hydro
Forest Mere, Liphook, Hants GU30 7JQ. *Principal:* Dr John Meehan. *Tel.:* Liphook (0428) 722051. *Capacity:* 79. *Fees:* £107.24 to £265.88 per week.

Treatment: Up-to-date equipment for osteopathy, dietetics, electrotherapy, massage, colonic lavage, neuro-muscular technique, remedial exercise, hydrotherapy, sauna and steam baths and physiotherapy. The physiotherapy department is fully equipped with all modern appliances: interferential therapy, rhythmic traction, infra red, ultrasonics, short wave diathermy, wax baths, faradism and remedial exercises. The department is under the supervision of a Member of the Chartered Society of Physiotherapists. Physiotherapy is free and if patients anticipate having this treatment during their stay they are asked to obtain a letter from their own doctor. State Registered Nurses and an attendant physician are on hand and arrangements can be made for special investigations like blood analysis, electro-cardiogram, X-rays and other tests.

Grange Health and Beauty Farm
Henlow, Bedfordshire. *Tel.:* Hitchin (0462) 811111.

Treatment: Special diets for reducing or gaining weight. Various types of massage provided, facial treatments, scalp massage, manicure, pedicure, volcanic mud treatment (Parafango), paraffin wax baths, hydrotherapy, ionized oxygen vapour bath and asynchrone. Amenities include tennis, badminton, archery, croquet, boating, indoor heated swimming pool, table tennis, billiards room, bridge room, library.

Location: Historic mansion in rural surroundings.

Grayshott Hall Health Centre
Headley Road, Grayshott, near Hindhead, Surrey GU26 6JJ. *Principal:* G. S. Stalbow. *Tel.:* Hindhead (042873) 4331. *Capacity:* 120. *Fees:* £89.25 to £367.20 per week.

Treatment: Concentrates on relaxation and weight adjustment. Each patient put on appropriate diet. Nursing staff on call 24 hours a day. Usual treatment involves a short period of fasting and rest combined with massage and heat therapy. May include osteopathy, physiotherapy, sauna or steam bath and group exercises. Described as being based on the concept of 'Positive Health' – a condition of body and mind. Computer-controlled solarium.

Location: A large Victorian house in 47 acres of landscaped and wooded grounds, near National Trust land which includes trout-fishing streams.

Green Pastures Home of Health and Healing
17 Burton Road, Branksome Park,

Bournemouth BH13 6DT. *Principal:* Rev. William E. Burridge. *Tel.:* Administrative, Bournemouth (0202) 764776; guests, Bournemouth 760958. *Fees:* £30 to £36 per week plus V.A.T.
Treatment: Private counselling and deep prayer relaxation therapy. Facilities include occupational therapy centre and outdoor swimming pool. A relay system to all public rooms and bedrooms calls guests to worship in the private chapel, and services can be heard in rooms.
Location: Set in Branksome Park, a wooded area on the borders of Bournemouth and Poole. One mile from sea.

Hygeia Clinic
Brook House, Avening, Tetbury, Gloucestershire. *Principal:* Theo Gimbel. *Tel.:* Dursley (045383) 2150. *Capacity:* 18. *Fees:* £43.50 to £58.50. per week
Treatment: Colour therapy and self-discipline in meditation for health. Instructions for the use of colours in daily life. Weekend courses in everyday language, each complete in itself. Courses are accumulative learning and will build up to a comprehensive training in colour therapy.
Location: The house stands in three and a half acres of garden in pretty Cotswold village. Central heating.

Inglewood Health Hydro
Kintbury, near Newbury, Berkshire. *Tel.:* Hungerford (048 86) 2022.
Treatment: Dieting, osteopathy, physiotherapy, remedial gymnastics, hydrotherapy, relaxation technique, massage, Slendertone, G5, salt, seaweed, mud, wax and Moor baths, sauna and steam cabinet, impulse shower, underwater massage, solarium (ultra-violet and infra red) ultrasonics. Special treatment for arthritis and rheumatism. Beauty department offers full range of hair treatment, facials and skin treatment. Amenities include organically grown food, own spring water, library, games room, Cellar Club, fruit juice bar, tennis, squash,

golf, horse-riding and hot-air ballooning. Heated indoor swimming pool and gymnasium. The unit is operated by a registered medical practitioner.

Lake District Health Centre
56 Gillingsgate, Kendal, Cumbria LA9 4JB. *Tel.:* Kendal (0539) 22208. *Fees:* £25 to £45 per week plus treatment fees.
Treatment: Includes relaxation, neuro-muscular massage, osteopathy and nutrition, naturopathy. Treatment administered by qualified staff and tailored to individual needs.
Accommodation: Self-catering double flats.

Maison de l'Hygiene Naturelle
10290 Marcilly le Hayer, Rigny-la-Nonneuse, Aube, France. *Principal:* Mr A. Mosséri. *Tel.:* 010 33 25 24–60–05. *Capacity:* 16. *Fees:* £56 to £84 per week.
Treatment: Supervised fasting without drugs. Also care and diet without fasting, remedial and convalescent medical treatment. English is spoken.
Location: Between Paris and Troyes.

Malvern Hydro
Mount Pleasant Hotel, Great Malvern. *Tel.:* Malvern (068 45) 61837.
Treatment: Various massages, sauna and steam baths, faradism, cosmetic sunray, facials, manicure, pedicure and wax depilation. Special diet provided, or guests can take the normal hotel meals.
Location: On the sheltered slopes of the Malvern Hills.

Metropole Health Hydro
Metropole Hotel, Kings Road, Brighton, Sussex BN1 2FU. *Principal:* Ian Scott O.B.E. *Tel.:* Brighton (0273) 775432. *Capacity:* 36. *Fees:* £102 to £114 per week, plus V.A.T.
Treatment: Diet control, osteopathic treatment, massage (hand, vibro and underwater), ultra sonic, inhalation therapy, infra red and ultra violet, vacuum Nemectron interferential treatment, hand and foot wax treatment, sauna, steam cabinet, colonic lavage, gymnasium, solarium, plus full range of beauty

treatments. Hairdressing salon within hydro.

Location: In the west wing of the Metropole Hotel in Brighton, opposite the West pier.

Mokoia Health Centre

11 Crosbie Road, Troon, Ayrshire, KA10 6HE. *Principal:* Jan de Vries. *Tel.:* Troon (0292) 311414. *Capacity:* 12. *Fees:* £80 per week.

Treatment: Each patient is given a private examination on arrival and prescribed a course of treatment and diet. If necessary, blood, urine tests and X-rays are taken. Treatments include acupuncture, balneotherapy (mineral water baths) a variety of diets, including a gluten-free diet for multiple sclerosis sufferers, fasting, physiotherapy, osteotherapy and massage. Most patients are put on a one-day fast. Yoga and breathing exercises are used for relaxation and a computer-controlled solarium gives guests the chance of getting a full-length tan.

Location: On the banks of the Clyde, with a view across the Firth to the Isle of Arran.

Nurtons Field Centre

Medhope Grove, Tintern, Chepstow, Gwent, Monmouthshire. *Principals:* Adrian and Elsa Wood.

Treatment: Vegetarian diet and naturopathy. Variety of natural history and cultural courses. Programme and terms on application.

Panarwel Health and Beauty Hydro

Llanbedrog, Gwynedd. *Principal:* Mrs J. H. Livingstone. *Fees:* From £75.00 per week.

Treatment: Finnish sauna baths, Turkish steam cabinets, Swedish massage, electro auto-slim, solarium. Treatment is given by qualified masseuses and beauty therapists. Special diets are available.

Ragdale Health Hydro

Ragdale, near Melton Mowbray. *Owners:* Slimming Magazine Ltd.

Treatment: Calorie-controlled diet, coupled with body massage, G5 massage, Slendertone, sauna, plunge pool, impulse shower, solarium and beauty treatment. Amenities include a swimming pool, putting, riding and archery.

Ramana Health Centre

Ludshott Manor Hospital, Bramshott, Liphook, Hants GU30 7RD. *Tel.:* Liphook (0428) 722993.

Treatment: Ramana Health Centre is a complete hospital, offering alternative medical care in every field. It aims to bring together a number of disciplines, each based on the concept of Natural Medicine and based on treating body, soul and mind as one. They include homoeopathy, Chinese medicine, dietetics and osteopathy. The hospital's facilities include a surgery unit, hydro-physiotherapy, general medicine (including laboratory and X-ray) and outpatients departments. Laboratory techniques include radiesthesic methods, which are used together with conventional techniques. Therapies are administered by a team of visiting and resident specialists and cater for cases of arthritis, cancer and various nervous and mental disorders. A sense of community among patients is encouraged as part of the treatment. The hospital includes a mother and baby unit. This provides for natural childbirth, plus care of the mother before the birth, and of mother and child after the birth. Fees vary. Further enquiries should be made to the secretary.

Shalimar Health Clinic

First Avenue, Frinton on Sea, Essex. *Principal:* Keki R. Sidhwa. *Tel.:* Frinton-on-Sea (02556) 2823. *Capacity:* 6. *Fees:* £46.50 to £52 per week.

Treatment: Does not offer quick 'cures' but guidance on the road to good health. Emphasis on education for health, with lectures, talks and discussions. Provides rest and relaxation with vegetarian reform food meals. Guests who may require constant nursing or attention are asked to bring a companion or nurse.

Location: Ten minutes' walk from beach,

promenade and shopping centre. Large country-style house with full central heating, two-acre grounds and sun-trap garden.

Sharnbrook Court

Sharnbrook, Bedford. *Tel.:* Bedford (0234) 781442.

Treatment: Full day treatments given on regular basis. Various types of massage, infra red, sauna, faradic toning, manicure, pedicure, facial treatment, electrolysis and hairdressing.

Shenley Lodge Health Resort

Ridge Hill, Shenley, Radlett, Herts. *Tel.:* Potters Bar 42424/5 and 43254.

Treatment: High protein diet provided. Various exercises, massage, facials, sauna baths, gymnasium.

Location: Situated in quiet Hertfordshire countryside surrounded by pleasant woodland. Accommodation in seventeenth-century house.

Shrubland Hall Health Clinic

Coddenham, Ipswich, Suffolk. *Principal:* Lady de Saumarez. *Tel.:* Ipswich (0473) 830404. *Capacity:* 44. *Fees:* £68.00 to £105 per week.

Treatment: Includes manipulation, sauna, steam cabinets, massage, under-water massage, vibro massage, sitz baths, Guss treatment, herbal and peat baths, colonic lavage. There is a fully-equipped physiotherapy and electro-therapy department. Specialized 'spot reducing' treatment. Diets are of fundamental importance and are individually prescribed to meet patients' needs. They mainly consist of raw fruits, salads, yoghourt, cheese, broths and other health foods. Patients are advised to adhere to their régime. Particular diet problems should be mentioned at the time of booking. There is a comprehensive range of treatment rooms, including a gymnasium.

Location and accommodation: Situated in the heart of the fen country, Shrublands has been designed to give the efficiency of a modern hydro with the atmosphere of a country house. Many of the fine paintings and furniture remain and there are spacious sitting and television rooms. A large orangery is flanked by a heated swimming pool.

Tyringham Naturopathic Clinic

Newport Pagnell, Buckinghamshire MK16 9ER. *Principal:* Sidney Rose-Neil. *Tel.:* Newport Pagnell (0908) 61045. *Capacity:* 85. *Fees:* £54 to £108 per week.

Treatment: A comprehensive range of naturopathic treatment is available, administered by qualified staff. State registered nurses are on call 24 hours. Specific treatments include: acupuncture, balneotherapy (mineral baths), breathing exercises, hydrotherapy, massage, osteopathy and physiotherapy. Diet is vegetarian and many of the vegetables are grown in the clinic's own organic garden. Close attention is paid to the principle of macrobiotic food preparation involving extensive use of whole cereals. Fasting is used to induce a physiological rest while allowing the body to begin its inner cleansing process. Psycho-counselling is available for patients suffering from tension, anxiety and depression, and relaxation is taught by methods which can be continued at home. Bio-feedback is used to monitor and encourage relaxation.

Location: Tyringham is situated about half-way between London and Birmingham The house is a Georgian mansion, standing in 30 acres of landscaped gardens and woodland. Officially classified as a property of outstanding architectural and historical interest, it has many interesting features. In the gardens are fountains, lawns, spinneys, a rose garden, swimming pool and Sir Edwin Lutyens's Temple of Music. The clinic is surrounded by hundreds of acres of parkland, formerly part of the estate.

Weymouth Hydro

Greenhill, Weymouth, Dorset DT4 7SU. *Principal:* D. C. Clarkson. *Tel.:* Weymouth (03057) 6893. *Capacity:* 32. *Fees:* £67.20 to £76.65 per week.

Treatment: The pattern of treatment is individually tailored and includes osteopathy, massage, hydrotherapy, steam and sauna baths, relaxation therapy and electro-therapy, in conjunction with a carefully planned dietetic regime to suit each patient. X-rays and blood tests are performed when necessary. Extra treatments are available at a nominal charge and include beauty therapy, hairdressing, Slenderstone, spot-reducing treatment and G5 vibratory massage.

Location: The house is situated in one of the best residential areas of Weymouth, overlooking the sea and with superb views of the bay.

Health Magazines

Others will be found in Associations and Societies, pp. 211–19.

Healthy Living
(*Monthly*)
Natural Food Publications, Unit 3,
Hertford Road, London E6 (01–591
0055)

Here's Health
(*Monthly*)
Newman Turner Publications, Beaver
House, York Close, Byfleet, Weybridge,
Surrey KT14 7HN (Byfleet (09323)
49123)

Homoeopathy
(*Bi-monthly*)
British Homoeopathic Association, 27a
Devonshire Street, London W1N 1RJ
(01–935 2163)

Jewish Vegetarian
(*Quarterly*)
The Jewish Vegetarian and Natural
Health Society, Bet Teva, 855 Finchley
Road, London NW11 (01–455
0692)

New Life Magazine
(*Bi-monthly*)
159 George Street, London W1 (01–723
7256)

New Vegetarian
(*Monthly*)
Parkdale, Dunham Road, Altrincham,
Cheshire WA14 4QG (Altrincham (061–
928) 0793)

Prevention
(*Monthly*)
Rodale Press, Chestnut Close, Potten End,
Berkhamsted, Herts. (Berkhamsted
(04427) 71313)

Seed
(*Monthly*)
269 Portobello Road, London W11
(01–229 4723)

Undercurrents
(*Bi-monthly*)
213 Archway Road, London N6 5DN
(01–340 1898)

The Vegan
(*Quarterly*)
47 Highlands Road, Leatherhead, Surrey
(Leatherhead (03723) 72389)

Yoga Today
(*Monthly*)
Harpdown Ltd, Hertford Road, Barking,
Essex.

Festival

Alternative medicine features strongly at The Festival for Mind and Body, held annually at Olympia, London. The first exhibition was in April 1977. It drew huge newspaper and television coverage, attracted 67000 visitors, and was an outstanding success. The Festival acts as a showcase for new ideas and developments, philosophies and lifestyles and expressions of people's creative energies that can be applied in a practical way to everyday living.

The exhibition includes non-stop lectures and demonstrations, small rooms set aside for private healing and a wholefood restaurant. Many associations and societies (pp. 211–19) are represented with interesting stands. Visitors may meet a number of the contributors to this encyclopedia. Admission is about £1.

Directors: Graham Wilson, Gay Wilson Smith
Festival for Mind and Body, 159 George Street, London w1 (01–723 7256)

Speakers

A number of contributors (pp. 220-3) may be willing to give talks to schools, conferences, groups and clubs. Many associations and societies (pp. 211-19) will gladly supply speakers.

Speakers International publish a directory of speakers, including photograph, name and address, biography, availability, radius of travel and fee. Fees range from £10 to £50, plus travel expenses. You get the directory then contact the speaker yourself. The directory comprises a classified index of subjects including alternative medicine, the arts, social. industrial, and New Age. It comes in a hard-backed ring binder for easy amendments and additions.

Speakers International Agency Ltd, 77 New Bond Street, London w 1 y 0 bp (01-493 3321)

Bibliography

Acupressure

Houston, Fred M., *The Healing Benefits of Acupressure*, Keats Pub. Inc./Thorsons, 1958

Lavier, Dr J., *Chinese Micro-Massage (Acupuncture without needles)*, Thorsons, 1977

Warren, Frank Z., *Freedom From Pain Through Acupressure*, Lorne, Caldough, 1976

Acupuncture

Austin, Mary, *Acupuncture Therapy*, Turnstone, 1974

Manaka, Yoshio, and Urquhart, Ian, *The Layman's Guide to Acupuncture*, Weatherhill, New York, 1972

Mann, Felix, *Acupuncture, Ancient Art of Chinese Healing*, Heinemann, 1971

Mann, Felix, *Acupuncture: Cure of Many Diseases*, Heinemann, 1971

Toguchi, Masaru, *The Complete Guide to Acupuncture*, Thorsons, 1974

Alexander technique

Alexander, F. Matthias, *Alexander Technique: Essential Writings of F. Matthias Alexander*, Thames & Hudson, 1974

Alexander, F. M., *The Universal Constant in Living*, Re-Educational Publications, 1942

Alexander, F. M., *The Use of Self*, Re-Educational Publications, 1957.

Barlow, Wilfred, *The Alexander Principle*, Gollancz, 1973

Jones, Frank Pierce, *Body Awareness in Action*, Schocken/Wildwood House, 1977

Aromathérapie

Maury, Marguerite, *The Secret of Life and Youth*, MacDonald, 1964

Tisserand, Robert B., *The Art of Aromatherapy*, C. W. Daniel, 1977

Astrology

Addey, John, *The Discrimination of Birthtype*, L. N. Fowler, 1974

Gauquelin, M., *Cosmic Influences on Human Behaviour*, Garnstone Press, 1975

Jenkyn, Richard, *Astrology and Diet*, Health Science Press, 1972

Jones, Marc, Edmund, *Astrology: How and Why it Works*, Routledge & Kegan Paul, 1977

Rudhyar, Dane, *The Pulse of Life – New Dynamics in Astrology*, Shambhala/Routledge & Kegan Paul, 1972

Autism

Bettelheim, B., *The Empty Fortress*, Collier-Macmillan, 1969

Kanner, L., *Childhood Psychosis*, Winston, 1973

Tinbergen, N., *The Animal in its World*, Allen & Unwin, 1973

Bach Flower Remedies

Bach, Edward, *Heal Thyself*, Fowler, 1931

Chancellor, Phillip, *Handbook of the Bach Flower Remedies*, C. W. Daniel, 1971

Bates method

Huxley, Aldous, *The Art of Seeing*, Chatto & Windus, 1943

Belly Dancing

Meilach and 'Dahlena', *Art of Belly Dancing*, Bantam, New York, 1975

'Soraya', *Slimming: An Oriental Approach*, Mayflower, 1974

Bio-energetics

Alexander, Lowen, *Bio-energetics*, Coventure, London, 1976

Biofeedback

Blundell, Geoffrey, *E.E.G. Measurement*, Audio Ltd, 1977

Blundell, Geoffrey, *The Omega 1 E.S.R. Meter*, 1977
(both available from Audio Ltd, 26 Wendell Road, London w12 9rt)

Breathing therapy

Knowles, William, P., *New Life Through Breathing*, Allen & Unwin, 1970

Cancer therapies

Anderson, G., and Woolley-Hart, A., *Relaxation Healing and Mind Training*, Anderson-Hart Cancer Research Project, 1977

Barrett, John, *Cancer and Cure*, Bachman & Turner, 1976

Bell, Robert, *Cancer: Its Cause and Treatment Without Operation*, G. Bell, 1903

Brandt, Johanna, *The Grape Cure*, Technical Press, Johannesburg, 1929

Gerson, Max, *A Cancer Therapy – Results of 50 Cases*, Totality Books, California, 1975 (distributed in U.K. by Margaret Straus, 97 Bedford Court Mansions, Bedford Avenue, London wc1b 3ae)

Issels, Josef, *Cancer, a Second Opinion*, Hodder & Stoughton, 1975

Kuhl, Johannes, *Checkmate to Cancer*, Humata-Verlag, Bern, Switzerland, 1954

Kuhl, Johannes, *Truth and Fantasy in the Cancer Sphere* (obtainable from Kilquade House, Newton, Mount Kennedy, Co. Wicklow, Ireland)

Ross, Forbes, *Cancer – the Problems of its Genesis and Treatment*, Methuen, 1912.

Schmidt, Siegmund, *Help for Cancer Sick Persons Through Biological Methods*, Helfer Verlag, 638 Bad Homburg, West Germany

Scott, Cyril, *Victory over Cancer*, Health Science Press, 1969

Thomas, Gordon, *Issels: The Biography of a Doctor*, Hodder and Stoughton, 1973

Warburg, Otto, 'The primary cause of cancer', *Energy and Character*, Vol. 4, No. 3, Abbotsbury, Dorset, 1973.

Childbirth

Brady, Margaret, *Having a Baby Easily*, Health for All, 1968

Dick-Reid, Grantly, *Childbirth Without Fear*, Heinemann, 1964

Kitzinger, Sheila, *The Experience of Childbirth*, Gollancz, 1972

Leboyer, Frederick, *Birth Without Violence*, Fontana, 1977

Children – health and psychology

Archard, Merry, *Kids, Bloody Kids: A Parent's Guide to Children*, Allen & Unwin, 1972

Brady, Margaret, *Children's Health and Happiness*, Health for All, 1948

Davis, Adelle, *Let's Have Healthy Children*, Allen & Unwin, 1974

LeShan, Eda L., *How to Survive Parenthood*, Penguin, 1967

Levy, Juliette de Bairacli, *Natural Rearing of Children*, Faber & Faber, 1970

Chiropractic

Scofield, A. G., *Chiropractic*, Thorsons, 1968

Colour healing

Anderson, Mary, *Colour Healing: Chromotherapy and How it Works*, Thorsons, 1975

Copen, Bruce, *A Rainbow of Health*, Academic Publications, 1975

Dianetics and Scientology

Garrison, Omar, V., *The Hidden Story of Scientology*, Arlington Books, 1974

Hubbard, L. Ron, *Dianetics, The Modern Science of Mental Health*, American Saint Hill Organization, 1950

Hubbard, L. Ron, *Scientology: A New Slant on Life*, American Saint Hill Organization, 1966

Hubbard, L. Ron, *The Volunteer Minister's Handbook*, Publications Organization of the Church of Scientology, 1976

Dowsing
Graves, Tom, *Dowsing Techniques and Applications*, Turnstone, 1976

Fasting
Cott, Allan, *Fasting: The Ultimate Diet*, Bantam, New York, 1975

Sinclair, Upton, *The Fasting Cure*, Heinemann, 1911

Wade, Carlson, *The Natural Way to Health Through Controlled Fasting*, Arco, New York, 1972

Feet
Williams, Paul C., M.D., *Low Back and Neck Pain*, University of Texas Press, 1975

Folk medicine
Jarvis, D. C., *Folk Medicine*, Pan, 1961

Food growing
Shewell-Cooper, W. E., *Vegetables: Growing and Cooking the Natural Way*, Allen & Unwin, 1975

Strandberg, Meta, *Food Growing Without Poisons*, Turnstone, 1976

General
Blythe, Peter, *Drugless Medicine*, Arthur Barker, 1974

Cornaro, Luigi, *How to Live 100 Years*, Thorsons

Dummer, Thomas G., and Mahé, André, *Out on the Fringe*, Max Parrish, 1963

Forbes, Alec, *Try Being Healthy*, Langdon Books, 1976

Illich, Ivan, *Limits to Medicine*, Pelican, 1977

Inglis, Brian, *Fringe Medicine*, Faber, 1964

Kingston, Jeremy, *Healing Without Medicine*, Aldus, 1976

Korth, Leslie O., *Some Unusual Healing Methods*, 2nd Edition, Health Science Press, 1967

Kushi, Michio, *An Introduction to Oriental Diagnosis*, Red Moon Press, 1976

Law, Donald, *A Guide to Alternative Medicine*, Turnstone, 1974

Massacrier, Jacques, *Another Way of Living*, Turnstone, 1977

Mellor, Constance, *How to be Healthy, Wealthy and Wise*, C. W. Daniel, 1976

Mellor, Constance, *Natural Remedies for Common Ailments*, Mayflower, 1975

Palaiseul, Jean, *Grandmother's Secrets: Her Green Guide to Health from Plants*, Penguin, 1976

Powell, Eric F. W., *The Natural Home Physician*, 2nd Edition, Health Science Press, 1975

The Staff of *Prevention Magazine*, *The Encyclopedia of Common Diseases*, Rodale Press Inc., U.S.A., 1976

Watson, Bill, *Health and Fitness for the Over Forties*, Stanley Paul, 1975

Gestalt therapy
Perls, Frederick, *Gestalt Therapy Verbatim*, Bantam, New York, 1971

Perls, F., Hefferline, R. F., Goodman, P., *Gestalt Therapy*, Souvenir Press, 1972

Perls, Frederick, *The Gestalt Approach and Eye Witness to Therapy*, Bantam, New York, 1976

Hair health
Law, Donald, *How to Keep Your Hair On*, Health Science Press, 1968

Steible, Daniel N., and McHale, Edward J., *You Don't Have to be Bald*, London Press, California, 1966

Thomson, J. C. and C. L., *Healthy Hair*, Thorsons, 1972

Herbs and herbalism
Conway, David, *The Magic of Herbs*, Mayflower, 1977

Genders, Roy, *A Book of Aromatics*, Darton, Longman & Todd, 1977

Hewlett-Parsons, J., *Herbs, Health and Healing*, Thorsons, 1968

Kloss, Jethro, *Back to Eden*, Lifeline Books, California, 1973

Law, Donald, *Concise Herbal Encyclopedia*, Bartholomew, 1973

Levy, Juliette de Bairacli, *The Illustrated Herbal Handbook*, Faber & Faber, 1974

Loewenfeld, Claire, *Herb Gardening*, Faber & Faber, 1964

High voltage photography

Burr, H. S., *Blueprint for Immortality*, Spearman, 1972

Dakin, H. S., *High Voltage Photography*, Metaphysicial Research Group, 1975

Kripner and Rubin, *Kirlian Photography*, Anchor Press, New York, 1974

Muftic, Mahmoud, *Researches on the Aura Phenomena*, Society of Metaphysicians, 1970

Pierrakos, J. C., *The Energy Field in Man and Nature*, Institute of Bio-energetics, 1971

Williamson, John J., *The Energised Aura: Papers*, Society of Metaphysicians, 1948

Williamson, John J., *Seeing the Aura: Lecture Report*, Society of Metaphysicians, 1948

Homoeopathy

Blackie, Margery Grace, *The Patient, Not the Cure: The Challenge of Homoeopathy*, MacDonald & Jane's, 1975

Chevanon, Paul and Levannier, René, *Emergency Homoeopathic First-Aid*, Thorsons, 1977

Sharma, C. H., *Manual of Homoeopathy and Natural Medicine*, Turnstone, 1974

Wheeler, C. E. and Kenyon, J. D., *An Introduction of the Principles and Practice of Homoeopathy*, Health Science Press, 1971

Human aura

Bagnall, Oscar, *Origin and Properties of the Human Aura*, Kegan Paul, Trench, Trübner, 1937

Kilner, W. J., *The Human Atmosphere*, Rebman, 1911

Williamson, John J., *Seeing the Aura: Lecture Report*, Society of Metaphysicians, 1948

Humanistic psychology

Bach, George, and Goldberg, Herbert, *Creative Aggression*, Coventure, 1977

Berne, Eric, *What Do You Say After You Say Hallo?*, Corgi, 1975

Bugental, James F. T. (ed.), *Challenges of Humanistic Psychology*, McGraw-Hill, New York, 1967

Faraday, Ann, *Dream Power*, Pan, 1972

Faraday, Ann, *The Dream Game*, Penguin, 1976

Howard, Jane, *Please Touch – A Guided Tour of the Human Potential Movement*, McGraw-Hill, New York 1970

Lewis, H. R., and Streitfield, H. S., *Growth Games*, Abacus, 1973

Rogers, Carl R., *Encounter Groups*, Penguin, 1975

Rowan, John, *Ordinary Ecstasy – Humanistic Psychology in Action*, Routledge & Kegan Paul, 1976

Schutz, William C., *Joy, Expanding Human Awareness*, Souvenir Press, 1971

Seaborn Jones, G., *Treatment or Torture*, Tavistock, 1968

Hypnosis

Blythe, Peter, *Hypnotism: Its Power and Practice*, Arthur Barker, 1971

Blythe, Peter, *Self-Hypnotism: Its Potential and Practice*, Arthur Barker, 1976

Hartland, J., *Medical and Dental Hypnosis and its Clinical Applications*, Bailliére, Tindall, 1971

Insomnia

Aitken, Ridwan, *Sleep Clinic*, Daily Express, 1976

Hoskisson, Jack Bradley, *What is This Thing Called Sleep?*, Davis-Poynter, 1976

Moyle, Alan, *Self-Treatment for Insomnia*, Thorsons, 1974

Rubenstein, Hilary, *The Complete Insomniac*, Jonathan Cape, 1974

Scott, Cyril, *Sleeplessness*, Thorsons, 1975

BIBLIOGRAPHY

Irisdiagnosis
Kriege, Theodor, *Fundamental Basis of Irisdiagnosis*, Fowler, 1969

Jogging
Harris, W. E., and Bowerman, W., *Jogging*, Grosset & Dunlop, New York, 1967
Maule, Tex, *Running for Life – The Odyssey of a Heart Attack Victim's Jogging Back to Health*, Pelham, 1973
Roby, Frederick B., *Jogging for Fitness and Weight Control*, W. B. Saunders, 1970

Lakhovsky's Multiple Wave Oscillator
Clement, Mark, *The Waves that Heal*, Health Science Press, 1965
Lakhovsky, Georges, *The Secret of Life*, Heinemann, 1939

Massage
Downing, George, *The Massage Book*, Penguin, 1974
Downing, George, *Massage and Meditation*, Random House/Bookworks, New York, 1974
Inkeles, Gordon, and Todris, Murray, *The Art of Sensual Massage*, Allen & Unwin, 1973
Leboyer, Frederick, *Loving Hands: The Traditional Art of Baby Massage*, Collins, 1977
Young, Constance, *Massage: The Touching Way to Sensual Health*, Bantam, New York, 1973

Meditation
Cooke, Grace, *The Jewel in the Lotus*, White Eagle Publishing Trust, 1973
Rieker, Hans-Ulrich, *The Secret of Meditation*, Rider, 1955
Russell, Peter, *The TM Technique*, Routledge and Kegan Paul, 1977

Multiple sclerosis
Evers, Joseph, *Directions for Treatment of Multiple Sclerosis*, Karl F. Haug, Ulm, Donau, West Germany, 1964
MacDougall, Roger, *My Fight Against Multiple Sclerosis*, Regenics Ltd, 1974

Music therapy
Alvin, Juliette, *Music for the Handicapped Child*, 2nd edition, Oxford University Press, 1976
Alvin, Juliette, *Music Therapy*, Hutchinson, 1975
Priestley, Mary, *Music Therapy in Action*, Constable, 1975.

Naturopathy
Benjamin, Harry, *Everybody's Guide to Nature Cure*, Thorsons, 1961
Moyle, Alan, *Natural Health for the Elderly*, Thorsons, 1975
Newman Turner, R., *Naturopathic First Aid*, Thorsons, 1969

Neometaphysical concepts of psychology
Mayne, A., *Creative Intelligence and Scientific Law – Towards a Unified Concept of Philosophy*, Report of Institute of Parascience, 1976.
Resser, Oliver, L., *The Psychosphere: A Holistic View of Psychic Phenomena*, Human Relations, 1974.
Williamson, John J., *The Cranwell Lectures: Infinitely Based General System*, Society of Metaphysicians, 1970
Williamson, John J., *Experiential Metaphysics, Mental Energy Studies*, Society of Metaphysicians, 1953
Williamson, John J., *An Outline of the Principles and Concepts of the New Metaphysics*, Society of Metaphysicians, 1967

Nutrition – cookery and nutrition
Bieler, Henry G., *Food is Your Best Medicine*, Spearman, 1968
Bircher, Ruth, *Eating Your Way to Health: The Bircher-Benner Approach to Nutrition*, Faber & Faber, 1961
Cavanagh, Ursula M., *The Wholefood Cookery Book*, Faber and Faber, 1974
Davis, Adelle, *Let's Eat Right to Keep Fit*, Allen & Unwin, 1971
Deadman, Peter, and Betteridge, Karen, *Nature's Foods*, Rider, 1977

Elliot, Rose, *Not Just a Load of Old Lentils*, Fontana, 1976

Ellis, Audrey, *Cooking to Make Kids Slim*, Stanley Paul, 1976

Farmilant, Eunice, *Macrobiotic Cooking*, Signet, New York, 1972

Hauser, Gayelord, *Look Younger, Live Longer*, Faber & Faber, 1960

Hunter, Beatrice Trum, *The Natural Foods Primer: Help for the Bewildered Beginner*, Allen & Unwin, 1973

MacAdie, Diane, *Healthy Eating*, Stanley Paul, 1977

Maury, E. A., *Wine is the Best Medicine*, Souvenir Press, 1977

Sams, Craig, *About Macrobiotics*, Thorson, 1973

Stanway, Andrew, *Taking the Rough With the Smooth: Dietary Fibre and Your Health, A New Medical Breakthrough*, Souvenir Press, 1976

Wordsworth, Jill, *Diet Revolution: Food Reform*, Gollancz, 1976

Orthomolecular psychiatry (Megavitamin therapy)

Adams, Ruth, and Murray, Frank, *Body, Mind and the B Vitamins*, Larchmont Books, New York, 1972

Hawkins, David, and Pauling, Linus (eds.), *Orthomolecular Psychiatry: Treatment of Schizophrenia*, W. H. Freeman, 1973

Hoffer, Abram, and Osmond, Humphre, *How to Live with Schizophrenia*, Johnson Publications

Ross, Harvey, *Fighting Depression*, Larchmont Books, New York, 1975

Vonnegut, Mark, *The Eden Express*, Bantam, New York, 1946

Osteopathy

Hoag, J. M., Cole and Bradford, *Osteopathic Medicine*, McGraw-Hill, 1969

Hoag, J. M., *Theory and Practice in Osteopathic Medicine*, McGraw-Hill, 1969

Stoddard, Alan, *Manual of Osteopathic Technique*, Hutchinson, 1962

Stoddard, Alan, *Manual of Osteopathic Practice*, Hutchinson, 1969

Phobia

Sharpe, Dr Robert, and Lewis, David, *Fight Your Phobia – and Win!*, Behavioural Press, available from Stresswatch, P.O. Box 4AR, London W1A 4AR

Physical culture

Cooper, Kenneth, *The New Aerobics*, Bantam, New York, 1970

Cooper, Mildred and Kenneth, *Aerobics for Women*, Bantam, New York, 1973

Fowler, Eileen, *Stay Young Forever*, Pan, 1975

Nottidge, Pamela, and Lamplugh, Diana, *Slimnastics*, Angus & Robertson, 1970

Royal Canadian Air Force, *Physical Fitness*, Penguin 1964

Primal therapy

Janov, Arthur, *The Primal Scream*, Abacus, 1973

Janov, Arthur, *The Primal Revolution*, Abacus, 1975

Janov, Arthur, and Holden, E. Michael, *Primal Man: The New Consciousness*, Thomas Crowell, New York, 1975

Psionic medicine

Reyner, Laurence and Upton, *Psionic Medicine*, Routledge & Kegan Paul, 1974

Psychic surgery

Chapman, George, *Extraordinary Encounters*, Lang Publishing, Aylesbury, 1973

Dooley, Anne, *Every Wall a Door*, Corgi, 1975

Fuller, John G., *Arigo – Surgeon of the Rusty Knife*, Panther, 1977

Miron, S. G., *The Return of Dr Lang*, 3rd ed., Lang Publishing, Aylesbury, 1973

Sherman, Harold, *Wonder Healers of the Philippines*, Psychic Press, 1967

Psychosynthesis

Assagioli, Roberto, *Psychosynthesis: A Manual of Techniques*, Turnstone, 1975

Assagioli, Roberto, *The Act of Will*, Wildwood Press, 1974

Psychotherapy

Hauck, Paul, *Overcoming Depression*, Sheldon Press, 1974

Powell, Milton, *An Outline of Naturopathic Psychotherapy*, British College of Naturopathy and Osteopathy, 1967

Weekes, Claire, *Peace from Nervous Suffering*, Angus & Robertson, 1972

Weekes, Claire, *Self-Help for Your Nerves*, Angus & Robertson, 1962

Radiesthesia

Benham, W., and Williamson, John, *Handbook of the Aura Biometer*, Society of Metaphysicians, 1968

Crawford, W. J., *The Reality of Psychic Phenomena*, Society of Metaphysicians, 1972

Reyner, Lawrence and Upton, *Psionic Medicine*, Routledge & Kegan Paul, 1974

Tansley, M., *Radionics and the Subtle Anatomy of Man*, Health Science Press, 1972

Williamson, John J., *An Outline of the Principles and Concepts of the New Metaphysics*, Society of Metaphysicians, 1967

Radionics

Russell, Edward, *Report on Radionics*, Spearman, 1973

Tansley, David V., *Radionics and the Subtle Anatomy of Man*, Health Science Press, 1972

Reflexology

Bergson, Anika and Tuchak, Vladimir, *Zone Therapy*, Pinnacle Books, New York, 1975

Ingham, Eunice D., *Stories the Feet have Told*, Eunice D. Ingham, Rochester, New York, 1951

Reichian therapy

Baker, Elsworth, *Man in the Trap*, Collier-Macmillan, New York, 1967

Boadella, David (ed.), *In the Wake of Reich*, Coventure, London, 1976

Boadella, David, *William Reich: The Evolution of His Work*, Vision Press, London, 1973

Boyesen, Gerda, 'Dynamic Relaxation', *Energy and Character*, Vol. 1, No. 1 (Abbotsbury, Dorset), 1970

Lowen, Alexander, *Bio-energetics*, Coventure, London, 1976

Mann, Edward, *Orgone, Reich and Eros*, Simon & Schuster, New York, 1973

Reich, Wilhelm, *The Cancer Biopathy*, Vision Press, 1973

Reich, Wilhelm, *Function of the Orgasm*, Panther, 1966

Relaxation

Benson, Herbert, *The Relaxation Response*, Collins, 1976

Fink, David, *Release from Nervous Tension*, Allen & Unwin, 1954

Hewitt, James, *Relaxation: Nature's Way with Tension*, Thorsons, 1968

Rosa, Karl Robert, *Autogenic Training*, Gollancz, 1976

Self-help

Self-Help Series – Natural Therapies for a Variety of Illnesses and Conditions (Thorsons)

Self-help for: Anaemia; Arthritis; Asthma and Hay Fever; Bronchitis and Emphysema; Catarrh; Cystitis; Digestive Troubles; Fatigue; Gain Weight; Gastric and Duodenal Ulcerations; Headaches and Migraine; Healthy Feet; Hernia; Painful Joints; Save Your Tonsils; Sinusitis; Weak Nerves

Sex

Berne, Eric, *Sex in Human Loving*, Penguin, 1973

Bieler, Henry G., *Dr Bieler's Natural Way to Sexual Health*, Bantam, New York, 1974

Chang, Jolan, *The Tao of Love and Sex*, Wildwood House, 1977

Scheimann, Eugene, *Sex can Save Your Heart and Life*, Bantam, New York, 1975

Shiatsu massage

Irwin, Yukiko, *Shiatzu, Japanese Finger Pressure for Energy, Sexual Vitality and*

Relief from Tension and Pain, Routledge & Kegan Paul, 1977
Namikoshi, Tokujiro, *Shiatsu, Japanese Finger-Pressure Therapy*, Japan Publications, California, 1973
Ohashi, Wataru, *Do-it-Yourself Shiatsu*, Mandala/Unwin Paperback, 1977

Spiritual healing
Edwards, Harry. *The Power of Spiritual Healing*, Herbert Jenkins, 1963
Hammond, Sally, *We are all Healers*, Turnstone, 1973
King, George, D.D., *You Too Can Heal*, The Aetherius Society, 1976
Ramacharaka, Yogi, *The Science of Psychic Healing*, Fowler, 1971
Turner, Gordon, *An Outline of Spiritual Healing*, Psychic Press, 1970
Turner, Gordon, *A Time to Heal*, Corgi, 1975
Worrall, Ambrose A., and Olga, N., *The Gift of Healing*, Rider, 1969

Stress
Blythe, Peter, *Stress, The Modern Sickness*, Pan, 1975
McQuade, Walter, and Aikman, Ann, *Stress: How to Stop Your Mind Killing Your Body*, Hutchinson, 1976
Selye, Hans, *Stress Without Distress*, Hodder & Stoughton, 1975

T'ai-chi Ch'üan
Cooper, J. C., *Taoism, the Way of the Mystic*, The Aquarian Press, 1972

Horwitz, Tom, and Kimmelman, Susan, *Tai Chi Ch'üan*, Chicago Review Press
Liu, Da, *T'ai Chi Ch'uan and I Ching A Choreography of Body and Mind*, Routledge & Kegan Paul, 1975

Urine therapy
Armstrong, J. W., *The Water of Life, A Treatise on Urine Therapy*, 2nd Edition, Health Science Press, 1971
Patel, R. M., *Manav Mootra (Human Urine as the Elixir of Life)*, Bharay Sevak Samaj Publications, Ahmabad, India, 1963

Wine
Maury, E. A., *Wine is the Best Medicine*, Souvenir Press, 1977

Wounds
Majno, Guido, *The Healing Hand: Man and Wound in the Ancient World*, Harvard University Press, 1975

Yoga
Bernard, Theos, *Hatha Yoga: The Report of a Personal Experience*, Rider, 1968
Crisp, Tony, *Yoga and Relaxation*, Collins, 1970
Hittleman, Richard, *Guide to Yoga Meditation,* Bantam, New York, 1969
Hittleman, Richard, *Introduction to Yoga,* Bantam, New York, 1969
Iyengar, B. K. S., *Light on Yoga*, Allen & Unwin, 1968
Lysbeth, André van, *Yoga Self-Taught*, Allen & Unwin, 1974
Volin, Michael, and Phelan, N., *Sex and Yoga*, Sphere, 1968.